CARDIOLOGY CLINICS

VOLUME 4 / NUMBER 1
FEBRUARY 1986

RISK OF DEVELOPING CARDIOVASCULAR RISK FACTORS AND ADVERSE EFFECTS OF RISK FACTOR REDUCTION

Franz H. Messerli, M.D., *Guest Editor*
Celso Amodeo, M.D., *Assistant Guest Editor*

W. B. SAUNDERS COMPANY
Philadelphia   London   Toronto   Mexico City
Rio de Janeiro   Sydney   Tokyo   Hong Kong

W. B. SAUNDERS COMPANY   West Washington Square
Philadelphia, PA 19105

The Cardiology Clinics is also published in translated editions
by the following:

Spanish   Nueva Editorial Interamericana S.A. de C.V., Cedro 512
06450, Mexico, D.F., Mexico

CARDIOLOGY CLINICS   ISSN 0733-8651
February 1986   **Volume 4—Number 1**

The Cardiology Clinics is published quarterly by W. B. Saunders Company, West Washington Square, Philadelphia, Pennsylvania 19105, at Hampton Road, Cherry Hill, New Jersey 08002. Subscription price is $55.00 per year. There is a postage charge of $5.00 for subscriptions billed to U.S. addresses and shipped outside the U.S. Application to mail at second class postage rates is pending at Cherry Hill, New Jersey 08002. POSTMASTER: Send address changes to W. B. Saunders Company, West Washington Square, Philadelphia, PA 19105.

The editor of this publication is Karen C. McFadden, W. B. Saunders Company, West Washington Square, Philadelphia, Pennsylvania 19105.

Contributors

Luis Alcocer, M.D.

Professor of Cardiology, Mexico National University, Tuxpan; Chief, Hypertension Clinic, Mexico City General Hospital, Mexico City, Mexico

Celso Amodeo, M.D.

Section on Hypertensive Diseases, Department of Internal Medicine, Ochsner Clinic and Alton Ochsner Medical Foundation, New Orleans, Louisiana

Gerald S. Berenson, M.D.

Professor, and Director, National Research and Demonstration Center—Arteriosclerosis, Department of Medicine, Louisiana State University Medical Center, New Orleans, Louisiana

Allan S. Brett, M.D.

Instructor, Department of Medicine, Harvard Medical School; Attending Physician, New England Deaconess Hospital, Boston, Massachusetts

Gregory L. Burke, M.D.

Assistant Professor, Departments of Medicine and Public Health and Preventive Medicine, Louisiana State University Medical Center, New Orleans, Louisiana

Trudy L. Bush, Ph.D., M.H.S.

Assistant Professor of Public Health (Epidemiology), Columbia University School of Public Health, New York, New York

James L. Cresanta, M.D.

Associate Professor, Department of Public Health and Preventive Medicine, Louisiana State University Medical Center, New Orleans, Louisiana

Jean Davignon, M.D.

Director, Department of Lipid Metabolism and Atherosclerosis Research, Clinical Research Institute of Montreal; Chief, Section of Vascular Medicine, Hôtel-Dieu Hospital; Professor of Medicine, University of Montreal, Montreal, Quebec, Canada

Contributors

Edward D. Frohlich, M.D.

Alton Ochsner Distinguished Physician and Vice-President for Academic Affairs, Alton Ochsner Medical Foundation; Professor of Medicine and Physiology, Louisiana State University; Adjunct Professor of Pharmacology, Tulane University, New Orleans, Louisiana

Paul N. Hopkins, M.D., M.S.P.H.

Resident in Preventive Medicine, Cardiology Division, Department of Internal Medicine, University of Utah Medical Center, Salt Lake City, Utah

Mark C. Houston, M.D., F.A.C.P.

Assistant Professor of Medicine; Co-Director, Medical Intensive Care Unit; and Medical Director, Cooperative Care Center, Vanderbilt University Medical Center, Nashville, Tennessee

Leslie J. Klaff, M.D., Ph.D.

Assistant Professor, Division of Metabolism, Endocrinology, and Nutrition, Department of Medicine, University of Washington School of Medicine, Seattle, Washington

M. Rene Malinow, M.D.

Professor, Division of Cardiology and Division of Metabolism and Clinical Nutrition, Oregon Health Sciences University, Portland; Senior Scientist, Division of Immune and Metabolic Diseases, Oregon Regional Primate Research Center, Beaverton, Oregon

Barry J. Materson, M.D.

Professor of Medicine, Department of Medicine, University of Miami School of Medicine; Acting Chief, Medical Service, Veterans Administration Medical Center, Miami, Florida

Franz H. Messerli, M.D.

Professor of Medicine, Tulane University; Section on Hypertensive Diseases, Department of Internal Medicine, Ochsner Clinic and Alton Ochsner Medical Foundation, New Orleans, Louisiana

Michael H. Miner, Ph.D.

Assistant Professor, Departments of Medicine and Psychiatry, Louisiana State University Medical Center, New Orleans, Louisiana

A. Christine Nestruck, M.Sc., Ph.D.

Senior Investigator, Department of Lipid Metabolism and Atherosclerosis Research, Clinical Research Institute of Montreal, Montreal, Quebec, Canada

Jerry P. Palmer, M.D.

Associate Professor, Division of Metabolism, Endocrinology, and Nutrition, Department of Medicine, University of Washington School of Medicine, Seattle, Washington

Ariel J. Reyes, M.D.

Chief of Clinical Research, Fundación Procardias, Montevideo, Uruguay

Heinz Ruddel, M.D.

Medizinische Universitatsklinik, Bonn-Venusberg, Federal Republic of Germany

Roland E. Schmieder, M.D.

Section on Hypertensive Diseases, Department of Internal Medicine, Ochsner Clinic and Alton Ochsner Medical Foundation, New Orleans, Louisiana

Charles L. Shear, D.P.H.

Assistant Professor, Departments of Medicine and Public Health and Preventive Medicine, Louisiana State University Medical Center, New Orleans, Louisiana

Roger R. Williams, M.D.

Professor, Cardiology Division, Department of Internal Medicine, University of Utah Medical Center, Salt Lake City, Utah

Kenneth G. Zahka, M.D.

Assistant Professor of Pediatrics, Division of Pediatric Cardiology, The Johns Hopkins University School of Medicine, Baltimore, Maryland

RECENT ISSUES

FORTHCOMING ISSUES

Contents

Roland E. Schmieder, Franz H. Messerli, and Heinz Ruddel

In this article, the most important risk factors that may predict the transition from borderline to established hypertension are reviewed. Primary prevention has to focus on identifying individuals who are at highest risk and delaying or reversing further elevation of arterial pressure levels. A review of the literature indicates that several environmental and congenital factors can be identified as risk factors for the development of hypertension, including family history of essential hypertension, age, race, obesity, alcohol consumption, salt intake, hormonal status, and some stress factors. Of all diagnostic approaches to predict the development of hypertension, measurements of resting heart rate and responses to dynamic exercise have some predictive value.

Leslie J. Klaff and Jerry P. Palmer

Cardiovascular disease is the major cause of morbidity and mortality in diabetics. In this article, the prevalence of cardiovascular disease in diabetes is described, and the factors that influence the development of cardiovascular disease are explored. The interaction of other risk factors for cardiovascular disease and glucose intolerance and the question of whether glucose intolerance is truly an independent risk factor are also discussed.

Celso Amodeo and Franz H. Messerli

Whether or not obesity per se is an independent risk factor remains controversial. However, a variety of studies have shown that obesity precipitates certain well-known risk factors, such as glucose intolerance, hyperlipidemia, hyperestrogenemia, hypertension, and left ventricular hypertrophy. Distribution of adipose tissue also seems to influence cardiovascular risk; patients with predominantly male-pattern obesity exhibit more profound risk for cardiovascular disease.

Kenneth G. Zahka

Left ventricular hypertrophy is a frequent finding in patients with essential hypertension. Increased afterload is the most important factor governing this hypertrophy. Systolic myocardial function is normal, and observed diastolic functional abnormalities are of uncertain importance. Measurement of left ventricular mass by echocardiography is useful for the diagnosis and management of patients with essential hypertension.

ADVERSE EFFECTS OF RISK FACTOR REDUCTION

M. Rene Malinow

A variety of treatments to lower elevated plasma lipid levels in patients with hyperlipidemia are available. Adverse side effects ranging from mere annoyances to uncommon serious consequences may be associated with dietary modification, recreational physical exercise, and drug intervention. As in other clinical circumstances, risk-to-benefit ratios must be taken into consideration in the management of hyperlipidemia.

Adverse effects of antihypertensive drugs usually can be avoided by selecting the best drug for a given patient, keeping the dose as low as possible, and avoiding overtreatment. Metabolic adverse effects of diuretics and beta-adrenergic antagonists have generated sufficient concern about drug-associated cardiac risk that attention is being directed toward single-drug therapy with newer drugs such as angiotensin-converting enzyme inhibitors and calcium entry–blocking agents.

Several antihypertensive drugs have an adverse effect on glucose tolerance that may partially or completely negate the beneficial effects of reducing blood pressure as it relates to the incidence of coronary heart disease and its complications. Diuretics (particularly high doses) and beta-blockers without intrinsic sympathomimetic activity have the greatest adverse effect on glucose intolerance. Central alpha-agonists, angiotensin-converting enzyme inhibitors, calcium channel blockers, and alpha-blockers do *not* adversely affect glucose and are preferred in diabetic hypertensive patients, selected hypertensive patients at risk for developing glucose intolerance, and probably most other patients with mild essential hypertension as initial and/or monotherapy compared with diuretics and beta-blockers.

Left ventricular hypertrophy is an adaptive structural cardiac response to the afterload imposed by the hypertensive (and other pressure overload) diseases. As such, it maintains a stable cardiac performance until further adaptation is no longer possible, and then cardiac failure supervenes. Offsetting this "beneficial" effect is a distinct risk demonstrated epidemiologically by a greater number of cardiovascular morbid and mortal events, more severe ischemic disease, cardiac dysrhythmias, and sudden death. The precise mechanisms are just beginning to be elucidated. Other new and intriguing areas related to ventricular hypertrophy include its regression with certain forms of pharmacologic therapy and not others. This problem is also being investigated further at this time.

This article reviews the risks and benefits of oral contraceptive therapy and menopausal hormonal therapy. It was seen that the adverse effects of oral contraceptive use in younger, nonsmoking women are minimal and may be outweighed by the benefits of such therapy.

Contents

However, among older women (older than 35 years of age) who smoke, the adverse effects of oral contraceptive use clearly outweigh any beneficial effects. Among menopausal women with intact uteri, hormonal therapy (estrogens and progestins) appears to offer significant therapeutic advantages without demonstrable risk. In women without intact uteri (prior hysterectomy), unopposed estrogen may actually reduce the risk of cardiovascular disease.

Some active interventions to modify risk factors paradoxically introduce new risk per se, but benefits in extensive populations vastly offset the proportionally small hazards introduced by these maneuvers. However, in daily practice, this potential source of danger can be crucial in a given patient in whom the new potential risk can be greater than the disease that one is trying to prevent or treat. Patients in whom risk factor modification introduces a new risk should be identified before it is decided who, when, and how to treat. The clinical profiles of these patients, with special reference to the negative effects of risk factor intervention on the heart, are discussed in this article.

Attempts to modify risk factors raise ethical questions. The ethical dimensions are heightened by uncertainties in the risk factor data base, the application of hypothetical probabilities to identified individuals, and the interaction between risk factors and values. The context of these issues varies from the isolated physician-patient relationship to the society as a whole.

Notice to Subscribers

Effective January 1, 1986, the subscription price of the *Cardiology Clinics* was increased to $55.00 per year. The increase is made necessary by the higher cost of paper and other materials used in printing. You may be sure that past efforts to keep expenses under control will continue. Your interest in the *Cardiology Clinics* is greatly appreciated.

Foreword

Morbidity and mortality of heart disease and stroke have declined dramatically over the past two decades in the United States. This indicates, at least to some extent, that we have become better at identifying and treating cardiovascular risk factors. However, for every stroke that we prevent by antihypertensive treatment, more than 900 patients with mild hypertension are treated in vain; that is, whether or not arterial pressure is lowered, these patients would never suffer a stroke. Clearly, identification of patients who are at highest risk becomes exceedingly important. Even more important than only treating established risk factors, however, is the identification of patients who are at the highest risk of developing these risk factors in the future.

As can be seen in the first part of this issue, several hereditary and environmental factors as well as provocative tests allow us to predict, at least to some extent, whether a given individual is at risk for a risk. Does early identification of these subjects allow us to hinder the development of a significant risk? Landmark studies from the Bogalusa and Framingham cohorts may provide an answer to this pertinent question within the next decade. Although prevention of cardiovascular risk factors is certainly a major goal in preventive cardiology, at present it still requires a lot of wishful thinking.

Fortunately, we have learned quite well during the last three decades how to reduce certain cardiovascular risk factors, such as obesity, hypertension, hyperlipidemia, and glucose intolerance, once they become manifest. However, we have become increasingly aware that the reduction of risk factors itself is not without risk. The studies documented in the second part of this volume point out that an attempt to reduce one risk factor may inadvertently increase others, so that the overall effect becomes nil or negative.

Treating or modifying risk factors is not synonymous with treating diseases. A disease commonly has symptoms that a patient perceives as disturbing, and the specific treatment is likely to relieve those symptoms. In contrast, most cardiovascular risk factors do not produce symptoms, and the patient may be worse off during and after the intervention than before. Clearly, an epidemiologic, clinical, and pathophysiologic "cost-benefit ratio" must be established before we embark on a program of risk factor reduction. Identifying the risk for cardiovascular risk factors before they become established and minimizing the risk of risk factor reduction will become increasingly important goals in preventive cardiology.

I appreciated the invaluable work of Susan Barker and the Medical Editing staff at the Alton Ochsner Medical Foundtion and Karen McFadden at W. B. Saunders.

FRANZ H. MESSERLI, M.D.

Guest Editor

Ochsner Clinic
1514 Jefferson Highway
New Orleans, Louisiana 70121

Identification and Relative Weight of Cardiovascular Risk Factors

Paul N. Hopkins, M.D., M.S.P.H.,*
and Roger R. Williams, M.D.†

OVERVIEW

Which cardiovascular risk factors are most important? Which can and should be modified according to current knowledge? Who needs risk factor reduction? Practicing physicians following the current medical literature often perceive conflicting answers to these practical questions. Details change somewhat with almost each new reported study. Amidst potential bewilderment, it is important for practicing physicians to recognize that assessing and modifying cardiovascular risk factors is a well-established part of clinical medicine. A few basic concepts probably represent a consensus of most experts in the field. Evolving studies and increased understanding will likely broaden that consensus to include powerful strategies for preventing the most common diseases afflicting modern man.

The most important risk factors for cardiovascular diseases include age, sex, strong positive family history, cigarette smoking, systolic and diastolic hypertension, plasma levels of total and high-density lipoprotein (HDL) cholesterol, diabetes, and obesity. Some would include the type A coronary-prone personality. All of these major factors should be considered in assessing any individual's risk. As much as 90 per cent of coronary heart disease (CHD) in the United States may be attributed to less-than-optimal exposure to risk factors that can be modified. Early or severe disease is usually associated with adverse levels of two or more factors operating in a multiplicative fashion. This implies an opportunity for magnified benefit of reducing risk factor levels in a person who has several risk factors. For example, smoking cessation is probably more useful for a person with a very high serum cholesterol level than for a person with a low cholesterol level.

Many investigators have their "favorite risk factor." Some published discussions of risk factors claim major predominance of some risk factors with minor importance of all others. It is our view that this is generally not a defensible position in view of current knowledge. All of the aforementioned major risk factors have substantial predictive value for cardiovascular diseases. Individual population studies may report one risk factor to be stronger than others. Variations in the relative predictive value of risk factors would be expected depending on differences in the characteristics of the populations studied and differences in risk factor definition. For example, because of the multiplicative effect of cholesterol level, hypertension is much more predictive of coronary disease in Finland, where cholesterol levels are high, than they are in Japan, where cholesterol levels are low. Some studies have shown a strong association of cigarette smoking with coronary disease in men but fail to find a significant association in women. This may be because relatively few women with long-term smoking habits were available in these studies. Yet other studies have clearly identified an important role for smoking precipitating coronary disease in women.

For a practicing physician, there is little purpose served by trying to rank the major risk factors in order of importance. Rather, it is important to recognize that all of them have a potential major role, and the *relative importance of risk factors in individual patients is the practical question of prime importance.* Furthermore, a broad knowledge of many risk factors, some less well recognized, may be useful in minimizing an individual's risk. For example, dialysis can cause carnitine deficiency, which may, in turn, lead to lipid abnormalities and increased CHD risk.

Age, sex, and a strong positive family history tend to be ignored because they cannot be changed.

---

*Resident in Preventive Medicine, Cardiology Division, Department of Internal Medicine, University of Utah Medical Center, Salt Lake City, Utah

†Professor, Cardiology Division, Department of Internal Medicine, University of Utah Medical Center, Salt Lake City, Utah

Nevertheless, they are particularly important risk factors because they help identify persons with the highest risk and the greatest need for risk factor modification. A 16-year-old boy with two brothers dead from coronary disease before age 45 has much greater need for evaluation of blood lipids, blood pressure, and smoking cessation than a 70-year-old woman with angina and a negative family history.

Smoking, hypertension, and hypercholesterolemia are the three risk factors for which intervention data clearly demonstrate decreased disease after risk reduction. A substantial number of persons with elevated risk due to hypertension or smoking can normalize their risk through physician encouragement and conscientious follow-up. Modification of the serum cholesterol level may be more difficult, but it is also justified based on current clinical trials. In any case, the relative benefits of risk reduction must be weighed against some potential risks, especially when medications are involved. Other articles in this issue describe the potential hazards of treatment of risk factors such as hypertension or cholesterol. To help the physician have a balanced approach to risk factors, we have tried to provide an in-depth understanding of some important methods of risk factor identification as well as means to assess relative risk factor weight.

INTRODUCTION

In a recent survey of the literature, we were able to locate supporting references for some 246 coronary risk factors.[75] Since that time, another 30 to 40 risk factors have come to our attention. The literature dealing with risk factors seems to expand at almost exponential rates. With so many risk factors vying for consideration, the assigning of "relative weight" takes on greater importance. In terms of relevance in public health planning, relative weight is also a primary concern. For the individual patient, on the other hand, any specific risk factor may be of major importance. For this reason, clinicians need to be aware of more than just a few "major" risk factors.

In this review, we will first consider general techniques for identifying cardiovascular risk factors and the assigning of relative weight. Public health implications will be discussed. We will then consider specific risk factors, focusing on recent insights into pathogenetic mechanisms and relationships to cardiovascular disease. A systematic approach to classification of cardiovascular risk factors will also be introduced that we find helps impart order to the otherwise bewildering array of physical measurements, blood values, personal traits, and environmental and genetic circumstances that have been found related to cardiovascular disease.

DEFINING AND IDENTIFYING RISK FACTORS

This is the realm of the epidemiologist, but not exclusively. In the epidemiologic sense, a risk factor is a statistical predictor of disease. It may or may not be causally related to the disease. Features that lend credence to a particular risk factor playing an etiologic role include (1) presence of the factor prior to disease onset, (2) strong, dose-related association with the disease, (3) consistent prediction in several studies with varying population composition, and (4) pathogenic plausibility.[96] It is in supplying the last evidence that the epidemiologist depends on experimental pathologists and a variety of other investigators. There has been a tremendous advance in the understanding of cardiovascular disease through the investigation of the detailed mechanism of atherogenesis. Many risk factors can be related to accelerated atherogenesis in animals, disturbances in arterial wall structure, or even perturbations in growth patterns of isolated vessel wall cells. Even with all the evidence marshalled in these areas, however, a risk factor cannot be proved causal without demonstration of risk reduction after intervention, that is, eliminating or reducing the risk factor in a controlled experiment.

The laboratory of the epidemiologist is a human population. Conceptually, the most direct means of identifying a risk factor is by a prospective study, as depicted in Figure 1. Persons free of disease are categorized by risk factor levels and followed, usually for several years. Of interest is the relative risk, which is the ratio of disease incidence (number of new cases per person-years) in the exposed versus the unexposed groups. Prospective studies are expensive and time-consuming. A more rapid means of identifying risk factors is by the case-control study. In this setting, the persons labeled "a" and "c" in Figure 1 are mixed together in the case sample, and the persons labeled "b" and "d" are controls. Note that an autopsy or angiographic study is essentially the same as a case-control study except that cases may be defined more objectively in terms of atherosclerosis involvement and controls are more truly free of disease. They are therefore somewhat more accurate studies in relating risk factors to disease occurrence. One assumption in the case-control study is that the risk factor in cases was present before the onset of the disease and that the ratio a/c would be similar among sampled cases compared with the same ratio if a prospective study had been done. The ratio may be artifactually

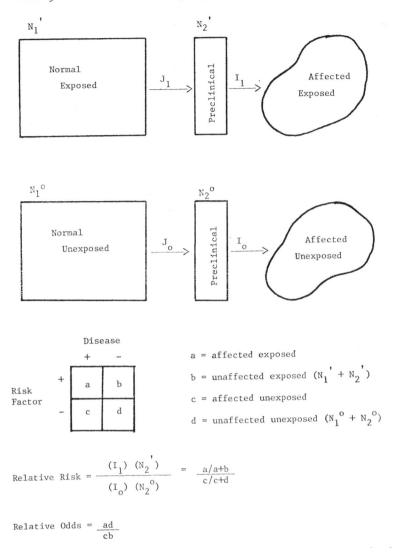

$$\text{Relative Risk} = \frac{(I_1)\ (N_2')}{(I_0)\ (N_2^0)} = \frac{a/a+b}{c/c+d}$$

$$\text{Relative Odds} = \frac{ad}{cb}$$

Figure 1. Conceptual model for a prospective study. N_1 and N_2 are number of persons in normal and preclinical pools shown. J_1 and J_0 are rate constants for passing from the normal to preclinical pools, and I_1 and I_0 are rate constants for incidence of clinical manifestations arising from the preclinical pools. Note that if $I_1 = I_0$, the relative risk equals N_2'/N_2^0.

high if the risk factor relates more to the *presence* of the disease than to its development. The ratio d/b is supplied by the control group. Here, the assumption is that d/b among controls represents the ratio of exposed to unexposed in the normal population if a prospective study were to be done. The relative risk cannot be calculated in a case-control study because incidence rates are unknown. A useful approximation of the relative risk is the relative odds, which is equal to ad/bc (see Fig. 1). The relative risk or relative odds gives a quantitative indication of the excess risk associated with exposure to a risk factor. It tells how many times higher an exposed person's risk is compared with his unexposed counterpart.

A useful means of determining relative odds for multiple risk factors in epidemiologic studies is logistic regression. In this method, the probability that an individual will develop disease is expressed by the equation $P = 1/1 + \exp[-f(x)]$, where $f(x) = \alpha + \beta_1 x_1 + \beta_2 x_2 \cdots + \beta_n x_n$. The α is the "intercept," x_1 to x_n are risk factor levels in the individual, and the coefficients β_1 to β_n relate the risk factor level to disease experience. One useful application of this expression is in the calculation of relative odds. If two levels of a risk factor, x_1 and x_0, are being compared, the relative odds is simply $\exp[\beta(x_1 - x_0)]$. If the risk factor is a yes/no variable, the relative odds is $\exp(\beta)$. Another method, the Cox proportional hazard model, generates coefficients with essentially equivalent values in most cases. In this case, $\exp(\beta)$ equals the relative risk.

Frequently, the logistic coefficient is expressed as the standardized coefficient β*. This standardized coefficient is equal to β (S.D.), with S.D. being the standard deviation of the risk factor in the particular population studied. Although the nonstandardized coefficients of different risk factors have very different values depending on the risk factor units, the standardized coefficients have values that can be compared roughly with each other in the same study. One can compare, for example, how strongly blood pressure and cholesterol predict disease outcome. The larger the absolute value of β*, the stronger the predictive power of that risk factor. Values of standardized logistic coefficients for major cardiovascular disease from the Framingham Study 20-year follow-up may be seen in Table 1. Values of multiple logistic regression coefficients from 11 other recent, large prospective studies are given in Appendix Table A–1.[14,16,23,59,60,71,81,131,156,168,182,214]

It should be noted that the reported logistic coefficients are not necessarily comparable in different populations and can vary widely in different age groups. If β* is large, presumably much could be gained by reducing the risk factor exposure in that population. There is a danger with this approach, however. If the entire population was at an elevated level of risk such that the standard deviation was small, the population could still gain much from reduction of risk exposure, but this would not be reflected in β*. One must know the risk factor distribution in the particular population to fully interpret β* and to predict the potential importance of risk factor modification. Unfortunately, few studies report risk factor distribution or even standard deviations along with β or β*.

Of note is the difficulty encountered in applying logistic regression coefficients derived from one population to another population, especially if risk factor prevalences are markedly different. For example, the Framingham Study logistic overestimates CHD rates in Japan, Honolulu, Puerto Rico, and the European countries of the seven-country study by twofold and in Yugoslavia by a factor of three.[61,100,108] This may be because the prevalence of risk factors, especially serum cholesterol, may have been much lower in the low-risk population before the baseline measures were made, that is, lifetime exposures may have been lower. In addition, the lack of fit may mean that risk factors other than serum cholesterol, hypertension, and cigarette smoking are largely responsible for the near sevenfold to tenfold higher CHD incidence rates in the United States or Finland compared with populations such as those of Japan and Yugoslavia.[100] On the other hand, the Framingham Study logistic predicted CHD rates accurately in men from the Western Collaborative Study,[16] a group with more similar risk background than the populations cited earlier.

Finally, it should be noted that actual values and statistical significance of logistic coefficients are highly sensitive to the risk factors entered into the risk equation. This is especially true if there are any correlations or interactions between the risk factors. This may explain why cholesterol, blood pressure, cigarette smoking, and even age may no longer be significant predictors when certain new risk factors are entered into a given logistic regression[14,71,156] (see Appendix Table A–1).

RELATIVE IMPORTANCE OF RISK FACTORS

Because of the limited utility of β* as an indicator of relative importance of risk factors,

Table 1. *Standardized Multiple Logistic Coefficients for Men and Women, Ages 45 to 74, in the Framingham Study, over a 20-Year Follow-up**

RISK FACTOR	CORONARY DISEASE		BRAIN INFARCTION		INTERMITTENT CLAUDICATION	
	Men	*Women*	*Men*	*Women*	*Men*	*Women*
Cigarettes	0.168	NS	NS	NS	0.372	NS
ECG-LVH	0.212	0.174	—	—	0.158	0.287
Serum cholesterol	0.255	0.314	NS	NS	0.271	0.244
Diabetes	0.117	0.201	0.244	—	0.316	0.358
Hypertension	0.338	0.483	0.682	0.717	0.362	0.529
Heart rate	0.125	NS	0.305	NS	NS	NS
Relative weight	0.206	0.223	NS	0.359	−0.192	NS
Vital capacity	−0.116	−0.292	NS	−0.264	0.264	−0.469
Proteinuria	0.094	0.120	—	—	NS	—

*Adapted from Kannel, W.B.: An overview of the risk factors for cardiovascular disease. *In* Kaplan, N.M., and Stamler, J. (eds.): Prevention of Coronary Heart Disease: Practical Management of the Risk Factors. Philadelphia, W.B. Saunders Company, 1983, pp. 1–19.
NS = not significant

other measures will be presented. The most relevant measure in public health planning is the fraction of disease that can be prevented by an alteration in risk factor exposure. Traditionally, this fraction has been called the population attributable risk. Attributable risk is the fraction of disease that would predictably be avoided if a risk factor were completely eliminated. A more general and elegant measure has been introduced recently—the impact fraction. The impact fraction allows calculation of the impact on disease outcome of a change in risk factor distribution. The expected reduction in CHD could be calculated, for example, for a 10 per cent decrease in serum cholesterol in the population or for eliminating hypertension. The impact fraction may be calculated from the following equation:

$$\frac{\Sigma \ (p_i' - p_i'')RR_i}{\Sigma \ p_i'RR_i}$$

where p_i' is the initial proportion of the population at a given risk factor level and p_i'' is the final or new proportion. RR_i is the relative risk at the given risk factor level relative to baseline. In the simple case in which the risk factor has only two levels (present/absent), the preceding equation reduces to the familiar expression for population attributable risk:

$$\frac{p \ (RR - 1)}{p \ (RR - 1) + 1}$$

where p is the prevalence of the risk factor in the population. The impact of multiple risk factors on total risk can be calculated by the following equation:

$$1 - (1 - IF_1) \ (1 - IF_2) \ (1 - IF_3) \cdots (1 - IF_n)$$

where IF_n is the individual risk factor impact fraction.[137]

Shown in Appendix Table A–2 are the actual population distributions and calculations of hypothetical impact fractions for serum cholesterol, diastolic blood pressure, and cigarette smoking derived from the pooled data of the Albany, Chicago Gas Company, Chicago Western Electric Company, Framingham, and Tecumseh Studies (pool 5 of the Pooling Project[11]). Based on calculations in Appendix Table A–2 and the equation for the total impact fraction given multiple risk factors, 80 per cent of all major coronary events in the Pooling Project population could be attributed to cigarette smoking, serum cholesterol above 160 mg per dl, and diastolic blood pressure above 80 mm Hg.

Verification of the Model. The problem of mass exposure to mildly elevated risk factors has been a subject of much discussion, especially as applied to serum cholesterol.[11,183] Indeed, each 1 per cent drop in serum cholesterol in the Pooling Project would be expected to result in a 1.3 per cent reduction in major coronary events. Part of the recent decline in CHD rates in the United States may be attributed to modest declines in serum cholesterol. One analysis predicted a 4.36 per cent decline in rates with the 5 mg per dl average reduction seen in the middle-aged United States population between 1960 and the early 1970s.[7] Finally, results of the Lipid Research Clinic intervention trial offer the strongest available evidence for the soundness of these projections.[121] In fact, that study documented a 19 per cent reduction of CHD rates in the cholestyramine group that achieved an 8 per cent decrease in total cholesterol (11 per cent decrease low-density lipoprotein [LDL] cholesterol) and a 50 per cent reduction in incidence among a subgroup that achieved a 25 per cent decrease serum cholesterol by careful adherence to the cholestyramine dosing schedule. The authors compared these results with those of seven prospective studies to show strong consistency with predicted effects. The mean nonstandardized logistic coefficient for serum cholesterol from these studies was 0.00899, predicting a 0.9 per cent decline in CHD incidence for each 1 mg per dl decrease in serum cholesterol. Intervention trials cited[121] reported a 15 to 20 per cent decline in CHD for each 10 mg per dl reduction in serum cholesterol, which was close to the effect observed in the Lipid Research Clinic trial. Therefore, *intervention trials have shown serum cholesterol to be causally related to CHD and at least as strong a CHD risk factor as predicted from prospective observational studies.*

The logistic coefficient for diastolic blood pressure from the Pooling Project predicts a 3 per cent decline in major coronary events for each 1 mm Hg decline in blood pressure. This predicted steep gradient for CHD risk has been difficult to demonstrate in intervention trials. In three major intervention trials, statistically significant declines in total CHD rates were not observed, although total cardiovascular end points and total mortality were significantly lowered in treatment groups.[83,160,202] In the Australian Trial, fatal CHD occurred in 5 of 1721 active drug recipients versus 11 of 1706 of those receiving placebo, and rates for total CHD were 56.9 and 63.9 per 1000, respectively. There was only a 5 to 7 mm Hg difference in diastolic blood pressure, which would be expected to result in a modest 14 per cent decline in incidence for major coronary events applying Pooling Project predictors. Such a small difference in rates is difficult to demonstrate, and it may not be ethical to do so. Most of the trials have been stopped when total end points were clearly greater in the control group. Because cerebrovascular disease is affected more strongly than CHD by blood pressure change and because total mortality has also been altered significantly before CHD rate changes reached statistical significance,[85] demonstration of significant CHD rate changes may be only of academic interest. We may have to be satisfied with the 45 per cent decline in total cerebrovascular events seen in the Australian Trial[160] or the 35 per cent reduction in strokes in the Hypertension Detection and Follow-up Program.[84] One recent intervention trial has noted a significant 38 per cent reduction of cardiac mortality among elderly treated hypertensives compared with a control group.[2] In that study, average diastolic blood pressure was reduced 5 to 10 mm Hg throughout the 7-year follow-up period.

The effect of cigarette smoking on cardiovascular disease has never been proved directly in an intervention trial. However, natural experiments have repeatedly demonstrated that CHD risk returns to that of a nonsmoker after smoking cessation during the course of a prospective study.[44,48,63,90] Some investigators reported that several years were required for risk to return to baseline after smoking cessation.[44] Nevertheless, others have reported that a rapid decrease in risk may occur, perhaps within 1 year.[44,48,90]

Application to Prevention Strategies. The impact fraction can be used to predict the beneficial effects of different intervention strategies. An interesting analysis was recently applied to data from the North Karelia Project.[107] Between 1972 and 1982, a vigorous attempt was made to reduce cigarette smoking, serum cholesterol level, and blood pressure by a comprehensive community-based education program in the county of North Karelia, Finland. After 10 years, there was a 36 per cent decrease in cigarette smoking, an 11 per cent decline in mean serum cholesterol, and a 5 per cent decrease in mean diastolic blood pressure.[155] During this period, cardiovascular death rates declined 24 per cent for men and 51 per cent for women. Although the rest of Finland also experienced declines in the prevalence of these risk factors and cardiovascular death rates, reductions in the county of North Karelia were significantly greater after 10 years.[169]

Between 1972 and 1978, there were 161 deaths from cardiovascular disease among a cohort of 5817 male participants aged 25 to 59 years examined at the beginning of the project. In the multiple logistic equation to model 6-year incidence of cardiovascular death in men, coefficients for age, diastolic blood pressure, and total serum cholesterol were 0.116, 0.025, and 0.009, respectively. The intercept (α) was -13.8. Applying this logistic model to the initial population distribution of risk factors, the authors examined expected outcomes for two different intervention strategies, a high-risk strategy and a population strategy. The results of their calculations are shown in Table 2. Approximately twice as many cardiovascular deaths could be prevented by intervening in the entire community rather than focusing exclusively in the high-risk group. The authors further point out the much greater cost-effectiveness of the community-based approach. The similar success of the Belgian arm of the WHO European Collaborative Trial further supports the usefulness of the community-based approach,[105] whereas the lack of significant sustained change in targeted baseline risks in the British arm of the same trial and the Multiple Risk Factor Intervention Trial may serve as an example of the dependency of such trials on the enthusiasm and vigor of educational messages[164] and the difficulty of maintaining a control group truly free from interventional effects.

Before leaving the subject of the public health impact of major risk factors, we should point out the potential importance of relatively rare risk factors that carry large relative risks. If a risk factor carries a relative risk of 20, a prevalence of only 4 per cent could still cause 40 per cent of the disease in the population. This relationship is shown graphically in Figure 2.

ATHEROGENESIS AND RISK FACTORS

Consistency with known principles of pathogenesis is a fundamental standard for evaluating cardiovascular risk factors. Although many features of atherogenesis and the development of complex, flow-impeding lesions have yet to be clarified, four general processes occur that seem fundamental. These processes serve as a means of classifying risk factors.

Initiators. Factors that injure or alter the integrity of the arterial endothelial lining may be considered initiators of atherosclerosis. Artificial damage by balloon catheterization, infusion of homocysteine or other noxious substances, and

Table 2. *Comparison of High-Risk Versus Population-Based Intervention Strategies
Based on Data From the North Karelia Project*

HIGH-RISK STRATEGY
(INTERVENTION ONLY IN HIGH-RISK GROUPS)

Target Group: Top 10% of risk factor distribution
Initial cholesterol levels > 325 mg/dl
Initial diastolic BP > 105 mm Hg

Cholesterol Reduction	*Diastolic BP Reduction*	*Impact on Population (Decline in CVD Deaths)*
By 10%	To 95 mm Hg	16%
By 20%	To 90 mm Hg	28%
To 190 mg/dl	To 80 mm Hg	33%

POPULATION-BASED STRATEGY
(INTERVENTION IN ENTIRE POPULATION)

Target Group: Entire population
Initial mean cholesterol = 263 mg/dl
Initial mean diastolic BP = 92 mm Hg

Cholesterol Reduction	*Diastolic BP Reduction*	*Impact on Population (Decline in CVD Deaths)*
By 10%	By 5% (regardless of initial BP)	31%
By 20%	By 10% (regardless of initial BP)	52%
Population mean of 190 mg/dl	Population mean of 80 mm Hg	70%

BP = blood pressure; CVD = cardiovascular disease
Adapted from Kottke, T.E., et al.: Projected effects of high-risk versus population-based prevention strategies in coronary
heart disease. Am. J. Epidemiol., *121*:697–704, 1985.

various other means has become a common maneuver to hasten the onset of experimental atherosclerotic lesions. A list of initiators is found in Table 3. References may be found in our previous survey.[75] Initiators noted since that survey include polychlorinated biphenyl, a correlate of elevated blood pressure,[110] increased sodium-lithium countertransport,[212] selenium,[203] superoxide, hydrogen peroxide, and fatty acid peroxides,[46,140] Kawasaki syndrome,[133] syphilis,[163] and certain viral infections.[127]

Promoters. Promoters are factors that primarily enhance deposition of lipids into the arterial wall or atheroma. Most familiar is elevated LDL and low HDL concentration. Other promoters may correlate with these or act independently. A list with proposed mechanisms of action and comments is presented in Table 4. Again, references for most are to be found in our previous survey of the literature.[75] Several subsequent reviews have been most enlightening.[65,126,184] Promoters not listed in our survey include elevated apo B/LDL cholesterol (see later section on serum cholesterol and LDL), decreased apo A_1 (see later section on HDL), overproduction of apo LDL (see later discussion), decreased total serum linoleic acid,[200] carnitine deficiency (see later section on HDL), the

assorted inborn errors of metabolism,[8,17,96] severe cystic acne,[201] and the three genetic polymorphisms.[47,82,128]

Potentiators. Factors that encourage platelet activity or enhance thrombosis are termed "potentiators." Although the role of the platelet and microthrombi in atherogenesis of early lesions has been well described and continues to be studied intensively, the role of the thrombotic process in the development of large, occlusive lesions is often neglected in reviews of atherogenesis. It is the process of building layer upon layer of thrombus that leads to clinical manifestations and often is the precipitating cause, especially in transmural myocardial infarction.[145,172] The direct angiographic demonstration of acute coronary thrombosis causing acute transmural myocardial infarction[42] instigated a flurry of activity in this area and generated hope that such clots might be dissolved acutely.

A list of potentiators is given in Table 5. Factors not cited in our previous review[75] are the inherited deficiencies in blood clotting inhibitors.[18,34,173] These latter risk factors are only theoretically related to cardiovascular disease, being primarily factors that predispose to venous thrombosis.

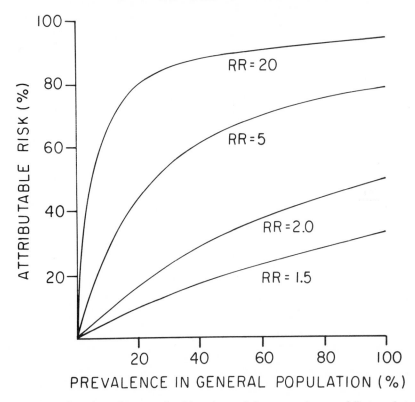

Figure 2. Relationship of population attributable risk to risk factor prevalence at differing relative risks.

Precipitators. Precipitators, as the name implies, precipitate acute clinical events. These factors relate primarily to coronary heart disease but, in some cases, may also cause stroke or peripheral arterial occlusion. Of special import is the induction of arrhythmia deaths. Although approximately 70 to 80 per cent of sudden arrhythmia death victims have advanced coronary artery disease[120,161] and risk factors for prospective prediction of sudden death are similar to other CHD manifestations,[171] many of the factors that precipitate these deaths act by means other than causing further coronary occlusion. Some precipitators increase myocardial oxygen demand, and some lower fibrillation thresholds by increasing electrical instability. It also should be noted that any potentiator can act as a precipitator by causing acute arterial thrombosis. A list of precipitators is found in Table 6.[32,75]

THE MAJOR RISK FACTORS

A distinguishing feature of major cardiovascular risk factors is their multiple roles as initiators, promotors, potentiators, and precipitators. Each factor will be discussed briefly, highlighting recent insights into pathogenetic relationships, unique contribution to different cardiovascular diseases, that is, CHD, stroke (cerebrovascular accident), and peripheral vascular disease, and important associated risk factors and interactions. Finally, the preventive potential or impact fraction for CHD will be estimated.

Age. Age is, of course, the strongest cardiovascular risk factor. Of interest here is the consistently reported inverse interaction of age with most cardiovascular risk factors. The recently reported outcome of the Tecumseh Study (Appendix Table A–1E) is a good example. It is this inverse interaction that causes the terms (age) × (risk factor) to be negative. Thus, all the risk factors in that study were less predictive of future events at older ages. This phenomenon has been reported most commonly for serum cholesterol. Cornfield and Detre published an insightful explanation.[35] We present here a clari-

Table 3. *Initiators of Atherosclerosis*

NATURALLY OCCURRING INITIATORS

Hypertension
  Lead, cadmium
  Polychlorinated biphenyl
  Increased sodium-lithium countertransport
  Excess dietary salt (NaCl)
  Low dietary potassium, magnesium, calcium
  Low dietary polyunsaturated/saturated fat ratio
Serum cholesterol above 300–400 mg/dl
Diabetes
Cigarette smoking, carbon monoxide
High-fat diet
Oxidized cholesterol derivatives
Epinephrine
Norepinephrine
Low blood oxygen
Serotonin
Angiotensin II
Vasopressin
Bradykinin
Cortisol
Prostaglandin E_2
Thromboxane A_2
Thrombin
Fibrin
Bile acids
Keto acids
Antigen-antibody complexes
Bacterial endotoxins
Viral infections
Deficiency of protein, choline, copper, selenium, magnesium, pyridoxine (vitamin B_6), tocopherol (vitamin E), and possibly chromium
Homocysteine, homocysteine conjugates, homocystinuria (heterozygotes and homozygotes)
Superoxide, hydrogen peroxide, fatty acid peroxides
Arteritides
  Kawasaki syndrome
  Syphilis
  Rheumatoid arthritis

LABORATORY INITIATORS

Vitamin D excess
Cyanide
Aminonitrile
Diethylstilbestrol
Allylamine
Glucosamine
Sodium caseinate—injected whole protein
Hematoporphyrin
Certain alkaloids
Various inorganic chemicals
Radiation
Mechanical injury—balloon catheter scraping, stretching, heat
Electrical stimulation of the central nervous system

fication of the mathematical basis for the inverse interaction between risk factors and age.

The conceptual basis for inverse age interaction can best be appreciated by a re-examination of Figure 1. The two-pool model shown represents a fundamental concept presented by Cornfield and Detre. *Observed* end points, such as acute myocardial infarction, occur among persons who already have advanced disease, namely those in the "preclinical" pool of Figure 1. Rates of progression from that pool to manifested clinical end points may not depend on factors that accelerate atherosclerosis per se, but rather on precipitators. Thus, cholesterol, a risk factor that promotes atherosclerosis and thus accelerates rates from the unaffected group to the preclinical group, may not affect rates of overt disease manifestation once the disease is fully developed.

The overall relative risk in a population study depends on combined exposure to initiators, potentiators, promoters, and precipitators. The mathematical model predicts that any risk factor that acts only to promote persons from the unaffected group to the preclinical group will have dramatically decreasing relative risk as the entire population ages. In fact, the model predicts that the relative risk will become less than 1 after persons in the exposed population are depleted from the unaffected pool. (The mathematical derivation may be found in the Appendix.) This in no way negates the importance of serum cholesterol or other risk factors as accelerators of atherosclerosis. It simply means that at older ages, the dirty work is done and precipitators become dominant factors.

There are two practical applications of this model. First, in older populations, precipitators (and potentiators) should be the main focus of preventive efforts. The natural corollary is that prevention of atherosclerosis must be started at early ages. The second application relates to recipients of cardiac aortocoronary bypass grafts. A patient who has undergone bypass graft surgery has a new vessel. That vessel must not be considered a member of an old population. Hence, even though the patient may be older, risk factors important at younger ages are still relevant to progression of atherosclerosis in the new artery graft. Thus, high LDL and low HDL were the factors that *best* predicted occlusion of saphenous-vein grafts in a 10-year study.[26] Vigorous attempts to minimize exposure to all major risk factors are therefore warranted in aortocoronary bypass graft recipients.

Family History. A complete discussion of the complex and major role of family history in cardiovascular disease is beyond the scope of this article.[17,211] Clearly, in conditions such as LDL pathway defects, familial combined hyperlipidemia, phenotypically expressed type III hyperlipidemia, and the various forms of genetic HDL deficiency,[170] family history is the overwhelming risk factor for the individual involved. Blood pressure, diabetes, and obesity, as well as total cholesterol and HDL cholesterol in the

Table 4. *Promoters of Atherosclerosis and Their Mechanism of Action*

PROMOTER	MECHANISM, COMMENTS
Elevated serum LDL	Endothelial cell–altered LDL are engulfed rapidly by macrophages to form foam cells; macrophages may be involved in initiation as well as promotion; LDL (possibly oxidized?) are toxic to smooth muscle cells; accumulation of cholesterol in arteries and lesions is directly proportional to concentration of LDL
Low serum HDL	HDL aids in removal of excess cholesterol; HDL_3 removes cholesterol actively from cultured cells, whereas HDL_2 does not
Elevated IDL or VLDL	May be atherogenic, especially for peripheral large arteries
VLDL	Generally thought to be a less atherogenic lipoprotein, although type IV individuals do have accelerated atherosclerosis
Altered apoprotein composition, overproduction of apo LDL	Lipoproteins with altered apoprotein composition implicated by epidemiologic evidence; primarily apo B/LDL cholesterol and apo A_1 in HDL fraction
Stress, type A personality	Both stress and type A personality are associated with increases in catecholamines, which may raise serum cholesterol levels (VLDL and LDL); certain individuals have especially labile cholesterol and cortisol levels
Low dietary P/S ratio	A high proportion of saturated (S) to polyunsaturated (P) fat raises LDL concentration in serum
High-fat diet, obesity, diabetes	All three tend to cause overproduction of VLDL and often result in high VLDL and LDL levels. Diabetes and obesity are especially associated with high VLDL and low HDL; central obesity (high waist/hip ratio) may be a stronger risk factor than body mass index or other measures of total adiposity
Lack of exercise	HDL is generally lower and VLDL generally higher in sedentary people; exercise will usually raise HDL and lower VLDL if sufficiently vigorous
Cigarette smoking, carbon monoxide	Low HDL levels are associated with cigarette use; carbon monoxide may cause smooth muscle cells to accumulate LDL cholesterol more rapidly; collagen content of atheromas is higher in smokers than nonsmokers
Low vitamin C intake	Smooth muscle cells deficient in vitamin C make a scar protein that binds LDL more avidly than normal; lesions in vitamin C–deficient animals are worse
Low silicon intake	Silicon supplements greatly reduced deposition of LDL in artery walls during experimental atherosclerosis in rabbits
Increased ratio of arterial wall sulfated/nonsulfated glycosaminoglycans	Altered proteins in intima can enhance LDL binding
Increased LDL affinity for artery wall glycoproteins	LDL from CHD cases tends to bind more avidly to arterial wall proteins
Decreased acid cholesterol ester hydrolase	A decrease in the ability to cleave incoming cholesterol esters in LDL to free cholesterol and a fatty acid may increase rates of cholesterol accumulation in the cell and cause cell death
Abstinence from alcohol	Alcohol consumption raises HDL; however, mortality from cancer and stroke offsets decreased risks from CHD at higher intakes
Increase in growth hormone	Frequently seen in diabetes; growth hormone stimulates proliferation of smooth muscle cells
Decreased serum cholesteryl linoleate	Probably reflects a high–saturated fat diet, which is a promoter by way of increased LDL and VLDL levels
Decreased total serum linoleic acid	Increased risk of reinfarction in a prospective study and accompanying CHD case-control study
Elevated serum disaturated lecithin	Lecithins with two saturated fatty acids are stickier than lecithins with a polyunsaturated fatty acid and a saturated fatty acid; may increase LDL binding to artery wall
Nephrotic syndrome	High LDL, low HDL
Chronic renal failure, dialysis	Increased LDL, low HDL; associated carnitine deficiency
Carnitine deficiency	Associated with low HDL levels that rapidly correct with supplementation; HDL raised in normals by supplementation as well

Inborn errors of metabolism
  Hunter's syndrome
  Hurler's syndrome
  Pseudoxanthoma elasticum
  Alkaptonuria
  Werner's syndrome
  Fabry's disease
  Cholesterol-ester storage disease
  Arterial calcification of infancy
  Cerebrotendinous xanthomatosis
  Progeria
  Friedreich's ataxia
	Possibly predispose to lipid accumulation in atheromatous plaques

Severe cystic acne	Associated with reduced HDL levels
Genetic polymorphism in apo AI/CIII gene cluster	Associated with elevated triglycerides but mechanism is unknown
Insertion of large DNA fragment by 5′ end of insulin gene	Unknown
DNA polymorphism near LDL receptor gene	May be used to track inheritance of LDL receptor defects within a pedigree line
Hypothyroidism	Elevated serum cholesterol

LDL = low-density lipoprotein; HDL = high-density lipoprotein; IDL = intermediate-density lipoprotein; VLDL = very-low-density lipoprotein

Table 5. *Potentiators of Atherosclerosis*

ENVIRONMENTAL POTENTIATORS

High dietary stearate-to-linoleate ratio (milk fats, beef fat, lard, or cocoa butter) or a high–saturated fat diet
Low intake of eicosapentaenoic acid (fish oils)
Low-fiber diet
Low-magnesium diet
Cigarette smoking
Estrogens (oral contraceptives)
Stress
Type A personality
High dietary arachidonic acid (peanut oil)
Dietary sucrose
Sudden violent exercise—a short, acute effect
Physical inactivity
Dietary cholesterol
Vitamin E deficiency

PHYSIOLOGIC AND EXPERIMENTAL POTENTIATORS

Collagen, injury to endothelial layer
Atheroma material, plasma from patients with heart disease
Thrombin
Elevated fibrinogen levels
Impaired fibrinolytic activity (associated with physical inactivity, high-fat meals)
Thromboxane A_2 (TXA$_2$), prostaglandin E_2 (PGE$_2$)
Platelet factor 3 (PF3), a clotting factor
Platelet factor 4 (PF4), heparin-neutralizing factor
Increased platelet aggregability
Decreased platelet survival time
Increased number of platelet aggregates
Adenosine diphosphate (ADP)
Epinephrine (adrenaline)
Norepinephrine
Vasopressin
Serotonin
Free fatty acids (especially if saturated)
Elevated serum disaturated lecithin
Reduced serum lysolecithin
Antigen-antibody complexes
Excessively turbulent blood flow
Slow blood flow or eddies
Increased blood or serum viscosity
High serum cholesterol (LDL)
Inherited deficiencies in blood clotting inhibitors
   Protein C deficiency
   Protein S deficiency
   Heparin cofactor II deficiency

"normal range," have strongly genetic determinants.[211] Cigarette smoking and diet as well as other shared environments also clearly play a role in the familiality of cardiovascular disease.

The strength of family history as an independent risk factor has only begun to be investigated.[174,182,191,192] These studies consistently show a significant impact of family history on CHD risk independent of known risk factors. To date, the most convincing of these studies is the Framingham Study on a sample of sibling pairs (Appendix Table A–1D).[182]

In Utah, a computer analysis linking 2504 male death certificates to 327 pedigrees from Mormon genealogy files suggested that up to 80 per cent of the early CHD deaths (in individuals under 55 years old) came from only 16 per cent of the families.[213] In a subsequent study, families of men dying at 45 years of age or younger were at a twofold to eightfold excess risk of premature CHD compared with in-law families.[78] Risk was most markedly elevated at younger ages. Other studies have likewise shown large relative risks (up to ninefold excess risk[211]) for early cardiovascular disease when family history has been defined as disease at an early age in first-degree relatives. Studies that have been less exacting in their definition of positive family history (disease at any age) show much lower relative risks.

Smoking appears to interact with family history in a synergistic fashion. In our study of families of early male CHD victims,[78] the relative risk of smoking depended on family history status. Among first-degree relatives of probands, the relative risk for smoking was 2.5, whereas among in-laws, it was 1.7 ($p < 0.05$). The effect was strongest at ages under 50 years. The combined effect of smoking with its exaggerated relative risk and the already high risk of a positive family history led to nearly 10-fold excess risk among smoking proband relatives compared with nonsmoking in-law controls. Indeed, fully one third of the proband families with multiple occurrences of early CHD reported cigarette smoking as the only known risk factor coincident with their CHD.

Applying data from our study of relatives of early male CHD victims to the population attributable risk formula given a prevalence equal to 8 per cent (percentage of control families with a positive family history) and relative risk for CHD under 60 years of age equal to 2.6 to 7.8 gives an attributable risk in the range of 11 to 35 per cent. Although not independent of other risk factors, this large attributable risk gives impetus to the need for screening high-risk families and, it is hoped, lowering their risk by intervention appropriate to their needs.

Serum Cholesterol and Low-Density Lipoprotein. The epidemiologies of serum total cholesterol and LDL cholesterol are statistically equivalent. That serum cholesterol is a significant risk factor for human cardiovascular disease has been shown in multiple prospective, case-control, autopsy, and angiographic studies.[75] The overwhelming evidence that LDL cholesterol plays a major causal role in cardiovascular disease is beyond refutation. Contrived controversy raised by a very few dissidents has been labeled unwarranted in a major policy review.[96] Much attention has been focused on the definition of an ideal cholesterol level. Very low

Table 6.   *Precipitators of Atherosclerosis and Their Mechanism of Action*

PRECIPITATOR	MECHANISM
All potentiators	Increase chance of arterial occlusion by thrombosis; also increased release of TXA_2 from platelets—a powerful vasoconstrictor
Excess thromboxane A_2 (TXA_2)	A potentiator from platelets and also a powerful vasoconstrictor
Impaired prostaglandin I_2 synthesis	This prostaglandin (also called prostacyclin) counteracts TXA_2 activity on vessel walls
Cigarette smoking	Acts as a potentiator; also, carbon monoxide decreases threshold for ventricular fibrillation; nicotine increases heart rate and heart's workload
Obesity	Increased cardiac output predisposes to ischemia
Overexertion	Increased workload on heart enhances risk of arrhythmias and ischemic events
Cold weather—blizzards	Probably related to strenuous activity such as shoveling snow
Type A personality, stress, pain	Elevated catecholamines and excitability increase risk of arrhythmia
Hypertension	Increased workload on heart; also increased size of left ventricle can lead to electrical instability
Increased blood or plasma viscosity	Decreased perfusion of tissues, may be especially associated with angina pain
Elevated hematocrit or hemoglobin	Increased blood viscosity
Elevated erythrocyte sedimentation rate	Increased blood viscosity
Red blood cell agglutination	Increased blood viscosity
High-fat meal	Actively induces red cell agglutination in susceptible persons
Potassium deficiency	Increases likelihood of arrhythmias; supplementation has a stabilizing effect
Magnesium deficiency	Increases likelihood of arrhythmias; supplementation has a stabilizing effect
Coffee	A vasoconstricting substance is found in coffee, including decaffeinated; drinking coffee, especially dark roasted and instant, was shown to cause extrasystoles (premature ventricular beats) in certain susceptible subjects
Nitrate withdrawal	Nitrates cause vasodilatation; after explosives factory workers exposed to nitrates for prolonged periods leave or retire, they often experience coronary artery spasms
Anaphylactic shock	Release of leukotrienes and other mediators of active immune response leads to increased AV conduction blocks and ventricular automaticity, decreased coronary blood flow, and negative inotropy in animals
Cocaine abuse	Can cause tachycardia, hypertension, ventricular arrhythmias, angina, and myocardial infarction
Hyperthyroidism	Tachycardia, increased susceptibility to arrhythmias

levels (an absence of promoters) may protect against the action of initiators and potentiators such as hypertension and cigarette smoking. Indeed, actual observed CHD rates in Framingham were less than predicted by the logistic regression coefficient in the lowest two serum cholesterol quintiles.[95] Extrapolation of results from several large angiographic studies suggests prevalence of significant lesions would reach 0 at a cholesterol level of about 150 mg per dl[75] (Fig. 3). Data from multiple international comparisons of CHD rates give similar estimates.[100]

As noted, low levels of cholesterol may even protect against other risk factors. In Japan and Puerto Rico, where the average serum cholesterol level approaches 160 mg per dl, systolic blood pressure and cigarette smoking are borderline or nonsignificant risk factors for predicting CHD.[61] This observation has clinical ap-

plication. Persons who smoke or have hypertension and also have high serum cholesterol levels should be treated more aggressively than persons with very low serum cholesterol levels. In fact, persons with multiple CHD risk factors should, in general, be approached more aggressively than patients with a single, isolated risk factor.

At very high levels of serum cholesterol, LDL becomes an initiator. In smooth muscle cell cultures, low-density lipoproteins are directly cytotoxic in a dose-dependent fashion.[73] The toxicity of LDL is enhanced by oxidative changes that may occur in vivo.[140] Some investigators report impaired endothelial regeneration in the face of experimental hypercholesterolemia.[159] In a study of primate atherogenesis induced by cholesterol feeding, the earliest changes that occurred were infiltration into the intima by mon-

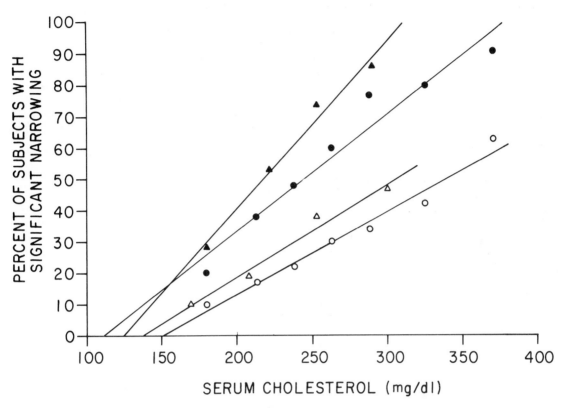

Figure 3. Angiographically determined "ideal" levels of serum cholesterol defined by extrapolation to zero prevalence of significant coronary narrowing. Significant narrowing was considered to be greater than 50 per cent occlusion in studies by Welch and associates,[75] represented here by *circles*. In studies by Cohn and colleagues,[75] shown as *triangles*, greater than 75 per cent occlusion was the criterion. *Closed symbols* represent men; *open symbols* represent women. A minimum of 16 and a maximum of 230 angiograms[75] are represented by each point. Age ranges: ● = men under 40 years old; ○ = women under 50 years old; ▲ = men 40 to 59 years old; △ = women 40 to 59 years old.

ocytes, which, in turn, imbibed lipid to become foam cells. It was only after these changes that endothelial consistency became disrupted over sites of engorged foam cells. Thereafter, atherosclerotic changes such as platelet adherence and smooth muscle cell migration occurred at an accelerated rate. Thus, the macrophage may play a supporting role with LDL in the initiation of atherosclerosis in hyperlipidemia.[46]

True to form as a major risk factor, an elevated LDL level acts in multiple phases of atherogen-

esis. It is a promoter sine qua non. Human arterial wall LDL concentration derived by immunofluorescence is directly proportional to serum LDL concentration.[10] Countless animal studies verify the promoting effect of high LDL levels on experimental atherosclerosis. Many studies are giving further insight into the role of endothelial altered LDL. These are taken up (primarily by macrophages) via a unique receptor that is different from the classic apo B-E receptor described by Goldstein and Brown.[46,184]

LDL may act as a potentiator by enhancing platelet aggregation, an effect possibly mediated by increasing cholesterol concentration in the platelet's outer membrane.[70,122] The nearly universal occurrence of clinically manifest CHD by the second decade of life in homozygote carriers of familial hypercholesterolemia genes gives solemn testimony to the atherogenicity of LDL.[17]

Recently, much attention has been given to LDL of altered composition. Specifically, an increased apo B–to–LDL cholesterol ratio is a risk factor independent of LDL concentration.[20,72,181] The altered composition may be an expression of increased apo B synthesis, which also appears to confer added CHD risk.[99] This may be a good argument for reduction of synthetic rates by means such as weight loss and low-fat diet.[77]

Although LDL plays a major role in CHD prediction, it is accorded a significantly lesser role in stroke[190] (see Table 1). The reason(s) for this difference in predilection for sites of atherosclerosis promotion is unknown. More data are needed before firm conclusions can be drawn. LDL is a strong risk factor for peripheral vascular disease, and here, apoproteins also seem to have important additional predictive power.[4,36,39,72,129,177]

Potential for prevention has already been discussed in considerable detail. The Lipid Research Clinic Trial firmly establishes the causal nature of elevated LDL levels and our ability to prevent CHD by altering cholesterol levels. The consensus of scientific opinion favors generalizing these results to other safe, effective means of lowering serum cholesterol such as dietary measures[96] (see later discussion). Results from the WHO clofibrate trial (increased total mortality in clofibrate group) do serve to caution against indiscriminate application of all available means to lower cholesterol.[33]

If serum cholesterol levels were lowered to 160 mg per dl in the Pooling Project population group, the impact fraction suggests a preventive potential of 44 per cent. If levels were lowered to under 220 mg per dl, the impact fraction becomes 25 per cent (see Appendix Table A–2).

High-Density Lipoprotein. Prospective data demonstrating a protective role for HDL are strong but very scarce. Only two prospective studies, one including only older men and women, have reported relative risks from a multiple logistic regression (the Framingham Study [Appendix Table A–1B] and the Israeli Ischemic Heart Disease Study [Appendix Table A–1K]). One small prospective study of younger men demonstrated that HDL was a stronger discriminatory factor than LDL for development of

CHD, but no relative risks were given.[138] Much confirmatory evidence comes from retrospective case-control, angiographic, and autopsy studies.[75] The largest of these is the Cooperative Lipoprotein Phenotyping Study.[29] In that study, LDL and HDL showed equal discriminating ability. CHD *prevalence* decreased progressively from 180 per 1000 to approximately 80 per 1000 as HDL levels increased from less than 25 mg per dl to values above 45 mg per dl. Data from other prospective studies are forthcoming and anxiously awaited. The LDL cholesterol–to–HDL cholesterol and total cholesterol–to–HDL cholesterol ratios have been proposed as the best risk indicators for CHD. Ratios and their associated risks derived from the Framingham Study are shown in Table 7.[59]

Recent insights into HDL metabolism have raised a number of questions. HDL occur in several subfractions. HDL_3 is the smallest particle and takes up cholesterol as cholesterol ester (via lecithin cholesterol acyl transferase–mediated exchange) to become HDL_2. HDL_2 apparently acquires more cholesterol esters and apoprotein E to become HDL_1 or HDL_c, which are considerably larger, highly cholesterol-enriched particles that are rapidly removed from circulation by the liver, primarily via an apo E receptor.[126] While HDL_3 avidly remove cholesterol from cultured cells and stimulate LDL receptor expression, HDL_2 and larger particles no longer do so and may actually deposit cholesterol, perhaps by attaching to the apo B-E receptor (LDL receptor).[148] HDL_c increase markedly after cholesterol feeding in humans and animals, independent from changes in total cholesterol concentration.[126] Interestingly, it is the HDL_2 rather than the HDL_3 subfraction that seems to be the strongest predictor of coronary artery disease.[5,139,148] HDL_2 levels are higher in women runners and are increased by various forms of exercise. Alcohol seems to raise HDL_3 at low to moderate intakes and both HDL_2 and HDL_3 at high intakes.[37,38,69] One investigator has reasoned that higher HDL_2 levels may reflect a more active cholesterol removal system.[126]

Population comparisons raise other perplexing questions. In a comparison of 13 countries, total cholesterol and HDL concentrations were strongly and *positively* correlated with each other. Low HDL levels were especially prevalent in slender African populations with low total cholesterol levels and low CHD incidence.[104] Japan may be an exception, especially in some areas.[80] However, differences in population

Table 7. *LDL Cholesterol–to–HDL Cholesterol and Total Cholesterol–to–HDL Cholesterol Ratios and Their Relative Risks—The Framingham Study*

	LDL CHOLESTEROL/ HDL CHOLESTEROL	TOTAL CHOLESTEROL/ HDL CHOLESTEROL	RELATIVE RISK
For Men	1.0	3.43	0.5
	3.55 (average)	4.97 (average)	1
	6.25	9.55	2
	7.99	23.39	3
For Women	1.47	3.27	0.5
	3.22 (average)	4.44 (average)	1
	5.03	7.05	2
	6.14	11.04	3

rates of CHD do not generally correlate with differences in HDL levels.

HDL apoprotein composition has become another area of debate. Several retrospective studies have suggested that apo A_1 is a better discriminator between CHD cases and controls than HDL cholesterol.[20,72] The only prospective study (Tromsø Heart Study) reported no improvement in discriminative power between HDL cholesterol and apo A_1 in cohort cases and selected controls.[88] At present, there is some suggestion that the particular batch of antibodies against the apo A_1 may make a difference in the predictive power of the apo A_1 radioimmunoassay determination. This may have accounted for the remarkable difference in apo A_1 levels between angiographically defined cases and controls in the Mayo Clinic Study[106,123] but not in other studies.

Interesting new insights into the risk of CHD associated with chronic renal dialysis relate to HDL. Dialysis depletes carnitine, a factor essential for fatty acid transport into mitochondria. Carnitine supplementation raised serum carnitine levels to normal in renal dialysis patients and concomitantly raised low HDL levels dramatically back into the normal range.[28,66,199] Other studies have demonstrated increases in HDL level (some marked, especially when initial HDL levels were low) in patients with hypertriglyceridemia who were given oral carnitine supplements (1 to 3 mg per day).[124,154]

Generally, results from epidemiologic studies confirm the strength of HDL as a protective factor in all forms of cardiovascular disease, including strokes and peripheral vascular disease.[15,166,178] This being the case, a moderate elevation of HDL would probably be desirable for preventive purposes. If running were the means of intervention, at least 20 to 23 miles per week would probably be required to raise HDL cholesterol 5 mg per dl.[98,209] Using the Framingham Study logistic, this would result in an 18 per

cent decrease in CHD incidence, other factors remaining constant.

Triglycerides. Serum triglycerides are generally considered weak or nonsignificant risk factors, especially when HDL is included in the multivariate equation[59,60] (see Appendix Table A–1). Some major prospective studies have reported a significant predictive value for triglycerides[14] (see Appendix Table A–1), but HDL was not measured. A strong, negative correlation between HDL and serum triglycerides may account for these observations.

Some lipoprotein abnormalities with elevated triglycerides are associated with markedly increased cardiovascular risk. Type IIb and familial combined hyperlipidemia are clear examples.[57] Hypertriglyceridemia without elevated serum cholesterol has been a controversial risk factor. Sporadically high triglyceride levels may be associated with higher CHD risk, but much of this risk may be mediated by associated low HDL levels (see preceding discussion). There are two genetically mediated forms of hypertriglyceridemia. Familial combined hyperlipidemia is a common autosomal dominant disorder. Affected relatives may express either pure hypertriglyceridemia (type IV phenotype), pure hypercholesterolemia (type IIa), or both (type IIb). Furthermore, individuals with familial combined hyperlipidemia may change phenotypic expressions at different times. A fundamental metabolic abnormality in familial combined hyperlipidemia appears to be over-production of very-low-density lipoprotein (VLDL) with normal composition. There is variability in conversion rates of VLDL to LDL and LDL fractional catabolic rates that appear to account for differences in phenotypic expression.[19,30,91,101,102] Myocardial infarction rates were about four times normal among persons affected with familial combined hyperlipidemia in one frequently quoted study.[21] In contrast, persons with familial hypertriglyceridemia did not appear to be at increased risk.[21] Familial hypertriglyceridemia is a distinct autosomal dominant defect in VLDL metabolism in which affected family members have elevated triglycerides exclusively. VLDL abnormally enriched in triglycerides are produced at excessive rates.[19,30,91,101,102] Some studies suggest a defect in VLDL catabolism as well.[91] Interestingly, elevated triglyceride levels (type IIb, type IV, type V, and type III) seem to promote atherosclerosis at peripheral sites more efficiently than in coronary arteries, possibly because of the associations of diabetes with increased triglycerides.[4,36,39,177,179]

New understanding of type III disease has emerged recently. The expression of the type III phenotype (1 in 10,000 persons in the general population) probably requires a combination of two genotypic patterns, each with a frequency of approximately 1 per 100.[67] The first requirement is a homozygous pattern for defective apolipoprotein E (E_2E_2). (There are three apo E alleles—E_2, E_3, and E_4. E_3 is the most common, normal allele.) The second requirement is for a defect causing increased production of VLDL. Homozygotes for apo E_2 are quite common, with a frequency of approximately 1 per 100, but persons with this defect alone or other genotypes, including apo E_2, tend to have low LDL levels and may actually have *lower*-than-expected risk for CHD.[67,134] If VLDL overproduction is present, the type III phenotype becomes expressed in the E_2E_2 homozygotes. Then, CHD risks are very high, as are risks for peripheral vascular disease.[141]

Blood Pressure. Blood pressure is one of the strongest CHD risk factors and clearly the strongest risk factor for stroke (see Table 1 and Appendix Table A–1). Although investigation of isolated systolic hypertension reveals that it is a reflection of stiffened arteries, casual systolic blood pressure, taken with a cuff, remains as predictive for future events as diastolic blood pressure.[54,97]

Insights into the interaction of blood pressure with atherogenesis have been forthcoming, but much remains to be learned. Early studies stressed the importance of increased flow rates at bifurcations and decreased lateral pressure as a cause of atherosclerosis initiation.[193] Later studies emphasized nonlaminar flow patterns resulting in eddies in which platelets might be given time to adhere to vessel walls and potentiate atherogenic processes.[114] Atherogenesis is accelerated in hypertensive animals.[75] Studies in Japan have explored possible causes for the observed high incidence of hemorrhagic strokes in that country while atherothrombotic stroke is

relatively rare. A condition called arterionecrosis, apparently caused by high cerebral perfusion pressures, has been described.[141] Medial necrosis, the hallmark of arterionecrosis, could weaken arterial walls and precipitate hemorrhagic strokes without an atherosclerotic lesion present.

Analysis of two large French prospective studies recently revealed a strong inverse relationship between hypertension and obesity. At comparable blood pressures, obese hypertensives were at significantly lower risk for cardiovascular disease than slender hypertensives.[25] In a clinical study, normal-weight hypertensives had more papilledema and nephrosclerosis than obese hypertensives.[150] Obesity has been associated with increased cardiac output. Thus, at comparable blood pressure, the obese person should have a lower peripheral resistance than a slender person. Along with blood pressure, increased peripheral resistance is possibly an important predictor of end-organ damage.[135]

A recent survey on changing blood lead levels deserves attention. A strong positive correlation between blood lead and systolic and diastolic blood pressure was observed among 564 men aged 40 to 59 years involved in the National Health and Nutrition Examination Survey (1976 to 1980). The correlation persisted after adjusting for 87 possibly related factors. An increase in blood lead from 10 to 20 μg per dl resulted in systolic and diastolic blood pressure elevation of 6 and 3 mm Hg, respectively. Between the years 1976 and 1980, mean blood lead levels were noted to drop 37 per cent. The authors then applied this change in blood lead levels to the regression for blood lead on blood pressure. Predicted changes in blood pressure were entered into the Pooling Project and Framingham multiple logistic equations. They calculated that the blood pressure decrement caused by lower blood lead levels would result in a 17.5 per cent decrease in the prevalence of hypertension (diastolic blood pressure of 90 mm Hg or greater), 4.7 per cent fewer fatal and nonfatal myocardial infarctions, and a 6.7 per cent decrease in fatal and nonfatal strokes over a 10-year period, as well as 5.5 per cent fewer deaths from all causes over 11.5 years. Decreasing blood lead levels may be making a substantial contribution to current favorable trends for cardiovascular disease in the United States population.[153]

The fraction of CHD attributable to hypertension (diastolic blood pressure above 90 mm Hg) is approximately 20 per cent. A 36 per cent decrease in risk could be achieved by lowering blood pressures to under 80 mm Hg (see Appendix Table A–2).

Cigarette Smoking. Cigarette smoking remains the single most preventable cause of excess death and disability from cardiovascular disease in the United States today. Mechanisms whereby cigarettes cause cardiovascular disease are likely multiple. Atherosclerotic lesions are more prevalent in smokers in autopsy and angiographic studies.[75] However, the rapid decrease in risk after terminating the habit suggests that precipitation of acute events is a major mechanism. Cigarette smoking increases platelet adhesiveness and aggregability and interacts strongly with oral contraceptives to increase risk from various thrombotic events.[3,89,172] As a potentiator, cigarette smoking could act both to thicken lesions with each layer of thrombus and to precipitate acute events. Furthermore, carbon monoxide, a major component of cigarette smoke, whether filtered or not, lowers the threshold for ventricular fibrillation, increasing the contribution of cigarettes to precipitating sudden death.[41,204] The facts that cigarette smoking continues to be a risk factor for cardiovascular death after a heart attack and that risk decreases rapidly to that of a nonsmoker after cessation at the time of a nonfatal myocardial infarction further support the role of cigarette smoking as a precipitator of acute events.[1,93,167,206]

An important new issue in research is the effect of cigarette smoking on bystanders, which is known as passive smoking. A recent prospective study compared the incidence of ischemic heart disease in nonsmoking women whose husband either did or did not smoke. There were 695 nonsmoking women aged 50 to 79 years. After adjusting for age and other risk factors, the incidence of ischemic heart disease among women with smoking husbands was 14.9 times that of women with nonsmoking husbands. Furthermore, all-cause mortality was significantly related to the husbands' smoking habits in a dose-dependent fashion.[55]

Cigarettes seem to accelerate peripheral vascular disease greatly. Some estimates of attributable risk are as high as 70 to 80 per cent.[205] The attributable risk of CHD from all tobacco use is 43 per cent, most of it from cigarette smoking (see Appendix Table A–2).

Stress and Type A Personality. Although retrospective studies have reported significantly greater life stress among survivors of myocardial infarction than among controls,[157,194] prospective studies have, for the most part, failed to do so.[94,195] However, type A personality and several interrelated risk factors have been accepted as prevalent, significant predictors of acute ischemic events.[162] The type A person is described as impatient, hostile, time- and deadline-conscious, aggressive, and excessively competitive. It is believed the distinction between A and B personality types is best made in a structured interview, although much prospective data was derived from questionnaires.[92] In fact, the Western Collaborative Study was the only prospective study demonstrating a relationship between type A behavior as assessed by structured interview and subsequent CHD.[16,165] Type A behavior assessed by either interview or Jenkins activity score was not associated with excess CHD risk in the Multiple Risk Factor Intervention Trial study.[176] However, several case-control and angiographic studies appear to favor type A behavior as a real risk factor.[75,210]

In a recent prospective Dutch study, self-employed men had 2.2 times and self-employed women had 6.8 times the risk of fatal CHD compared with men and women who were employees. In the same study, a retrospective analysis revealed relative odds of 7 and 3.3 for men and women, respectively, for those who answered the following question in the affirmative: "Is your nature such that you feel driven to do all your work with great intensity and against the clock?"[125] Interestingly, general practitioners have more than twice the risk of CHD compared with specialists.[143] Investigations in mechanisms for the excess risk associated with type A personality have stressed increased cortisol and catecholamine levels and more labile cholesterol levels, especially during times of stress.[49] The fact that type A personality is a predictor of CHD[165] and that intervention may prevent secondary myocardial infarction[51] suggest its role as a precipitator.

Most prospective studies[16,71] (see Appendix Table A–1) estimate the relative risk between type A and type B persons to be approximately 2.0. Although this is a relatively small relative risk, a prevalence of 50 per cent among American men[165] results in an estimated attributable risk of 33 per cent.

Another class of risk factors probably interrelated with type A behavior and/or stress may be termed "social support indicators." Increased risk from myocardial infarction has been reported for not attending church, inactivity in work or nonwork organization, and having a nonsupportive boss, divorced parents, and frequent feelings of loneliness.[75] Most of these studies have been retrospective. Men who reported less love and support from their wives had a greater incidence of angina pectoris but not myocardial infarction in a prospective Israeli study.[132] Prospectively determined CHD rates among widows and widowers and single persons are significantly higher than among their married counterparts.[109,149,158] Furthermore, married persons are more likely to survive longer after an acute myocardial infarction.[31] Recent prospective analyses of Framingham spouse pairs showed a strong increased risk for CHD in men whose wives were working in white collar professions, had 13 or more years of education (independent of husband's educational status), were more angry and ambitious, or had more children[71] (see Appendix Table A–1). Elevated risk among men with more educated wives has been confirmed in two other prospective studies.[27,186] In the latter study, the excess risk was confined to men with type A personality.

Diabetes. Diabetes is a strong risk factor for cardiovascular disease. It may act as an initiator and a promoter of atherosclerosis.[75] Arteriosclerosis obliterans and peripheral microvascular disease are especially difficult problems for diabetics.

Risk from cardiovascular disease attributed to diabetes is said to be greater among women than men[59,60] (see Appendix Table A–1). Indeed, female diabetics have lower HDL and higher VLDL levels and modest elevation in total cholesterol, which may eliminate their protected status compared with men. However, two recent studies suggest that diabetes carries an equal, strong risk for both men and women.[6,23] Estimated relative risks are approximately 3 to 4. In the Tecumseh Study[23] (see Appendix Table A–1E), the prevalence of diabetes was 4.7 per cent and 7.5 per cent among men and women, respectively, aged 40 to 79+ years. The relative risk for a diabetic was 3.9. Applying these numbers to the population attributable risk equation, 12 per cent of CHD mortality in men and 18 per cent of the CHD mortality in women can be attributed to diabetes. In the prospective study at Rancho Bernardo, California, an interaction of diabetes with cigarette smoking was reported that potentially could account for 65 per cent of the CHD cases among diabetics in that study.[187]

Obesity and Physical Activity. Obesity and physical activity, adjusted for other factors, are minor CHD risk factors. Only after 26 years of follow-up in Framingham did obesity become significantly and independently related to future cardiovascular disease end points[81] (see Appendix Table A–1A). A woman 100 per cent over desirable weight by Metropolitan Life Insurance tables carried a 2.5-fold excess risk for all cardiovascular disease. Because these 26-year results could not include HDL or LDL, their interpretation must be guarded.

Interesting new observations regarding adipose distribution are appearing. Measures of central or abdominal obesity (male-type pattern, late-onset pattern) are better predictors of cardiovascular risk and metabolic derangement than previous measures of total adiposity.[12,68,113,116,117] In women, in whom the relationship seems strongest, there was a fourfold increase in risk of new myocardial infarction, going from the smallest to highest tertile of waist-to-hip ratio.[116] This measure was a significant predictor for strokes and total mortality as well, even after correcting for traditional risk factors, age, and body mass index (weight/height^2).

Problems in assigning significant, independent risk to physical activity levels remain. Are low activity levels the result or cause of disease? This question is still debated, and no prospective study has answered it irrefutably. Nevertheless, the weight of opinion and evidence supports physical inactivity as a bona fida CHD risk factor with a contribution to risk similar to that of obesity (RR of about 2 between inactive and active persons[75,96]).

Because of significant correlations with other risk factors, especially blood pressure, HDL, LDL, and diabetes, it is difficult to assess the independent contribution of obesity and physical activity to cardiovascular disease. However, because these risk factors do have important and, at times, major effects on known strong risk factors, they deserve deliberate attention in any effort to reduce cardiovascular risk.

Thrombotic Tendencies. Risk factors relating to thrombotic tendencies are potentiators of atherosclerosis. However, limited information is available supporting their role in predicting new disease in normal people. Because atheromatous plaque and fibrin itself are strong platelet activators, it is not surprising that measures such as platelet survival, numbers of platelet aggregates, platelet adhesiveness or aggregability in vitro, and platelet factor or prostaglandin levels all should be abnormal in persons with significant atherosclerotic disease. A risk factor associated with the *presence* of the disease more than with prediction of disease will give exaggerated estimates of relative odds in retrospective studies. This clearly seems to be the case in a number of studies.[75] In one recent study, platelet survival in normal persons under 50 years of age was decreased in 56 per cent who smoked cigarettes or had a strong family history of coronary disease versus only 14 per cent of persons without a family history and who did not smoke.[52] Nevertheless, *presence* of the disease could not be ascertained.

Recently, prospective studies with long follow-up periods have indicated some potentiators as significant, predictive risk factors for CHD. The Stockholm Prospective Study[14] reported erythrocyte sedimentation rate as a significant risk factor (see Appendix Table A–1F). Because the erythrocyte sedimentation rate is largely a reflection of fibrinogen levels, these results are in harmony with a report from Gothenberg, Sweden,[207] in which higher fibrinogen levels were prospectively associated with myocardial infarction and stroke. Fibrinolytic activity is reportedly lower in survivors of myocardial infarction, but prospective data are still lacking.[75]

Diet. A thorough discussion of diet interrelations with atherogenesis and manifestations of cardiovascular disease is clearly beyond the scope of this article. A few salient points need emphasis, however.

For many years, international correlations between saturated fat or cholesterol intakes have led investigators to suspect diet as a leading cause of CHD. Indeed, recent correlations between trends in CHD and changing food consumption patterns in various countries support earlier static observations.[24] Generally, the relationship between diet and CHD has emphasized serum cholesterol as the mediating risk factor. It is less well appreciated that diet has a strong potential influence on every phase of atherogenesis.

The "typical" American diet is laden with fats (especially saturated fats), high in cholesterol, high in salt, and depleted of fiber, potassium, and essential trace minerals by overrefining. This diet pattern may be implicated as an initiator because fatty acids, during the absorption phase, may disrupt endothelial cell integrity,[215] and such a diet can raise cholesterol in susceptible persons to such high levels that initiation becomes likely. In addition, saturated fat tends to raise blood pressure, whereas polyunsaturated fats lower blood pressure,[180,185] not to mention well-known relationships between sodium, potassium, and magnesium and blood pressure.[130] The typical American diet acts as a promoter by increasing LDL and VLDL, as well as inducing increases in atherogenic lipoproteins such as beta VLDL.[126] A high-cholesterol diet may impede HDL cholesterol removal independent of its effect on serum cholesterol.[126] A diet with a high ratio of saturated to polyunsaturated fat is a strong potentiator, because plate-

lets become much more susceptible to aggregating agents.[79,122] Fish oils, which are rich in eicosapentaenoic acid, have the opposite effect and markedly lower VLDL.[152] Persons consuming at least 30 gm of fish per day had 50 per cent fewer CHD deaths than persons who did not eat fish in the 20-year follow-up of the Zutphen study.[112] A high-fat meal acutely lowers fibrinolytic activity,[13,22] induces red cell agglutination,[45,50,115,118,189,208] and can cause angina in susceptible persons,[115] thus qualifying as a precipitator of acute events. Persons with angina starting a very-low-fat diet and stress modification program reported over 90 per cent fewer anginal episodes within 3 weeks and had objective improvements in cardiac function indices.[146] Other dietary precipitating factors may be low potassium and magnesium intakes, both of which strongly relate to myocardial irritability.[45,86,87]

Evidence is accumulating that dietary patterns can help predict an individual's risk of disease within a population, despite inherent difficulties in measuring individual dietary habits within a population. The Honolulu Heart Study (see Appendix Table A–1G) provides particularly strong evidence. Dietary factors most strongly predictive of future CHD in prospective studies include *low* daily total caloric intake,[111,131,141,214] a low proportion of calories from starch,[131,144,214] low fiber (correlated highly with starch intake),[144] and higher intakes of saturated fat,[53,62,131,144,175] cholesterol,[53,131,175,214] and animal protein.[131,214] This is essentially a description of the typical American diet. Male vegetarians may have CHD rates as low as one-third to one-eighth the rates of the general American population.[151]

Alcohol has quite consistently been shown to protect against CHD. However, because total mortality and cancer risk increase above just two to three drinks per day, as well as the obvious social ramifications, alcohol cannot be recommended as a means to prevent CHD in the general population.[75,96]

The potential for prevention of CHD by diet is enormous. The major CHD risk factors, cholesterol, blood pressure, and diabetes, are clearly related to diet. Many intervention studies, including the prospective Oslo Study,[74] the North Karelia Project,[107] the Belgian WHO Collaborative Study,[105] and several older studies, especially the Finnish Mental Hospital Study by Miettinen and associates,[136] among others,[9,40,119,198] have consistently demonstrated a significant reduction in CHD end points when baseline characteristics (for example, serum cholesterol) are significantly altered compared with control groups. Young subjects have especially benefited. In Great Britain, where dietary measures to prevent CHD have not been encouraged, CHD incidence has remained static, whereas other countries have experienced significant declines. Reluctance to recommend general dietary guidelines aggressively has been blamed for this lack of progress.[197] Indeed, opposition to or ambivalence toward the prevention of CHD by dietary means can no longer be considered a scientifically tenable position.[96,184a] Given a relative risk of up to 7 to 8 (Japanese or Seventh-Day Adventist strict vegetarians versus average Americans), a prevalence of perhaps 80 per cent of persons eating the typical American diet, the attributable risk is approximately 83 per cent. Thus, more than 80 per cent of heart attacks may potentially be prevented by dietary means.

PERSPECTIVE ON PREVENTION

Prevention is, of course, the goal and justification for risk factor identification. Assigning relative weight allows objective apportioning of limited resources to areas that promise the greatest returns. We have discussed the potential for prevention, the impact fraction, or attributable risk for each of the major coronary risk factors. Prevention of other cardiovascular disease reflects a similar pattern, with a few exceptions noted. The total percentage of disease preventable by reducing risk exposure to more nearly optimal levels may be calculated to be 90 per cent by the multiple factor impact fraction equation. The following independent risk factors, with attributable risk or impact fraction (IF) in parentheses, were included in the calculation: total serum cholesterol, reduced to ideal levels of 160 mg per dl (IF = 44 per cent); HDL cholesterol, raising mean levels by 5 mg per dl through exercise or weight loss (IF = 18 per cent); blood pressure, reducing all diastolic pres-

sures to less than 80 mm Hg (IF = 36 per cent); cigarette smoking, discontinuing all tobacco smoking (IF = 43 per cent); type A personality, changing to B personality types or reduction of related social stressors (IF = 33 per cent); and diabetes (mean IF = 15 per cent). Thus, 90 per cent of CHD is potentially preventable by intervention to optimize known coronary risk factors. Most of this potential appears to be realizable by cessation of cigarette smoking and comprehensive dietary reform.

Recommended guidelines to reduce risk factor exposure should be promoted for the entire population. Laboratory screening of all persons and intervention only in those found to be at high risk is too expensive and less effective. However, a very inexpensive screening method that will identify a sizable number of high-risk persons is the family history. Attributable risk, or the proportion of early CHD cases in the general population from high-risk families, may be as high as 35 per cent. Many of these families will have traits or habits that are amenable to intervention. A combination of enthusiastically endorsed recommendations for the entire population and more detailed screening and intervention among high-risk families may be the most cost-effective means to prevent CHD.

Although much of this discussion has been idealistic, sound data are available to support the conclusions drawn. The potential for prevention of cardiovascular disease is enormous. We believe that there is more enthusiasm in the general population to reduce exposure to risk factors than generally acknowledged by the medical profession—witness trends of cardiovascular death rates accompanied by greater awareness of diet, reductions in saturated fat, cholesterol, and salt intakes, and the exercise craze, all of which are part of the contemporary American scene. The continuation of these favorable trends depends, in part, on strong, positive support from the medical profession. It is hoped that this article will be useful in the dissemination of information so necessary for that support.

APPENDIX

Table A–1. *Multiple Logistic or Cox Regression Coefficients from Several Recent,*
Large Prospective Studies*

A. FRAMINGHAM STUDY[81]
> *Follow-up:* 26 years
> *Population:* men (n = 2197), women (n = 2714)
> *Age at baseline:* 28–62 years
> *End point:* all CVD (866 men, 688 women developed CHD, congestive heart failure, stroke, or intermittent claudication)

RISK FACTOR	β* Men	β* Women
Age	0.469	0.390
Systolic BP	0.311	0.332
% Metropolitan Life Insurance desirable weight	0.143 (15.9)	0.199 (22.1)
Cholesterol	0.309	0.197
Cigarettes/day	0.232	0.139
Glucose intolerance	0.220	0.100
ECG-LVH	0.215	NS

B. FRAMINGHAM STUDY[59,60]
> *Follow-up:* 4 years from 11th biannual exam
> *Population:* men (n = 1025), women (n = 1445)
> *Age at baseline:* 49–82 years
> *End point:* all CHD (138 cases)

RISK FACTOR	β* Men	β* Women
Systolic BP	0.327 (26)	NS
Relative weight	NS	NS
LDL cholesterol	0.332 (46)	0.260 (39)
HDL cholesterol	−0.610 (15)	−0.650 (15)
Triglycerides	NS	NS
Cigarettes/day	NS	NS
Diabetes	NS	0.390
ECG–LVH	0.245	0.159

C. FRAMINGHAM STUDY[71]
> *Follow-up:* 10 years
> *Population:* men (n = 285)
> *Age at baseline:* 45–64 years
> *End point:* all CHD (44 cases)

RISK FACTOR	β*
Age	NS
Systolic BP	NS
Cholesterol	NS
Cigarettes/day	NS
Framingham type A	0.368 (0.50)
Wife's occupation	
White collar vs clerical	0.669
White collar vs blue collar	0.762
White collar vs housewife	0.821
Wife's years of education: (1 = ≤ 8; 2 = 9–12; 3 = 13+)	0.414
Wife's ambitiousness	−0.490
Wife's anger symptoms	0.382
Number of children	0.365

D. FRAMINGHAM STUDY[182]
> *Follow-up:* 26 years
> *Population:* brother-brother pairs (n = 169)
> *Ages at baseline:* 28–62 years
> *End point:* CHD death (46 events)

RISK FACTOR	β*
CHD in older brother	0.440
Age	0.546
Systolic BP	0.749
Cholesterol	0.342
Metropolitan Life Insurance relative weight	NS
Smoking (yes/no)	NS

E. TECUMSEH STUDY[23]
> *Population:* men (n = 921), women (n = 937)
> *Age at baseline:* 40–70+ years
> *End point:* CHD mortality (161 cases in men, 88 cases in women)

RISK FACTOR	COX REGRESSION COEFFICIENT
Age (0 = women, 1 = men)	0.103
Sex (0 = women, 1 = men)	1.119
Cholesterol	0.008
Systolic BP	0.024
Cigarettes/day	0.022
Diabetes (0 = no, 1 = yes)	1.349
Age × cholesterol	−0.0003
Age × systolic BP	−0.0007
Age × cigarettes	−0.0011
Age × diabetes	−0.353

F. STOCKHOLM PROSPECTIVE STUDY[14]
> *Follow-up:* 14.5 years
> *Population:* healthy men (n = 2961)
> *Age at baseline:* 15–77 years
> *End point:* Ischemic vascular deaths (184 cases)

RISK FACTOR	β
Age	0.114
Systolic BP	0.0231
Smoking (1 = yes, 0 = no)	0.491
Serum cholesterol	NS
Serum triglycerides†	0.435
Weight-height index	NS
Hemoglobin	0.0220
ESR	0.357
Intercept (α)	−16.68

†In units of ln (100 × mmol/liter), where ln is the natural logarithm

G. HONOLULU HEART PROGRAM[131,214]
Follow-up: 10 years
Population: Japanese men (n = 7705)
Age at baseline: 45–68 years
End point: Total CHD (511 cases)

RISK FACTOR	β*
Age	0.186
Systolic BP	0.401
Physical activity index	−0.117
Serum cholesterol	0.222
Serum triglycerides	NS
Serum uric acid	0.43
Serum glucose	0.158
Vital capacity/height	−0.133
Cigarettes/day	−0.264
Alcohol consumption	−0.264
Daily caloric intake	−0.1057 (711)
Starch (g)	0.1136 (71.4)
Alcohol (g)	−0.1978 (29.2)
Protein % calories	0.1273 (3.8)
Fat % calories	0.1308 (9.3)
Cholesterol/1000 calories	0.0962 (130.1)

H. WESTERN COLLABORATIVE GROUP STUDY[16]
Follow-up: 8.5 years
Population: men (n = 3154)
Age at baseline: 39–59 years
End point: Total CHD (257 cases)

RISK FACTOR	β Men 39–49	β Men 50–59
Age	0.0902	0.0615
Cholesterol	0.0120	0.0086
Systolic BP	0.0150	0.0202
Relative body weight	NS	NS
Hematocrit	NS	NS
Cigarette smoking†	0.2429	0.2990
Type A personality	0.6396	0.7430
Intercept (α)	−14.62	−13.46

†Cigarette smoking category codes: 0 = no smoking; 1 = < 1 pack/day; 2 = 1 pack/day; 3 = > 1 pack/day

I. HELSINKI POLICEMEN STUDY[156]
Follow-up: 5 years
Population: men (n = 1042)
Age at baseline: 30–59 years
End point: CHD death = nonfatal (36 cases)

RISK FACTOR	β*
Age	0.725
Diastolic BP	NS
Cholesterol	0.536
Triglycerides	NS
Cigarettes/day	NS
Body mass index	NS
2-hour plasma insulin	0.420
2-hour plasma glucose	NS

J. NORTH KARELIA PROJECT[168]
Follow-up: 7 years
Population: men (n = 4057)
Age: 30–59 years
End point: Acute myocardial infarction (211 cases)

RISK FACTOR	β*
Serum cholesterol	0.43
Serum triglycerides	NS
Age	0.71
Smoking	0.35
Casual diastolic BP	0.29
History of myocardial infarction or angina in parents < 50 years	NS
History of stroke in parents	NS
Body mass index	NS
History of diabetes	NS
Years of education	NS

K. THE ISRAELI ISCHEMIC HEART DISEASE STUDY[56]
Follow-up: 5 years
Population: Men (n = 6547)
Age at baseline: 40–64 years
End point: Myocardial infarction (141 cases)

RISK FACTOR	β (BY AGE AT BASELINE) 40–44	45–54	55–64
Age	0.0378	0.0634	0.0603
Systolic BP	0.0139	0.0181	0.0304
Total cholesterol	0.0074	0.0107	0.0068
HDL cholesterol	NS	−0.0331	−0.0338
Smoking†	0.5582	0.3575	0.1516
Diabetes‡	1.3460	0.5068	0.2562
Quitelet index (kg/m²)	0.0331	−0.0084	−0.0278
Intercept (α)	−12.3502	−11.2673	−11.1460

†Coded 0 = never smoked; 1 = past smoker; 2 = 1–10 cigarettes/day; 3 = 11–20 cigarettes/day; 4 = > 20 cigarettes/day
‡Coded 0 = no diabetes; 1 = abnormal glucose tolerance but no diabetes; 2 = diabetes at baseline

*All coefficients shown are statistically significant at p < 0.05.
CVD = cardiovascular disease; BP = blood pressure; NS = not significant; ESR = erythrocyte sedimentation rate.
β = nonstandardized logistic coefficient; β* = standardized logistic coefficient

Table A–2. *Calculating the Impact of Three Major Coronary Risk Factors on Risk of Coronary Heart Disease From a Large, Representative U.S. Population*[196]

DIASTOLIC BP (n = 7066)			SERUM CHOLESTEROL (n = 6983)			CIGARETTE SMOKING (n = 6975)		
level	p_i'	p_i''	*level*	p_i'	p_i''	*level*	p_i'	p_i''
<60	0.0011	0.0011	<160	0.0309	0.0309	0	0.3361	1.0
60–64	0.0011	0.0113	160–179	0.0664	0.0664			
65–69	0.0154	0.154	180–199	0.1275	0.4345	0.5	0.1204	0
70–74	0.1144	0.486	200–219	0.1612	0.4681			
75–79	0.0507	0.486	220–239	0.1866	0	1	0.0778	0
80–84	0.2829	0	240–259	0.1562	0			
85–89	0.1044	0	260–279	0.1107	0	2	0.3127	0
90–94	0.1886	0	280–299	0.0696	0			
95–99	0.0500	0	300–319	0.0412	0	3	0.1530	0
100–104	0.0804	0	320–339	0.0242	0			
100–109	0.0181	0	340–359	0.0105	0			
100–114	0.0299	0	360–379	0.00066	0			
115–119	0.0064	0	380–399	0.0040	0			
≥120	0.0164	0	≥400	0.0043	0			
$\Sigma\ p_i'RR_i$ = 2.66		IF$_o$ = 0.62	$\Sigma\ p_i'RR_i$ = 1.774		IF$_o$ = 0.44	$\Sigma\ p_i'RR_i$ = 1.76		IF$_o$ = 0.43
$\Sigma\ p_i''RR_i$ = 1.70		IF$_h$ = 0.36	$\Sigma\ p_i''RR_i$ = 1.3379		IF$_h$ = 0.25			

Risk of major coronary event in 10 years in men aged 40–59 years at entry = $1/1 + \exp(f(x))$, where $f(x) = \alpha + \beta_1$ (age) + β_2 (diastolic BP) + β_3 (serum cholesterol) + β_4 (cigarette smoking code). Major coronary events are nonfatal myocardial infarction, fatal myocardial infarction, and sudden CHD death.

Codes for cigarette smoking: never smoked, past smoker, or smoking < ½ pack/day = 0; cigar or pipe only = 0.5; ½ pack/day = 1.0; 1 pack/day = 2.0; > 1 pack/day = 3.0

α = −10.328; β_1 = 0.0685; β_2 = 0.0304; β_3 = 0.00614; β_4 = 0.385
p_i' = proportion of men currently at stated risk factor level
p_i'' = hypothetical new distribution
RR_i = relative risk above baseline (see text)
IF_o = ideal impact fraction if the entire population were at baseline risk
IF_h = the hypothetical impact fraction given the p_i'' distribution shown

AGE AND RELATIVE RISK

Referring to Figure 1, the relative risk is equal to $\dfrac{IN_2}{IN_{2^o}}$, or the ratio of the incidence rates in the exposed versus unexposed population. Risk factors that affect only the rate of progression from the unaffected to the preclinical pool affect only the rate constant J. Thus, if $I_1 = I_o = I$, the relative risk would depend only on the relative sizes of the preclinical pools, N_2' and N_{2^o}.

Differential equations describing the rates of change for the two pools are as follows:

$$dN_1 = -\ J(x)\ N_1\ dt \qquad [1]$$

and

$$dN_2 = +\ J(x)\ N_1\ dt\ -\ N_2\ I\ dt \qquad [2]$$

where J (x) denotes the dependence of J on risk factor level x.

Solution of equation 1 yields $N_1 = N \exp(-Jt)$, where N equals the entire population size (as $N_1 + N_2 = N$ and $N_2 = 0$ at time 0). Substitution into the second equation and rearrangement gives

$$\frac{dN_2}{dt} + IN_2 = NJ \exp(-Jt) \qquad [3]$$

Solutions of the homogeneous and nonhomogeneous equations may be combined, given the starting conditions described above, to yield

$$N_2 = \frac{J\ N}{I\text{-}J} \exp(-Jt)\ -\ \exp(-It) \qquad [4]$$

Applying this equation to the formula for relative risk (N_2'/N_{2^o}) yields

$$\frac{J_1\ (I - J_o)\ (\exp((I-J_1)t)\ -\ 1)}{J_o\ (I - J_1)\ (\exp((I-J_o)t)\ -\ 1)} \qquad [5]$$

where $J_1 = J$ at some arbitrary risk factor exposure level, and $J_o = J$ at baseline risk. Note that the relative risk given by equation 5 is strongly dependent on time and not just $\dfrac{J_1}{J_o}$ as it would be in a one-pool model.

Let us suppose that J_1 was equal to 25 per 1000 person-years and J_o was 5 per 1000 person-years and that I equaled 100 per 1000 person-years. At t = 5 years, the relative risk would be 4.7. At t = 30 years, the relative risk would be 3.3. By 65 years of age, the relative risk would be only 1.7, and by age 95 it would actually be 0.95! Therefore, the powerful effect of age must always be considered when judging the importance of a cardiovascular risk factor.

REFERENCES

1. Aberg, A., Bergstrand, R., Johansson, S., et al.: Cessation of smoking after myocardial infarction—effects

on mortality after 10 years. Br. Heart J., *49*:416–422, 1983.

2. Amery, A., Birkenhager, W., Brixko, P., et al.: Mortality and morbidity results from the European Working Party on High Blood Pressure in the Elderly Trial. Lancet, 2:1349–1354, 1985.

3. Arthes, F.G., and Masi, A.T.: Myocardial infarction to younger women—associated clinical features and relationship to use of oral contraceptive drugs. Chest, 70:574–583, 1976.

4. Avogaro, P., Cazzolato, G., Taroni, G.C., et al.: Chemical composition of ultracentrifugal fractions in different patterns of human atherosclerosis. Atherosclerosis, *26*:163–172, 1977.

5. Ballantyne, F.C., Clark, R.S., Simpson, H.S., et al.: High density and low density lipoprotein subfractions in survivors of myocardial infarction and in control subjects. Metabolism, 31:433–437, 1982.

6. Barrett-Connor, E., and Wingard, P.L.: Sex differential in ischemic heart disease mortality in diabetics: A prospective population-based study. Am. J. Epidemiol., *118*:489–496, 1983.

7. Beaglehole, R., LaRosa, J.C., Heiss, G., et al.: Serum cholesterol, diet, and the decline in coronary heart disease mortality. Prev. Med., 8:538–547, 1979.

8. Berginer, V.M., Salen, G., and Shefer, S.: Long-term treatment of cerebrotendinous xanthomatosis with chemodeoxycholic acid. N. Engl. J. Med., *311*:1649–1652, 1984.

9. Bierenbaum, M.L., Fleischman, A.I., Raichelson, R.I., et al.: Ten year experience of modified fat diets on younger men with CHD. Lancet, 1:1404–1407, 1973.

10. Bierman, E.L., and Ross, R.: Aging and atherosclerosis. Atheroscl. Rev., 2:79–111, 1977.

11. Blackburn, H.: Diet and mass hyperlipidemia: A public health view. *In* Larry, K., Rifkind, B., Dennis, B., et al. (eds.): Nutrition, Lipids, and Coronary Heart Disease. New York, Raven Press, 1979, pp. 309–347.

12. Blair, D., Habicht, J.-P., Sims, E.A.H., et al.: Evidence for an increased risk for hypertension with centrally located body fat and the effect of the race and sex on this risk. Am. J. Epidemiol., *119*:526–540, 1984.

13. Bordia, A., Paliwal, D.K., Jain, K., et al.: Acute effect of ascorbic acid on fibrinolytic activity. Atherosclerosis, *30*:351–354, 1978.

14. Bottiger, L.-E., and Carlson, L.A.: Risk factors for ischaemic vascular death for men in the Stockholm Prospective Study. Atherosclerosis, 36:389–408, 1980.

15. Bradby, G.V.H., Valente, A.J., and Walton, K.W.: Serum high-density lipoprotein in peripheral vascular disease. Lancet, 2:1271–1274, 1978.

16. Brand, R.J., Rosenman, R.H., Sholtz, R.I., et al.: Multivariate prediction of coronary heart disease in the Western Collaboraative Group Study compared to the findings of the Framingham Study. Circulation, 53:348–355, 1976.

17. Braunwald, E. (ed.): Heart Disease. Edition 2. Philadelphia, W.B. Saunders Company, 1984, pp. 1606–1640.

18. Broekmans, A.W., Veltkamp, J.J., and Bertina, R.M.: Congenital protein C deficiency and venous thromboembolism. A study of three Dutch families. N. Engl. J. Med., 309:340–344, 1983.

19. Brunzell, J.D., Albers, J.J., Chait, A., et al.: Plasma lipoproteins in familial combined hyperlipidemia and monogenic familial hypertriglyceridemia. J. Lipid Res., 24:147–155,, 1983.

20. Brunzell, J.D., Sniderman, A.D., Albers, J.J., et al.: Apoproteins B and A-1 and coronary artery disease in humans. Arteriosclerosis, 4:79–83, 1984.

21. Brunzell, J.P., Schrott, H.G., Motulsky, A.G., et al.: Myocardial infarction in the familial forms of hypertriglyceridemia. Metabolism, 25:313–320, 1976.

22. Burkitt, D.B., and Trowell, H.C.: Refined Carbohydrate Foods and Disease. London, Academic Press, 1975, pp. 195–226.

23. Butler, W.J., Ostrander, L.D., Carman, W.J., et al.: Mortality from coronary heart disease in The Tecumseh Study. Long-term effect of diabetes mellitus, glucose tolerance and other risk factors. Am. J. Epidemiol., *121*:541–547, 1985.

24. Byington, R., Dyer, A.R., Garside, A.R., et al.: Recent trends of major coronary risk factors and CHD mortality in the United States and other industrialized countries. *In* Havlik, R.J., and Feinleib, M. (eds.): Proceedings of the Conference on the Decline in Coronary Heart Disease Mortality. U.S. Department of Health, Education and Welfare, Public Health Service. NIH Publication No. 79-1610, 1979, pp. 340–380.

25. Cambien, F., Chretien, J.M., Ducimetiere, P., et al.: Is the relationship between blood pressure and cardiovascular risk dependent on body mass index? Am. J. Epidemiol., *122*:434–442, 1985.

26. Campeau, L., Enjolbert, M., Lesperance, J., et al.: The relation of risk factors to the development of atherosclerosis in saphenous-vein bypass grafts and the progression of disease in the native circulation. A study 10 years after aorto-coronary bypass surgery. N. Engl. J. Med., *311*:1329–1332, 1984.

27. Carmelli, D., Swan, G.F., and Rosenman, R.H.: The relationship between wives' social and psychologic status and their husbands' coronary heart disease: A case-control family study from the Western Collaborative Group Study. Am. J. Epidemiol., *122*:90–100, 1985.

28. Casciani, C.U., Caruso, U., et al.: Effect of L-carnitine on lipid pattern in hemodialysis. Lancet, 2:1309–1310, 1980.

29. Castelli, W.P., Doyle, J.T., Gordon, T., et al.: HDL cholesterol and other lipids in CHD. The Cooperative Lipoprotein Phenotyping Study. Circulation, 55:767–772, 1977.

30. Chait, A., Albers, J.J., and Brunzell, J.D.: Very low density lipoprotein overproduction in generic forms of hypertriglyceridemia. Eur. J. Clin. Invest., *10*:17–22, 1980.

31. Chandra, V., Szklo, M., Goldberg, R., et al.: The impact of marital status on survival after an acute myocardial infarction: A population based study. Am. J. Epidemiol., *117*:320–325, 1983.

32. Coleman, D.L., Ross, T.F., and Naughton, J.L.: Myocardial ischemia and infarction related to recreational cocaine use. West. J. Med., *136*:444–446, 1982.

33. Committee of Principal Investigators: WHO Cooperative trial on primary prevention of ischaemic heart disease using clofibrate to lower serum cholesterol: Mortality follow-up. Lancet, 2:379–385, 1980.

34. Comp, P.C., and Esmon, C.T.: Recurrent venous thromboembolism in patients with a partial deficiency of protein S. N. Engl. J. Med., *311*:1525–1528, 1984.

35. Cornfield, J., and Detre, K.: Selection on atheroscle-

rosis as an explanation of the attenuated cholesterol-mortality relation in coronary heart disease populations. Am. J. Epidemiol., *110*:716–723, 1979.

36. Crepaldi, G., Fellin, R., Briani, G., et al.: Prevalence of CHD and peripheral artery disease with different types of primary hyperlipidemia. Atherosclerosis, *26*:593–602, 1977.

37. Dai, W.S., LaPorte, R.E., Horn, D.L., et al.: Alcohol consumption and high density lipoprotein cholesterol concentration among alcoholics. Am. J. Epidemiol., *122*:620–627, 1985.

38. Danielsson, B., Ekman, R., Fox, G., et al.: Changes in plasma high density lipoproteins in chronic male alcoholics during and after abuse. Scand. J. Clin. Lab. Invest., 38:113–119, 1978.

39 Davignon, J., Lussier-Cacan, S., Ortin-George, M., et al.: Plasma lipids and lipoprotein patterns in angiographically graded atherosclerosis of the legs and in CHD. Calif. Med. Assoc. J., *4*:1245–1250, 1977.

40. Dayton, S., Pearce, M.L., Hashimoto, S., et al.: A controlled clinical trial of diet high in unsaturated fat in preventing complications of atherosclerosis. Circulation, *39,40*:1–63, 1969.

41. DeBias, D.A., Banerjee, C.M., Birhead, N.C., et al.: Effects of carbon monoxide inhalation on ventricular fibrillation. Arch. Environ. Health, *31*:38–42, 1976.

42. DeWood, M.A., Spores, J., Notske, R., et al.: Prevalence of total coronary occlusion during the early hours of transmural myocardial infarction. N. Engl. J. Med., *303*:897–902, 1980.

43. Dintenfass, L.: Erythrocyte sedimentation rates—a tentative correction for haematocrit. Rheol. Acta, *13*:936–943, 1974.

44. Doll, R., and Peto, R.: Mortality in relation to smoking: 20 years' observation on male British doctors. Br. Med. J., *2*:1525–1536, 1976.

45. Dyclener, T., and Wester, P.O.: Clinical significance of diuretic-induced magnesium loss. Pract. Cardiol., *10*:125–133, 1984.

46. Faggiotto, A., Ross, R., and Harker, L.: Studies of hypercholesterolemia in the nonhuman primate. Arteriosclerosis, *4*:323–356, 1984.

47. Ferns, G.A.A., Ritchie, C., Stocks, J., et al.: Generic polymorphisms of apolipoprotein C-III and insulin in survivors of myocardial infarction. Lancet, *2*:300–303, 1985.

48. Friedman, G.D., Petitti, D.B., Bawol, R.D., et al.: Mortality in cigarette smokers and quitters. Effect of baseline differences. N. Engl. J. Med., *304*:1407–1410, 1981.

49. Friedman, M.: Type A behavior pattern: Some of its pathophysiological components. Bull. N.Y. Acad. Med., *53*:593–604, 1977.

50. Friedman, M., Byers, S.O., and Rosenman, R.H.: Effect of unsaturated fats upon lipemia and conjunctival circulation—a study of coronary-prone (pattern A) men. J.A.M.A., *193*:882–886, 1965.

51. Friedman, M., Thoresen, C.E., Gill, J.J., et al.: Feasibility of altering type A behavior pattern after myocardial infarction. Recurrent Coronary Prevention Project Study: Methods, baseline results and preliminary findings. Circulation, *66*:83–92, 1982.

52. Fuster, V., Chesebro, J.H., Brye, R.L., et al.: Platelet survival and the development of coronary artery disease in the young adult: Effects of cigarette smoking, strong family history and medical therapy. Circulation, *63*:546–551, 1981.

53. Garcia-Palmieri, M., Sorlie, P., Tillorson, J., et al.: Relationship of dietary intake to subsequent coronary heart disease. Am. J. Clin. Nutr., *18*:149, 1966.

54. Garland, C., Barrett-Connor, E., Suarez, L., et al.: Isolated systolic hypertension and mortality after age 60 years: A prospective population-based study. Am. J. Epidemiol., *118*:365–376, 1983.

55. Garland, C., Barrett-Connor, E., Suarez, L., et al.: Effects of passive smoking on ischemic heart disease mortality of nonsmokers: A prospective study. Am. J. Epidemiol., *121*:645–650, 1985.

56. Goldbourt, R., and Medalie, J.H.: High density lipoprotein cholesterol and incidence of coronary heart disease: The Israeli Ischemic Heart Disease Study. Am. J. Epidemiol., *109*:296–308, 1979.

57. Goldstein, J.L., Schrott, H.G., and Hazzard, W.R.: Hyperlipidemia in coronary heart disease. II. Genetic analysis of lipid levels in 176 families and delineation of a new inherited disorder, combined hyperlipidemia. J. Clin. Invest., *52*:1544–1568, 1973.

58. Gordon, D.J., Probstfield, J.L., Rubenstein, C., et al.: Coronary risk factors and exercise test performance in asymptomatic hypercholesterolemic men: Application of proportional hazards analysis. Am. J. Epidemiol., *120*:210–224, 1984.

59. Gordon, T., and Kannel, W.B.: Multiple risk function for predicting heart disease: The concept accuracy and application. Am. Heart J., *103*:1031–1039, 1982.

60. Gordon, T., Castelli, W.P., Hjortland, M.C., et al.: Predicting coronary heart disease in middle-aged and older persons. The Framingham Study. J.A.M.A., *238*:497–499, 1977.

61. Gordon, T., Garcia-Palmieri, M.R., Kagan, A., et al.: Differences in coronary heart disease in Framingham, Honolulu and Puerto Rico. J. Chronic Dis., *27*:329–344, 1974.

62. Gordon, T., Kagan, A., Garcia-Palmieri, M., et al.: Diet and its relation to coronary heart disease and death in three populations. Circulation, *63*:500–515, 1981.

63. Gordon, T., Kannel, W.B., McGee, D., et al.: Death and coronary attacks in men after giving up cigarette smoking. Lancet, *2*:1345–1348, 1974.

64. Green, M.S., and Symons, M.J.: A comparison of the logistic risk function and the proportional hazards model in prospective epidemiologic studies. J. Chronic Dis., *36*:715–724, 1983.

65. Grundy, S.M.: Absorption and metabolism of dietary cholesterol. Am. Rev. Nutr., *3*:71–96, 1983.

66. Guarnieri, G.F., Raniers, F., and Toigo, G.: Lipid-lowering effect of carnitine in chronically uremic patients treated with maintenance hemodialysis. Am. J. Clin. Nutr., *33*:1489–1492, 1980.

67. Hanel, R.J.: Familial dysbetalipoproteinemia. New aspects of pathogenesis and diagnosis. Med. Clin. North Am., *66*:441–454, 1982.

68. Hartz, A.J. Rupley, D.C., and Rimm, A.A.: The association of girth measurements with disease in 32,856 women. Am. J. Epidemiol., *119*:71–80, 1984.

69. Haskell, W.I., Camargo, C., Williams, P.T., et al.: The effect of cessation and resumption of moderate alcohol intake on serum high density lipoprotein subfractions: A controlled study. N. Engl. J. Med., *310*:805–810, 1984.

70. Hassall, D.G., Forrest, L.A., Bruckdorfer, K.R., et al.: Influence of plasma lipoproteins on platelet aggregation in a normal male population. Arteriosclerosis, *3*:332–338, 1983.

71. Haynes, S.G., Eaher, E.D., and Feinleib, M.: Spouse behavior and coronary heart disease in men: Pro-

spective results from The Framingham Heart Study. 1. Concordance of risk factors and the relationship of psychosocial status to coronary incidence. Am. J. Epidemiol., *118*:1–22, 1983.

72. Heiss, G., and Tyroler, N.A.: Are lipoproteins useful for evaluating ischemic heart disease? A brief overview of the literature. *In* Lippel, K. (ed.): Proceedings of the Workshop on Apolipoprotein Quantification. U.S. Department of Health and Human Services. Public Health Service. NIH Publication No. 83-1266, August 1983, pp. 7–24.

73. Henricksen, T., Evensen, S.A., and Carlander, B.: Injury to human endothelial cells in culture induced by low density lipoproteins. Scand. J. Clin. Lab. Invest., *39*:361–368, 1979.

74. Hjermann, I., Holme, I., Byre, K.V., et al.: Effect of diet and smoking intervention on the incidence of coronary heart disease. Report from the Oslo Study Group of a randomised trial in healthy men. Lancet, *2*:1303–1310, 1981.

75. Hopkins, P.N., and Williams, R.R.: A survey of 246 suggested coronary risk factors. Atherosclerosis, *40*:1–52, 1981.

76. Hopkins, P.N., and Williams, R.R.: Response to letter to the editor. West. J. Med., *143*:681, 1985.

77. Hopkins, P.N., and Williams, R.R.: A simplified approach to lipoprotein kinetics and factors affecting serum cholesterol and triglyceride concentrations. Am. J. Clin. Nutr., *34*:2560–2590, 1981.

78. Hopkins, P.N., Williams, R.R., and Hunt, S.C.: Magnified risks from cigarette smoking for coronary prone families in Utah. West. J. Med., *141*:196–202, 1984.

79. Hornstra, G., and Ules, R.: Effects of dietary fats on atherosclerosis and thrombosis. *In* Carlson, L.A., et al. (eds.): International Conference on Atherosclerosis. New York, Raven Press, 1978, pp. 471–476.

80. Hosaki, S., Kishimoto, T., Yamauchi, M., et al.: Serum lipoproteins in Japanese rural community with low cardiovascular mortality. Atherosclerosis, *54*:43–47, 1985.

81. Hubert, H.B., Feinleib, M., McNamara, P.M., et al.: Obesity as an independent risk factor in the Framingham Heart Study. Circulation, *67*:968–977, 1983.

82. Humphries, S.E., Kessling, A.M., Horsthemke, B., et al.: A common DNA polymorphism of the low-density lipoprotein (LDL) receptor gene and its use in diagnosis. Lancet, *1*:1003–1005, 1985.

83. Hypertension Detection and Follow-up Program Cooperative Group: Five-year findings of the Hypertension Detection and Follow-up Program. J.A.M.A., *242*:2562–2577, 1979.

84. Hypertension Detection and Follow-up Program Cooperative Group: Five-year findings of the Hypertension Detection and Follow-up Program. II. Reduction in stroke incidence among persons with high blood pressure. J.A.M.A., *247*:633–638, 1982.

85. Hypertension Detection and Follow-up Program Cooperative Group: The effect of treatment on mortality in "mild" hypertension. Results of the Hypertension Detection and Follow-up Program. N. Engl. J. Med., *307*:976–980, 1982.

86. Iseri, L.T., and French, J.H.: Magnesium: Nature's physiologic calcium blocker. Am. Heart J., *106*:188–194, 1984.

87. Iseri, L.T., Chung, P., and Tobis, J.: Magnesium therapy for intractable ventricular tachyarrhythmias in normomagnesemic patients. West. J. Med., *138*:823–828, 1983.

88. Ishikawa, T., Fidge, N., Thelle, D.S., et al.: The Tramso Heart Study: Serum apolipoprotein A-1 concentration in relation to future coronary heart disease. Eur. J. Clin. Invest., *8*:179–182, 1978.

89. Jain, A.K.: Cigarette smoking, use of oral contraceptives, and myocardial infarction. Am. J. Obstet. Gynecol., *126*:301–307, 1976.

90. Jajick, C.L., Ostfeld, A.M., and Freeman, D.H.: Smoking and coronary heart disease mortality in the elderly. J.A.M.A., *252*:2831–2834, 1984.

91. Janus, E.D., Nicoll, A.M., Turner, P.R., et al.: Kinetic bases of the primary hyperlipidaemias: Studies of apolipoprotein B turnover in genetically defined subjects. Eur. J. Clin. Invest., *10*:161–172, 1980.

92. Jenkins, C.D., Rosenman, R.H., and Zyzanski, S.J.: Prediction of clinical coronary heart disease by a test for the coronary-prone behavior pattern. N. Engl. J. Med., *290*:1271–1275, 1974.

93. Johansson, S., Bergstrand, R., Pennert, K., et al.: Cessation of smoking after myocardial infarction in women: Effects on mortality and reinfarctions. Am. J. Epidemiol., *121*:823–831, 1985.

94. Kannel, W.B.: Some lessons in cardiovascular epidemiology from Framingham. Am. J. Cardiol., *37*:269–282, 1976.

95. Kannel, W.B., and Gordon, T.: The search for an optimum serum cholesterol. Lancet, *2*:374–375, 1982.

96. Kannel, W.B., Doyle, J.T., Ostfeld, A.M., et al.: Optimal resources for primary prevention of atherosclerotic disease. Circulation, *70*:157A–205A, 1984.

97. Kannel, W.B., Dawker, T.R., and McGee, D.L.: Perspectives on systolic hypertension. The Framingham Study. Circulation, *61*:1179–1182, 1980.

98. Kavanagh, T., Shephard, R.J., Lindley, L.J., et al.: Influence of exercise and life-style variables upon high density lipoprotein cholesterol after myocardial infarction. Arteriosclerosis, *3*:249–259, 1983.

99. Kesaniems, Y.A., and Grundy, S.M.: Overproduction of low density lipoproteins associated with coronary heart disease. Arteriosclerosis, *3*:40–46, 1983.

100. Keys, A.: Seven Countries: A Multivariate Analysis of Death and Coronary Heart Disease. Boston, Harvard University Press, 1980, p. 65.

101. Kissebah, A.H., Alfarsi, S., and Adams, P.W.: Integrated regulation of very low density lipoprotein triglyceride and apolipoproteins—B kinetics in man: Normolipidemic subjects, familial hypertriglyceridemia and familial combined hyperlipidemia. Metabolism, *30*:856–868, 1981.

102. Kissebah, A.H., Alfarsi, S., and Evans, D.J.: Low density lipoprotein metabolism in familial combined hyperlipidemia. Mechanism of multiple lipoprotein phenotypic expression. Arteriosclerosis, *4*:614–624, 1984.

103. Kleinbaum, D.G., Kupper, L.L., and Morgenstern, H.: Epidemiologic Research: Principles and Quantitative Methods. Belmont, California, Lifetime Learning Publications, 1982.

104. Knuiman, J.T., West., C.E., and Burema, J.: Serum total and high density lipoprotein cholesterol concentrations and body mass index in adult men from 13 countries. Am. J. Epidemiol., *116*:631–642, 1982.

105. Kornitzer, M., DeBacker, G., and Dramaix, M.: Belgian heart disease prevention project: Incidence and mortality results. Lancet, *1*:1066–1070, 1983.

106. Kottke, B.: Personal communications. September 1985.

107. Kottke, T.E., Puska, P., Salonen, J.T., et al.: Projected effects of high-risk versus population-based prevention strategies in coronary heart disease. Am. J. Epidemiol., *121*:697–704, 1985.

108. Kozarevic, D., Pirc, B., Dawber, T.R., et al.: The Yugoslavia Cardiovascular Disease Study. 2. Factors in the incidence of coronary heart disease. Am. J. Epidemiol., *104*:133–140, 1976.

109. Kraus, A., and Lilenfeld, A.: Some epidemiologic aspects of the high mortality rate in the young widowed group. J. Chronic Dis., *10*:207–217, 1959.

110. Kreiss, K., Zack, M.M., Kimbrough, R.D., et al.: Association of blood pressure and polychlorinated biphenyl levels. J.A.M.A., *245*:2505–2509, 1981.

111. Kromhout, D., and Coulander, C.: Diet, Prevalence and 10-year mortality from coronary heart disease in 871 middle-aged men: The Zutphen Study. Am. J. Epidemiol., *119*:733–741, 1984.

112. Kromhout, D., Bosschieter, E.B., and Coulander, C.: The inverse relation between fish consumption and 20-year mortality from coronary heart disease. N. Engl. J. Med., *312*:1205–1209, 1985.

113. Krotkiewski, M., Bjorntorp, P., Sjostrom, L., et al: Impact of obesity on metabolism in men and women. Importance of regional adipose tissue distribution. J. Clin. Invest., *72*:1150–1162, 1983.

114. Ku, D.N., and Giddens, D.P.: Pulsatile flow in a model carotid bifurcation. Arteriosclerosis, *3*:31–39, 1983.

115. Kuo, P.T., and Joyner, C.R.: Angina pectoris induced by fat ingestion in patients with coronary artery disease. J.A.M.A., *158*:1008–1013, 1955.

116. Lapidus, L., Bengtsson, C., Larsson, B., et al., Distribution of adipose tissue and risk of cardiovascular disease and death: A 12 year follow up of participants in the population study of women in Gothenburg, Sweden. Br. Med. J., *289*:1257–1261, 1984.

117. Larsson, B., Svardsudd, K., Welin, L., et al.: Abdominal adipose tissue distribution, obesity, and risk of cardiovascular disease and death: 13 year follow up of participants in the study of men born in 1913. Br. Med. J., *288*:1401–1404, 1984.

118. Lee, E.T.: Statistical Methods for Survival Data Analysis. Belmont, California, Lifetime Learning Publications, 1980.

119. Leren, P.: The effect of plasma cholesterol lowering diet in male survivors of MI. Acta Med. Scand. Suppl. *466*:1–92, 1966.

120. Liberthson, R.R., Nagel, E.L., Hirschman, J.C., et al.: Pathophysiologic observations in prehospital ventricular fibrillation and sudden cardiac death. Circulation, *49*:790–798, 1974.

121. Lipid Research Clinic Program: The Lipid Research Clinic Coronary Primary Prevention Trial results. II. The relationship of reduction in incidence of coronary heart disease to cholesterol lowering. J.A.M.A., *251*:365–374, 1984.

122. Luscher, E.F.: The effects of lipids and fatty acids on blood coagulation and platelets in relation to thrombosis. Adv. Exp. Med. Biol., *60*:107–118, 1975.

123. Maciejko, J.J., Holmes, D.R., Kottke, B.A., et al.: Apolipoprotein A-I as a marker of angiographically assessed coronary-artery disease. N. Engl. J. Med., *309*:385–389, 1983.

124. Maebashi, M., Kawanura, N., Sato, M., et al.: Lipid-lowering effect of carnitine in patients with type-IV hyperlipoproteinaemia. Lancet, *2*:805–807, 1978.

125. Magnus, K., Matroos, A.W., and Strackee, J.: The self-employed and the self-driven: Two coronary-prone subpopulations from The Ziest Study. Am. J. Epidemiol., *118*:799–805, 1983.

126. Mahley, R.W.: Atherogenic hyperlipoproteinemia. The cellular and molecular biology of plasma lipoproteins altered by dietary fat and cholesterol. Med. Clin. North Am., *66*:375–402, 1982.

127. Malinow, M.R., and Blaton, V.: Regression of atherosclerosis lesions. Atheriosclerosis, *4*:292–295, 1984.

128. Mandrup-Poulsen, T., Mortensen, S.A., Meinertz, H., et al.: DNA sequences flanking the insulin gene on chromosome 11 confer risk of atherosclerosis. Lancet, *1*:250–252, 1984.

129. Mann, J.I., and Hughson, W.G.: Intermittent claudication—a preventable condition? Am. Heart J., *98*:666–668, 1979.

130. McCarron, D.A., and Kotchen, T.A., (eds.): Nutrition and blood pressure control. Current status of dietary factors and hypertension. Ann. Intern. Med., *98*:697–884, 1983.

131. McGee, D.L., Reed, D.M., Yano, K., et al.: Ten-year incidence of coronary heart disease in The Honolulu Heart Program. Relationship to nutrient intake. Am. J. Epidemiol., *119*:667–676, 1984.

132. Medalie, J.H., and Goldbourt, U.: Angina pectoris among 10,000 men. Part 2 (Psychosocial and other risk factors as evidenced by a multivariate analysis of a five year incidence study). Am. J. Med., *60*:910–921, 1976.

133. Melish, M.E., Hicks, R.V., and Reddy, V.: Kawasaki syndrome: An update. Hosp. Pract., *17*:99–106, 1982.

134. Menzel, H.-J., Kladetzky, R.-G., and Assmann, G.: Apolipoprotein E polymorphism and coronary artery disease. Arteriosclerosis, *3*:310–335, 1983.

135. Messerli, F.H.: Obesity in hypertension—how innocent a bystander. Am. J. Med., 1984.

136. Miettinen, M., Karvonen, M., Turpeinen, O., et al.: Effect of cholesterol-lowering diet on mortality from coronary heart disease and other causes. A twelve-year clinical trial in men and women. Lancet, *2*:835–838, 1972.

137. Miettinen, O.S.: Proportions of disease caused or prevented by a given exposure, trait or intervention. Am. J. Epidemiol., *99*:325–332, 1979.

138. Miller, N.E., Forde, O.H., Thelle, D.S., et al.: The Tromso Heart Study. HDL and CHD: A prospective case-control study. Lancet, *1*:965–967, 1977.

139. Miller, N.E., Hammett, F., Saltissi, S., et al.: Relation of angiographically defined coronary artery disease to plasma lipoprotein subfractions and apolipoproteins. Br. Med. J., *282*:1741–1744, 1981.

140. Morel, D.W., DiCorleto, P.E., and Chisohm, G.M.: Endothelial and smooth muscle cells alter low density lipoprotein in vitro by free radical oxidation. Arteriosclerosis, *4*:357–364, 1984.

141. Morganroth, J., Levy, R.I., and Frederickson, D.S.: The biochemical, clinical, and genetic features of type III hyperlipoproteinemia. Ann. Intern. Med., *82*:158–174, 1975.

142. Morgenstern, H., and Bursic, E.S.: A method for using epidemiologic data to estimate the potential impact of an intervention on the health status of a target population. J. Commun. Health, *7*:292–309, 1982.

143. Morris, J.N., Heady, J.A., and Barley, R.G.: Coronary heart disease in medical practitioners. Br. Med. J., *1*:503–517, 1952.

144. Morris, J.N., Marr, J.W., and Clayton, D.G.: Diet and heart—a postscript. Br. Med. J., *2*:1307–1314, 1977.

145. Mustard, J.F., Packam, M.A., and Kimlough-Rath-

bone, R.: Platelets, thrombosis and atherosclerosis. Adv. Exp. Med. Biol., *104*:127–144, 1978.

146. Oestrogens, calcium transport, and coronary spasm. (Editorial.) Lancet, *1*:229–230, 1977.

147. Ooneda, G., and Yoshida, Y.: Atherosclerosis in Japan: Pathology. Atheroscl. Rev., *2*:223–232, 1977.

148. Oram, J.F.: Effects of high density lipoprotein subfractions on cholesterol homeostasis in human fibroblasts and arterial smooth muscle cells. Arteriosclerosis, *3*:420–432, 1983.

149. Parkes, C.M., Benjamin, B., and Fitzgerald, R.G.: Broken heart: A statistical study of increased mortality among widowers. Br. Med. J., *1*:740, 1969.

150. Perrera, G.A., and Damon, A.: Height, weight, and their ratio in the accelerated form of hypertension. Arch. Intern. Med., *100*:263, 1957.

151. Phillips, R.L., Lemmon, F.R., Beeson, W.L., et al.: Coronary heart disease among Seventh-Day Adventists with differing habits—a preliminary report. Am. J. Clin. Nutr., *31*:5191–5198, 1978.

152. Phillipson, B.E., Rothrock, D.W., Conner, W.E., et al.: Reduction of plasma lipids, lipoproteins, and apoproteins by dietary fish oils in patients with hypertriglyceridemia. N. Engl. J. Med., *312*:1210–1216, 1985.

153. Pirkle, J.L., Schwartz, J., Landis, J.R., et al.: The relationship between blood lead levels and blood pressure and its cardiovascular risk implications. Am. J. Epidemiol., *121*:246–258, 1985.

154. Pola, P., Savi, L., Grilli, M., et al.: Carnitine in the therapy of dyslipidemic patients. Curr. Ther. Res., *27*:208–216, 1980.

155. Puska, P., Salonen, J.T., Nissinen, A., et al.: Change in risk factors for coronary heart disease during 10 years of a community intervention program (North Karelia Project). Br. Med. J., *287*:1840–1844, 1983.

156. Pyorala, K.: Relationship of glucose tolerance and plasma insulin to the incidence of coronary heart disease: Results from two population studies in Finland. Diabetes Care, *2*:131–141, 1979.

157. Rake, R.H., Bennett, L., Rom, M., et al.: Subjects' recent life changes and coronary heart disease in Finland. Am. J. Psychiatry, *130*:1222, 1973.

158. Rees, W.D., and Lutkins, S.G.: Mortality of bereavement. Br. Med. J., *4*:13, 1967.

159. Reidy, M.A., and Bowyer, D.E.: Distortion of endothelial repair. The effect of hypercholesterolaemia on regeneration of aortic endothelium following injury by endotoxin—a scanning electron microscope study. Atherosclerosis, *29*:459–466, 1978.

160. Report by the Management Committee: The Australian Therapeutic Trial in Mild Hypertension. Lancet, *1*:1261–1267, 1980.

161. Retchembach, D.D., Moss, N.S., and Meyer, E.: Pathology of the heart in sudden cardiac death. Am. J. Cardiol., *39*:865, 1977.

162. Review Panel on Coronary-Prone Behavior and Coronary Heart Disease: Coronary-prone behavior and coronary heart disease: A critical review. Circulation, *63*:1199–1215, 1981.

163. Robbins, S.L., and Cotran, R.S.: Pathologic Basis of Disease. Edition 2. Philadelphia, W.B. Saunders Company, 1979, p. 687.

164. Rose, G., Tunstall-Pedoe, H.D., and Heller, R.F.: UK Heart Disease Prevention Project: Incidence and mortality results. Lancet, *1*:1062–1066, 1983.

165. Rosenman, R.H., Brand, R.J., Jenkins, C.D., et al.: Coronary heart disease in the Western Collaborative Group Study. Final follow-up experience of 8½ years. J.A.M.A., *233*:872–877, 1975.

166. Rossner, S., Kjellin, K.G., Mettinger, K.L., et al.: Dyslipoproteinemia in patients with ischemic cerebrovascular disease. A study of stroke before the age of 55. Atherosclerosis, *30*:199–209, 1978.

167. Salonen, J.T.: Stopping smoking and long-term mortality after acute myocardial infarction. Br. Heart J., *43*:463–469, 1980.

168. Salonen, J.T., and Puska, P.: Relation of serum cholesterol and triglycerides to the risk of acute myocardial infarction, cerebral stroke and death in eastern Finnish male population. Int. J. Epidemiol., *12*:26–31, 1983.

169. Salonen, J.T., Puska, P., Kottke, T.E., et al.: Decline in mortality from coronary heart disease in Finland from 1969 to 1979. Br. Med. J., *286*:1857–1860, 1983.

170. Schaefer, E.J.: Clinical, biochemical, and genetic features in familial disorders of high density lipoprotein deficiency. Arteriosclerosis, *4*:303–322, 1984.

171. Schatzin, A., Cupples, L.A., et al.: Sudden death in the Framingham Heart Study. Differences in incidence and risk factors by sex and coronary disease status. Am. J. Epidemiol., *120*:888–899, 1984.

172. Schwartz, C.V., Chandler, A.B., Gerrity, R.T., et al.: Clinical and pathological aspects of arterial thrombosis and thromboembolism. Adv. Exp. Med. Biol., *104*:111—126, 1978.

173. Seligsohn, U., Berger, A., Abend, M., et al.: Homozygous protein C deficiency manifested by massive venous thrombosis in the newborn. N. Engl. J. Med., *310*:559–562, 1984.

174. Shea, S., Ottman, R., Gabriel, C., et al.: Family history as an independent risk factor for coronary artery disease. J. Am. Coll. Cardiol., *4*:793–801, 1984.

175. Shekelle, R., MacMillan, S., Shryoch, R., et al.: Diet, serum cholesterol and death from coronary heart disease: The Western Electric Study. N. Engl. J. Med., *304*:65–70, 1981.

176. Shekelle, R.B., Hulley, S.B., Neaton, J.D., et al.: The MRFIT Behavior Pattern Study. II. Type A behavior and incidence of coronary heart disease: Am. J. Epidemiol., *122*:559–570, 1985.

177. Sirtori, C.R., Biasi, G., Vercellio, G., et al.: Diet, lipids and lipoproteins in patients with peripheral vascular disease. Am. J. Med. Sci., *268*:325–332, 1974.

178. Sirtori, C.R., Gianfranceschi, G., Gritti, I., et al.: Decreased high density lipoprotein cholesterol levels in male patients with transient ischemic attacks. Atherosclerosis, *32*:205–211, 1979.

179. Slack, J.: Risks of ischaemic heart-disease in familial hyperlipoproteinaemic states. Lancet, *2*:1380–1382, 1969.

180. Smith-Barbaro, P.A., and Pucak, G.J.: Dietary fat and blood pressure. Ann. Intern. Med., *98*:828–831, 1983.

181. Sniderman, A., Shapiro, S., Marpole, D., et al.: Association of coronary atherosclerosis with hyperapobetalipoproteinemia [increased protein but normal cholesterol levels in human plasma low density (β) lipoproteins]. Proc. Natl. Acad. Sci. USA, *77*:604–608, 1980.

182. Snowden, C.B., McNamara, P.M., Garrison, R.J., et al.: Predicting coronary heart disease in siblings—a multivariate assessment. The Framingham Heart Study. Am. J. Epidemiol., *115*:217–222, 1982.

183. Stamler, J.: Lifestyles, major risk factors, proof and public policy. Circulation, 58:3–19, 1978.
184. Steinberg, D.: Lipoproteins and atherosclerosis. A look back and a look ahead. Arteriosclerosis, 3:283–301, 1983.
184a. Steinberg, D., et al.: Consensus Conference: Lowering blood cholesterol to prevent heart disease. J.A.M.A., 253:2080, 1985.
185. Stern, B., Heyden, S., Miller, D., et al.: Intervention study in high school students with elevated blood pressures. Dietary experiment with polyunsaturated fats. Nutr. Metab., 24:137–147, 1980.
186. Suarez, L., and Barrett-Connor, E.: Is an educated wife hazardous to your health? Am. J. Epidemiol., 119:244–249, 1984.
187. Suarez, L., and Barrett-Connor, E.: Interaction between cigarette smoking and diabetes mellitus in the prediction of death attributed to cardiovascular disease. Am. J. Epidemiol., 120:670–675, 1984.
188. Swank, R.L.: Blood viscosity in cerebrovascular disease—effects of low fat diet and heparin. Neurology (Minneap.), 9:553–560, 1959.
189. Swank, R.L.: The influence of ecologic factors on blood viscosity and sedimentation and on serum cholesterol—ecology and blood viscosity. Am. J. Clin. Nutr., 19:418–432, 1962.
190. Szatrowski, T.P., Peterson, A.V., Shimizu, Y., et al.: Serum cholesterol, other risk factors, and cardiovascular disease in a Japanese cohort. J. Chronic Dis., 37:569–584, 1984.
191. ten Kate, L.P., Boman, H., Daiger, S.P., et al.: Familial aggregation of coronary heart disease and its relation to known genetic risk factors. Am. J. Cardiol., 50:945–953, 1982.
192. ten Kate, L.B., Boman, H., Daiger, S.P., et al.: Increases frequency of coronary heart disease in relatives of wives of myocardial infarct survivors: Assortative mating for lifestyle and risk factors? Am. J. Cardiol., 53:399–403, 1984.
193. Texon, M.: Atherosclerosis. Its hemodynamic basis and implication. Med. Clin. North Am., 58:257–268, 1974.
194. Theorello, T.: Psychosocial factors and myocardial infarction—why and how? Adv. Cardiol., 8:117–131, 1973.
195. Theorello, T., Lind, E., and Floderus, B.: The relationship of disturbing life changes and emotions in the early development of myocardial infarction and other serious illnesses. Int. J. Epidemiol., 4:281, 1975.
196. The Pooling Project Research Group: Relationship of blood pressure, serum cholesterol, smoking habit, relative weight and ECG abnormalities to incidence of major coronary events: Final report of the Pooling Project. J. Chronic Dis., 31:201–306, 1978.
197. Truswell, A.S.: End of a static decade for coronary disease? Br. Med. J., 289:509–510, 1984.
198. Turpeinen, O.: Effect of cholesterol-lowering diet on mortality from coronary heart disease and other causes. Circulation, 59:1–7, 1979.
199. Vacha, G.M., Giorcelli, G., Siliprandi, N., et al.: Favorable effects of L-carnitine treatment on hypertriglyceridemia in hemodialysis patients: Decisive role of low levels of high-density lipoprotein-cholesterol. Am. J. Clin. Nutr., 38:532–540, 1983.
200. Valek, J., Hammer, J., Kohow, M., et al.: Serum linoleic acid and cardiovascular death in postinfarction middle-aged men. Atherosclerosis, 54:111–118, 1985.
201. Vergani, C., Finzi, A.F., Pigatto, P.D., et al.: Low levels of HDL in severe cystic acne. (letter.) N. Engl. J. Med., 307:1151–1152, 1982.
202. Veterans Administration Cooperative Study Group on Antihypertensive Agents: Effects of treatment on morbidity in hypertension. II. Results in patients with diastolic blood pressure averaging 90–114 mm Hg. J.A.M.A., 213:1143–1152, 1970.
203. Virtamo, J., Valkeila, E., Alfthan, G., et al.: Serum selenium and the risk of coronary heart disease and stroke. Am. J. Epidemiol., 122:276–282, 1985.
204. Walker, A.R.P., and Arvidsson, U.B.: Fat intake, serum cholesterol concentration and atherosclerosis in the South African Bantu. Part 1 (Low fat intake and the age trend of serum cholesterol concentration in the South African Bantu). J. Clin. Invest., 33:1358–1365, 1954.
205. Weiss, N.S.: Cigarette smoking arteriosclerosis obliterans: An epidemiologic approach. Am. J. Epidemiol., 95:17–25, 1972.
206. Wilhelmson, C., Vedin, J.A., Elmfeldt, E., et al.: Smoking and myocardial infarction. Lancet, 1:415, 1975.
207. Wilhelmsen, L., Svardsudd, K., Karsan-Bengtsen, K., et al.: Fibrinogen as a risk factor for stroke and myocardial infarction. N. Engl. J. Med., 311:501–505, 1984.
208. Williams, A.V., Higginbotham, A.C., and Knisely, M.H.: Increased blood cell agglutination following ingestion of fat, a factor contributing to cardiac ischemia, coronary insufficiency, and anginal pain—a contribution to the biophysics of disease. Angiology, 8:29–39, 1957.
209. Williams, P.T., Wood, P.D., Krause, R.M., et al.: Does weight loss cause the exercise-induced increase in plasma high density lipoproteins? Atherosclerosis, 47:173–185, 1983.
210. Williams, R.B.: Behavioral factors in cardiovascular disease: An update. *In* Hurst, J.W. (ed.): The Heart. Update V. New York, McGraw-Hill, 1979, pp. 219–230.
211. Williams, R.R.: The role of genes in coronary atherosclerosis. *In* Hurst, J.W. (ed.): Update for The Heart. New York, McGraw-Hill, 1979, pp. 89–118.
212. Williams, R.R., Hunt, S.C., Kuida, K., et al.: Sodium-lithium countertransport in erythrocytes of hypertension prone families in Utah. Am. J. Epidemiol., 118:338–344, 1983.
213. Williams, R.R., Skolnick, M., Carmelli, D., et al.: Utah pedigree studies: Design and preliminary data for premature male CHD deaths. *In* Sing, C.F., and Skolnick, M. (eds.): The Generic Analysis of Common Diseases. New York, Alan R. Liss, Inc., 1979, pp. 711–721.
214. Yano, K., Reed, D.M., and McGee, D.L.: Ten-year indicence of coronary heart disease in The Honolulu Heart Program. Relationship to biologic and lifestyle characteristics. Am. J. Epidemiol., 119:653–661, 1984.
215. Zilversmit, D.B.: A proposal linking atherogenesis to the interaction of endothelial lipoprotein lipase with triglyceride-rich lipoproteins. Circ. Res., 33:633–638, 1973.

Cardiology Division
Department of Internal Medicine
University of Utah Medical Center
Salt Lake City, Utah 84132

Cardiovascular Risk Factors and Their Modification in Children

Gregory L. Burke, M.D.,* James L. Cresanta, M.D.,†
Charles L. Shear, D.P.H.,‡ Michael H. Miner, Ph.D.,§
and Gerald S. Berenson, M.D.‖

More than 50 per cent of all mortality in the United States and other Western countries can be directly attributed to cardiovascular disease. Epidemiologic studies of adults have established the causal relationships between cardiovascular disease and antecedent risk factors such as hypertension, diabetes mellitus, dyslipidemia, and cigarette smoking.[14,25,53] More recently, attention has been directed toward the study of the early natural history of cardiovascular disease.[7,8,52]

Although the etiologic link between childhood cardiovascular disease risk factors and the early onset of atherosclerotic events remains to be clarified, there are strong, consistent relationships between childhood risk factor levels and adult cardiovascular disease. The determinants of the traditional risk factors for adult cardiovascular disease such as obesity, smoking, carbohydrate metabolism abnormalities, alcohol intake, and oral contraceptive usage also are determinants of risk factors in childhood.[13,27,37,48,60,61] In addition, a positive family history of cardiovascular disease is associated with elevated risk factors in childhood.[29,57]

New evidence from autopsy studies of children from the Bogalusa Heart Study[8,52] demonstrates the adverse effects of elevated risk factor levels in enhancing an accelerated development of atherosclerotic fatty streaks and fibrous plaques during the first two decades of life. Tracking, or the persistence of levels of risk factors over time in childhood,[7,9,16,36] when linked to studies of young adults, such as naval aviators[34] and those from Evans County,[64] supports the concept of risk factors in children predicting adult cardiovascular disease.

Primary prevention has the greatest potential to interrupt the early natural history and course of atherosclerosis. Because the initiation of healthy lifestyles is adopted more easily than the alteration of established unhealthy lifestyles, primary prevention should occur in early life.[73]

Intervention during childhood and adolescence requires either benign treatment modalities (if the intervention is geared toward all children) or more aggressive therapy in high-risk patients (in which the benefits derived from early intervention would outweigh the risk of treatment). In light of the recent evidence of atherosclerosis beginning early in life, which correlates with clinical risk factors in children,

*Assistant Professor, Departments of Medicine and Public Health and Preventive Medicine, Louisiana State University Medical Center, New Orleans, Louisiana

†Associate Professor, Department of Public Health and Preventive Medicine, Louisiana State University Medical Center, New Orleans, Louisiana

‡Assistant Professor, Departments of Medicine and Public Health and Preventive Medicine, Louisiana State University Medical Center, New Orleans, Louisiana

§Assistant Professor, Departments of Medicine and Psychiatry, Louisiana State University Medical Center, New Orleans, Louisiana

‖Professor, and Director, National Research and Demonstration Center—Arteriosclerosis, Department of Medicine, Louisiana State University Medical Center, New Orleans, Louisiana

standards for abnormal cardiovascular disease risk factor levels in children need to be defined; certainly, levels used in adults must be adjusted downward.[6,50]

In this article, we present current concepts and recommendations concerning the natural history of arteriosclerosis in childhood. Concepts discussed include target organ changes in early life that are associated with traditional risk factors, levels of risk factors, and their tracking (or persistence) throughout childhood. The majority of the data presented are from the Bogalusa Heart Study, a long-term epidemiologic study of cardiovascular disease risk factors in childhood.[7] We have studied children from this biracial community for 12 years, focusing on the specific methods required for measuring cardiovascular disease risk factors and their distribution and persistence over time in childhood. Currently accepted recommendations concerning the measurement of and intervention on blood pressure, lipids and lipoproteins, and obesity in childhood are also presented.

TARGET ORGAN CHANGES IN EARLY LIFE

Studies of children and young adults by both echocardiography and necropsy have demonstrated target organ changes. These investigations provide valuable evidence of early manifestations of cardiovascular disease in healthy free-living populations. The findings of prospective, community-based studies (such as the Bogalusa Heart Study) are extrapolated more easily to larger populations because they establish a temporal relationship between cause and effect without subject-selection biases. Most autopsy series come from hospital-based populations and limit the generalizability of findings.

Several investigators have noted increased echocardiographically measured left ventricular mass in children with high levels of blood pressure.[23,40,55,75] We have noted an increase in left ventricular size with higher levels of blood pressure across the entire blood pressure distribution. In addition, we have documented a relationship between vascular changes in renal arteries and antemortem blood pressure levels from autopsy studies of children.[8] Although no specific lesion serves as a precise sign of early hypertensive disease, tissue alterations related to blood pressure levels provide evidence of early target organ changes from high blood pressure during early life.

Autopsy studies provide the best evidence to validate clinical measurements and the cardiovascular risk factor concept in childhood. The high prevalence of coronary artery lesions seen in young soldiers serving in the United States military during the Korean War[24] and Vietnam War,[47] along with the early age of onset for cardiovascular lesions noted in the Community Pathology Study in the greater New Orleans area,[62,63] documents a high degree of atherosclerosis in relatively young populations. Atherosclerotic fatty streak and fibrous plaque development in the aorta and coronary arteries is strongly related to antemortem serum lipid and lipoprotein levels.[8,52] In autopsy studies of young Bogalusa children and adolescents dying in motor vehicle accidents and from other violent causes, there was a direct, linear relationship between the percentage of total surface involvement of atherosclerotic fatty streaks in the aorta and both antemortem total cholesterol and low-density lipoprotein (LDL) cholesterol levels. Those youngsters with antemortem serum total cholesterol levels between 140 and 170 mg per dl had more than 25 per cent total surface involvement with fatty streaks, whereas those with antemortem serum total cholesterol levels above 200 mg per dl had 50 per cent total surface involvement (Fig. 1). The relationship was even stronger between total surface involvement and LDL cholesterol levels. In the coronary arteries, antemortem very-low-density lipoprotein (VLDL) cholesterol levels were related to the percentage of fatty streak involvement. Young decedents with atherosclerotic fibrous plaques in the coronary arteries had higher antemortem systolic blood pressure levels and tended to have higher serum triglyceride levels than those decedents without raised lesions.[8,52] These findings clearly demonstrate adverse manifestations of high blood pressure in combination with abnormal lipids and lipoprotein levels early in life in an at-risk population. The need for primary prevention and early intervention to retard atherosclerotic lesion progression during the first two decades of life is evident.

BLOOD PRESSURE IN CHILDREN

Blood pressure levels in adulthood have been related to increased cardiovascular disease morbidity and mortality.[14,25,26,53,65] The significance of an elevated blood pressure level in childhood remains a controversial issue owing to the lack of morbid events noted in childhood populations and inadequate information pertaining to the risk-to-benefit ratio of hypertension interven-

ATHEROSCLEROTIC FATTY STREAK INVOLVEMENT OF THE AORTA RELATED TO SERUM TOTAL CHOLESTEROL IN THE YOUNG (n = 30)

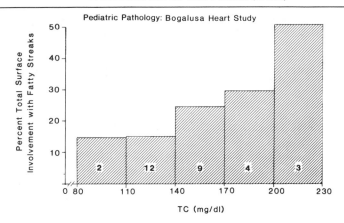

Figure 1. Atherosclerotic fatty streak involvement of the aorta related to serum total cholesterol in the young. (Pediatric Pathology Study: Bogalusa Heart Study.)

tion programs in rapidly growing individuals. On the other hand, early intervention using both pharmacologic and nonpharmacologic measures not only could act to prevent future target organ damage but also may preclude the subsequent development of adult hypertensive disease in an at-risk population. This section will describe normal levels of blood pressure in a biracial population of children and the trends in blood pressure levels in a cohort of individuals followed over time.

Normal Levels of Blood Pressure. Studies of blood pressure levels and problems in diagnosing hypertension in children and young adults are complicated by inconsistent methods.[9] Systolic and diastolic blood pressure levels in boys aged 5 to 20 years from numerous epidemiologic studies are listed in Table 1. In general, systolic blood pressure levels increase approximately 1.5 mm Hg per year in growing children, with diastolic levels increasing by approximately 0.7 mm Hg per year. Although trends with increasing age are similar among studies, significant differences in actual blood pressure levels among these studies are observed. The marked differences are likely related to methodology, even though the observations are on different populations. Only slight differences in population groups have been noted when studied by the same investigators under similar circumstances.[39]

In the measurement of blood pressure levels in children, close attention should be paid to the technique of measurement.[8–10,38,44,54,72] We be-

lieve that in order to obtain reliable estimates of an individual child's blood pressure status, multiple blood pressure measures should be taken, and if possible, they should be taken by two different well-trained examiners. This can be accomplished easily in an office setting, where, in addition, serial measurements can be obtained to determine sustained elevations in blood pressure levels over time. Because reported levels of indirect blood pressure vary considerably among epidemiologic studies of populations of children,[9] it is important that the reference percentiles or cut points used are based on population norms that employ methodology similar to that used in the physician's office (right arm, sitting, and relaxed measurements are usually reported). We recommend replicate measurements recorded by two different observers (as we have noted that measurements from two observers, when averaged, provide a better representative measurement than replicate readings by one observer).

Changes in blood pressure levels with age reflect, in part, the rapid increase in body size throughout childhood. Both systolic and diastolic blood pressure levels exhibit a consistently stronger relationship with height and weight than with age.[67] Figure 2 shows normal levels of blood pressure at a given height for Bogalusa boys aged 2 to 18 years (although weight is important, height is a better anthropometric measure). These data emphasize the importance of considering the relative height and weight of a particular child before classification of an indi-

Table 1. *Blood Pressure Levels in Boys by Age for Selected Surveys*

	N	5	6	7	8	9	10	11	12	13	14	15	16	17	18	19	20
									AGE (years)								
SYSTOLIC BLOOD PRESSURE (mm Hg) (means)*																	
Southern CA (W)	2249		96	98	102	102	104	106	110	114	117	121	122				
Southern CA (B)	797	95	98	97	102	101	105	108	112	115	115	120	122				
Muscatine, IA (W)	2240	96	97	99	100	102	103	106	109	114	117	122	122	125	125		
Bogalusa, LA (W)	2430	93	95	97	97	99	102	103	104	108	109	112	113	113	117	116	121
Bogalusa, LA (B)	1228		93	96	97	100	100	102	102	107	111	113	114	115	118	119	
Minneapolis, MN (B & W)	5046		103	104	106	107											
Rochester, MN (W)	1842		106	108	112	114	114	116	118	120	122	125					
St. Louis, MO (B & W)	3494								110	111	114	117	131	134	133		
New York, NY (B & W)	1844										114	116	120	121	121		
DIASTOLIC BLOOD PRESSURE (mm Hg) (means)*																	
Southern CA (W)	2249		62	62	64	64	64	66	66	67	67	70	70				
Southern CA (B)	797	62	64	62	65	65	68	67	66	68	67	69	68				
Muscatine, IA (W)	2240	57	64	64	66	66	68	69	71	73	75	78	79	80	82		
Bogalusa, LA (W)	2430	57	57	58	59	60	63	62	63	65	67	68	70	70	73	74	77
Bogalusa, LA (B)	1228		57	60	58	61	62	63	64	64	67	68	70	70	72	72	
Minneapolis, MN (B & W)	5046		65	66	68	69											
Rochester, MN (W)	1842		67	70	71	73	72	75	72	71	74	72					
St. Louis, MO (B & W)	3494								71	72	64	67	73	76	78		
New York, NY (B & W)	1844										73	73	69	70	72		

*Average of replicate readings

N = number of boys; W = white; B = black

Adapted from Berenson, G.S., et al.: High blood pressure in the young. Annu. Rev. Med., 35:535, 1984; with permission.

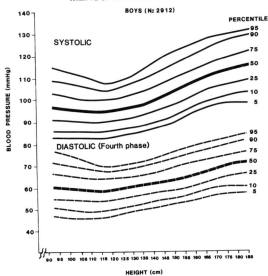

Figure 2. Indirect blood pressure measurement by height in boys. (Bogalusa Heart Study.) (*From* Berenson, G.S., et al.: Cardiovascular Risk Factors in Children—The Early Natural History of Atherosclerosis and Essential Hypertension. New York, Oxford University Press, 1980; with permission.)

vidual into a high-risk category based on age-specific blood pressure grids (for example, a tall and heavy 6-year-old child with height and weight at the fiftieth percentile for the 10-year-old group would be expected to exhibit a blood pressure level similar to that seen in the 10-year-old group). Height- and gender-specific blood pressure grids should be used to plot an individual's blood pressure measurements over time in the same way that physicians currently plot weight and linear growth increments in a child's permanent medical record.

Figure 3 depicts the blood pressure levels of children followed over a 6-year period based on their initial age. Black children, especially black male children, have a greater increase in blood pressure levels when compared with white children of the same age. Subtle racial differences in blood pressure levels have been observed in younger children (2 to 14 years old)[11]; however, as our cohort is followed into the midteens and beyond, the classic picture of an increased proportion of black children in the upper distribution of systolic and diastolic blood pressure becomes more evident.[70]

Tracking of Blood Pressure. Because adverse effects of hypertensive disease have been documented in adult studies, if blood pressure levels can be shown to persist at high levels (track-

ing) through childhood and early adulthood, high-risk individuals can be identified prior to their development of target organ damage. We have measured children's blood pressure levels in Bogalusa, Louisiana, since 1973. Table 2 shows the high correlation between initial and subsequent measurements of children followed for 8 years.[56] Initial blood pressure levels are significant predictors of blood pressure in late childhood or early adulthood.[66,70,71] These data show the persistence of blood pressure rankings of children in relation to their peers and demonstrate the ability to predict subsequent blood pressure status based on readings taken during early childhood. For example, of those children with a prior measurement of systolic blood pressure in the upper decile, 41.3 per cent remained in the upper decile 3 years later. However, more than 61 per cent of those children with three prior measurements in the upper decile remained in the upper decile 3 years later, showing the importance of serial measurements.[56]

Recommendations for Blood Pressure. We believe that accurate determination of blood pressure levels in childhood can be accomplished using well-trained observers. In an epidemiologic setting, basal resting blood pressures taken by at least two different observers are the best predictors of subsequent blood pressure levels in children. Proper cuff sizes should be used and the fourth Korotkoff phase is recommended as a measure of diastolic blood pressure in childhood.[69] Serial blood pressure measurements increase the physician's prognostic ability to discriminate which individuals are more likely to have elevated blood pressure levels in later life. These findings document the importance of monitoring blood pressure levels in children and comparing the results with previously defined gender- and height-specific population norms. Blood pressure rank and trends can be assessed accurately and efficiently with multiple measures taken during routine office visits to a child's primary care physician. Plotting on standard grids (such as that shown in Figure 2) adjusts for differences in body size and provides a rapid visual assessment of blood pressure tracking in an individual child.

As an exploratory study, we conducted a clinical trial in a small rural and biracial community to study the effectiveness of low-dose antihypertensive medication on a group of children tracking at or above the ninetieth percentile.[10a,26a] The objective was to control blood pressure at a lower percentile and attempt to prevent blood pressure rises over time. A beta-blocker and a diuretic were given along with dietary instruc-

SYSTOLIC AND DIASTOLIC BLOOD PRESSURES OF THREE COHORTS OVER TIME BY RACE, SEX, AND INITIAL BIRTH COHORT

BOGALUSA HEART STUDY, 1973–1980

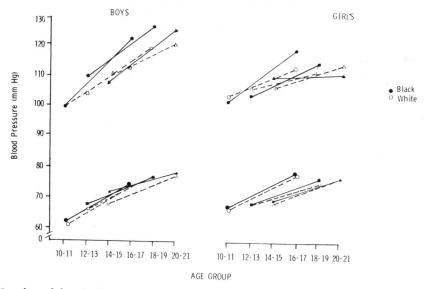

Figure 3. Systolic and diastolic blood pressures of three age cohorts by race and sex. (Bogalusa Heart Study.) (*From* Berenson, G.S., (ed.): Causation of Cardiovascular Risk Factors in Childhood. New York, Raven Press, 1986; with permission.)

tion, an exercise program, and training in blood pressure recording. Parents were provided with cooking classes and low-sodium food products. Programs in the school cafeteria, community restaurants, and grocery stores were also conducted. Obesity was present in about 20 per cent of the children, mainly white, and a strong family history was noted in the blacks. Most impressive among the results was the response to the low-dose medication. Approximately 10 per cent of the children did not respond to the treatment program, and in general, blood pressure

decreases were less in the blacks. Little or no side effects occurred with the drug treatment. These observations suggest an approach to consider in the control of early hypertension to have an impact on the initiating factors of hypertension and interrupt its natural course.

With regard to follow-up and treatment for elevated values, the Joint National Committee on Detection, Evaluation, and Treatment of High Blood Pressure and the Task Force on High Blood Pressure in Children both recommend nonpharmacologic intervention in chil-

Table 2.   *Tracking Coefficients for Blood Pressure in Childhood Through 8 Years of Follow-up—Bogalusa Heart Study, 1973–1982*

	SYSTOLIC			DIASTOLIC		
	Yr 1 vs. Yr 9	Yr 4 vs. Yr 9	Yr 6 vs. Yr 9	Yr 1 vs. Yr 9	Yr 4 vs. Yr 9	Yr 6 vs. Yr 9
All children	0.51	0.58	0.61	0.44	0.48	0.55
White						
Male	0.52	0.59	0.67	0.46	0.51	0.60
Female	0.47	0.56	0.59	0.41	0.43	0.54
Black						
Male	0.51	0.56	0.55	0.45	0.46	0.47
Female	0.49	0.55	0.62	0.38	0.47	0.55

$p < 0.001$ for all correlation coefficients
Adapted from Shear, C.L., et al.: The value of childhood blood pressure measurements and family history in predicting future blood pressure status: Results from eight years of follow-up in the Bogalusa Heart Study. Pediatrics, in press.

dren with blood pressure levels persisting at or above the ninety-fifth percentile and pharmacologic intervention in those children who are resistant to the initial intervention.[50,51] In addition, recommendations for weight reduction in obese children are presented in a later section.

LIPIDS AND LIPOPROTEINS IN CHILDREN

There is now overwhelming evidence that coronary artery disease and atherosclerosis are related to the serum total cholesterol level.[6,52,58,62,73] Research and clinical emphasis have shifted during the past decade from total cholesterol to focus more sharply on its three components, high-density lipoprotein (HDL) cholesterol, LDL cholesterol, and VLDL cholesterol. Elevated levels of LDL cholesterol are atherogenic, but elevated levels of HDL cholesterol apparently provide some protection against coronary atherosclerosis.[15,32,58] The ratio of LDL cholesterol to HDL cholesterol or the ratio of total cholesterol to HDL cholesterol has been used to estimate the risk for future coronary morbidity and mortality in adults.[32] Large collaborative studies such as the Lipid Research Clinics[42,43] have shown the benefits gained from treatment of hyperlipidemia in adults. This section will describe the normal levels and trends of lipids and lipoproteins in children.

Normal Levels of Lipids and Lipoproteins. In the first two decades of life, average levels of serum total cholesterol are remarkably similar in white male children throughout the United States, but they are somewhat higher in European children.[6] In all race and gender groups of American children, mean serum total cholesterol levels are relatively stable near 160 mg per dl from age 2 years until the onset of sexual maturation (Fig. 4).[6,19,22] They decline during adolescence but increase sharply after maturation is completed.[10,19,21,22] Total cholesterol levels are slightly higher in black children because they have higher HDL cholesterol levels than white children,[19,22] but when screening patients for hypercholesterolemia in a clinical setting, total cholesterol levels in black and white children are close enough to use a single reference grid for all American children under age 20 years (Fig. 5).[22]

The stability and changes in total cholesterol levels with age and maturation are related to similar changes in LDL cholesterol, which composes the major proportion of total cholesterol

at all ages.[19] The simple correlation between total cholesterol and LDL cholesterol ranges from 0.73 to 0.82.[20] Both total cholesterol and LDL cholesterol decline during adolescence but increase dramatically after age 17 years.[22] Dynamic changes in HDL cholesterol levels during sexual maturation,[6,10,19,21,70] especially in white male adolescents,[28] also contribute significantly to the adolescent decline in serum total cholesterol levels. The ratio of LDL cholesterol to HDL cholesterol is relatively stable in all race and gender groups from 2 years of age through adolescence, at which time a dramatic increase begins in white male adolescents (Fig. 6).[6] The late adolescent rise of this ratio in white male teenagers results from a longitudinal mean increase of 13 mg per dl in LDL cholesterol levels, coupled with a simultaneous mean decrease of 11 mg per dl in HDL cholesterol levels,[70] placing the white male population at an extraordinarily high risk for premature coronary artery disease.[19,28,58]

There are much larger racial differences in serum triglyceride, VLDL cholesterol, and HDL cholesterol levels,[22] probably related to a greater body fatness in white children.[27] Over a 5-year interval, mean changes in serum lipid and lipoprotein levels were strongly related to tertile of change in triceps skinfold thickness, that is, those with the greatest increase in body fat over time had the greatest increase in both LDL cholesterol and VLDL cholesterol levels. Although female children have the greatest absolute increase in triceps skinfold thickness over time, associations between body fat and serum lipids and lipoproteins were stronger in male children.[27]

Persistence of Levels of Lipids and Lipoproteins. Persistence of lipid and lipoprotein levels was examined in 2236 children who were screened three times over a 5-year interval.[71] Pearson correlation coefficients between initial and subsequent levels were highest for LDL cholesterol, ranging from 0.62 to 0.78, and nearly as high for serum total cholesterol. Both LDL cholesterol and total cholesterol tracked to a similar degree even after 8 years of follow-up.[29] Tracking was of similar magnitude in all race and gender groups.

For those children at or above the ninetieth percentile for LDL cholesterol during the first examination, 47 per cent of those with initially high measurements were also at or above the ninetieth percentile 3 years later. In this same group, 73 per cent and 41 per cent were at or above the eightieth and ninetieth percentiles, respectively, 5 years after the initially high

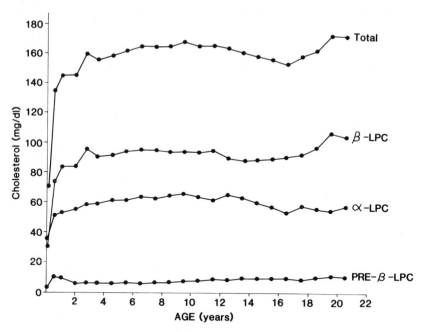

Figure 4.   Mean serum total and lipoprotein cholesterol (LPC) levels from birth to young adulthood. (Bogalusa Heart Study.) (*From* Berenson, G.S., and Epstein, F.H. (Chairmen): Conference on Blood Lipids in Children: Optimal Levels for Early Prevention of Coronary Artery Disease. Workshop Report: Epidemiologic Section, American Health Foundation. Prev. Med., *12*:741, 1983; with permission.)

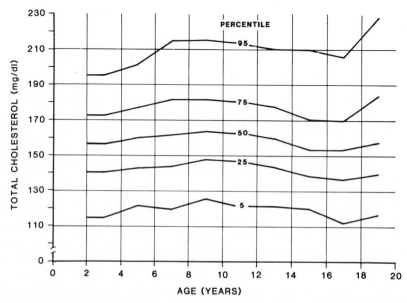

Figure 5.   Serum total cholesterol by age. (Bogalusa Heart Study.) (*From* Cresanta, J.L., et al.: Serum lipid and lipoprotein cholesterol grids for cardiovascular risk screening of children. Am. J. Dis. Child., *138*:379, 1984; with permission.)

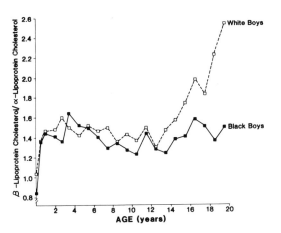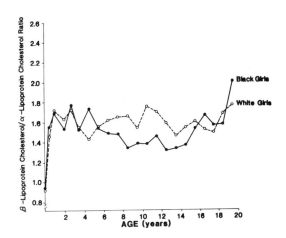

Figure 6. Beta-lipoprotein–to–alpha-lipoprotein cholesterol ratio by race and age. (Bogalusa Heart Study.) (*From* Berenson, G.S., et al.: Black-white contrasts as determinants of cardiovascular risk in childhood: Precursors of coronary artery and primary hypertensive disease. Am. Heart J., *108*:672, 1984; with permission.)

measurement. Persistence at extreme levels was nearly as good for serum total cholesterol and was equally good at both high and low extremes. Persistence at extreme levels was less consistent for serum triglycerides, VLDL cholesterol, and HDL cholesterol.[71]

A linear discriminant function model was developed to distinguish characteristics of children who persisted at high levels for lipids and lipoproteins from those who did not. The best predictor of future levels of serum total cholesterol and LDL cholesterol was the previous level of the variable of interest. Other concomitant variables helped determine whether a child will track. For example, in children younger than 9 years of age at the time of the initial measurement, an initially high LDL cholesterol level coupled with a low HDL cholesterol level best discriminated between trackers and nontrackers for elevated LDL cholesterol. In addition, obesity and increases in body size also contribute to persistence at high levels of LDL cholesterol.[71]

Recommendations for Lipids and Lipoproteins. Serum total cholesterol should be measured routinely at a child's annual physical examination, but a screening test procedure, the serum turbidity index,[22] is equally effective in identifying individuals with elevated LDL cholesterol and VLDL cholesterol levels and requires only 0.5 ml of serum.[59] In much the same way as physicians screen for anemia with hemoglobin determinations, the turbidity index could be used as a rapid, inexpensive, and convenient screening tool for identifying those with hyperlipoproteinemias.

Serum lipid and lipoprotein data were pooled from Bogalusa Heart Study examinations of pre-

schoolers, school-aged children, and post–high school young adults to develop percentile grids for children and young adults in the first two decades of life.[22] Just as pediatricians and family practitioners use growth grids for monitoring a child's linear growth and weight increments, these grids provide handy reference tools for physicians interested in preventing coronary artery disease. Because heart disease begins in childhood,[46,52,62] primary prevention and very early intervention can begin to reduce the high mortality rates from cardiovascular disease.

An easy five-step format has been outlined for routine office use of percentile grids to prevent hypercholesterolemia and hyperlipoproteinemias in childhood.[22] Any child with a serum total cholesterol level above the age-specific seventy-fifth percentile on two occasions deserves medical attention. Any child with a serum total cholesterol level above 170 mg per dl is at greater risk for premature atherosclerosis,[52] because ideal total cholesterol levels in children are much lower.[6] A 1983 conference on blood lipid levels in children recommended an ideal population mean total cholesterol level of 110 mg per dl to prevent premature atherosclerosis and coronary artery disease and concluded that a population mean level of 140 mg per dl was feasible and achievable in the near future.[73]

OBESITY IN CHILDREN

Obesity is quite prevalent in adults in the United States, with 20 to 30 per cent of adults being moderately to markedly obese and 3 to 10 per cent being massively obese.[1] These percentages would be even greater if established norms were used from less industrialized cultures.

Measurements for body habitus and fatness in children are made easily, and population data have been available for many years; however, the specific determinants of obesity are unclear.[30,41] The relative impact of genetic versus environmental factors is still debated, but obesity probably begins in infancy.[31,35] Although obesity has not been documented conclusively as an independent risk factor for cardiovascular disease, the interrelationships between obesity and other cardiovascular risk factor variables and subtle metabolic abnormalities related to insulin resistance are just beginning to be understood.

As with other cardiovascular risk factor variables, the prevalence of obesity depends on the criteria for definition of excess weight or body fatness. Obesity begins to accelerate in the high school age group, with a particularly rapid increase in black girls.[70] Careful monitoring of body habitus and composition during childhood is particularly important because of the interrelationships of obesity with atherosclerotic and hypertensive disease.

Tracking of Obesity. The persistence of height, weight, and triceps skinfold thickness levels in children followed longitudinally over 5 years is presented in Table 3. Body size variables track very well in children from ages 2 to 14 years. These data indicate a maintenance of obesity levels during childhood. Because obesity persists to a great extent from childhood, primary prevention of obesity and habits that lead to weight gain may be the best modality to reduce the prevalence of obesity and its correlated risk factors in adulthood.

As has been seen in adults, obesity is related to elevated blood pressure and abnormal lipid and lipoprotein levels in children.[2,27] Figure 7

shows the mean blood pressure levels of individuals by level of obesity (based on triceps skinfold thickness). Those individuals with the highest skinfold levels had significantly higher levels of blood pressure when compared with the midrange or lowest obesity groups. In addition, we have noted similar increases in levels of total cholesterol, LDL cholesterol, VLDL cholesterol, plasma insulin, and plasma glucose and decreases in levels of HDL cholesterol in obese children.[13,27]

Thus, although it remains controversial as to whether obesity is an independent risk factor for cardiovascular disease in adults, the relationship with traditional cardiovascular risk factors is clear. This relationship between obesity and risk factors and the high degree of tracking for obesity from early life make prevention or reduction of obesity in childhood, especially in those who are markedly obese, a high priority.

Intervention Strategies. In the following sections, we will concentrate our review on methods for the physician to intervene in the areas of diet and activity modification. This strategy is recommended not only for obesity but also for elevated blood pressure and hyperlipidemia.

In general, strategies for treating obesity have produced very modest outcomes.[18,74] The most promising intervention strategies have been those that involve behavioral modification approaches coupling changes in diet with increased physical activity.[18] The major problem with these forms of intervention has been that weight loss is maintained only while the patient is actively involved in the program. After the formal program ends, individuals do not continue to exercise.[18,45]

Some recent projects have aimed at changing children's eating and activity behaviors using a set of concepts drawn from social learning theory. These programs are based on the premise

Table 3. *Tracking Coefficients for Body Size in Childhood Through 5 Years of Follow-up—*
Bogalusa Heart Study, 1973–1979

AGE (YEARS) (Year 1)	N	YR 1 HEIGHT VS YEAR 6 R	YR 1 WEIGHT VS YEAR 6 R	YR 1 TRICEPS SKINFOLD VS YEAR 6 R
2–4	402	0.91	0.84	0.64
5–6	471	0.88	0.83	0.73
7–8	419	0.84	0.85	0.71
9–10	391	0.66	0.79	0.64
11–12	359	0.47	0.70	0.69
13–14	188	0.69	0.82	0.77

$p < 0.0001$ for all correlation coefficients
N = number of patients
Adapted from Webber, L.S., et al.: Tracking of cardiovascular disease risk factor variables in school-age children. J. Chronic Dis., 36:647, 1983; with permission.

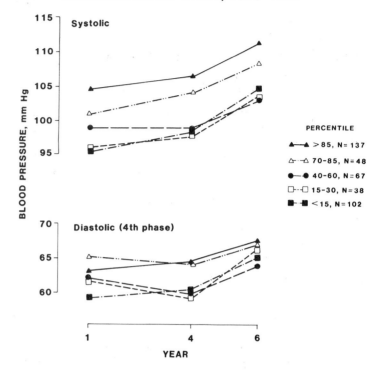

Figure 7. Blood pressure levels of individuals who consistently maintain obesity ranking across three total community screenings. (Bogalusa Heart Study.) (*From Aristimuno, G.G., et al.: Influence of persistent obesity in children on cardiovascular risk factors—The Bogalusa Heart Study. Circulation, 69:895, 1984; with permission.)

that behaviors are hard to change and that an individual requires support and mastery experiences in order to adopt and sustain a new behavior. Nader and associates[49] attempted to change eating and exercise patterns of third through sixth graders in a program that involved record keeping, various rewards for goal attainment, individual goal setting, and the involvement of the parents in the behavioral change program. They found that the program was successful in modifying the consumption of saturated fat and salt, but no change in exercise activity occurred. Using similar techniques, Coates and colleagues[17] were able to increase the amount of heart-healthy foods that children brought to school for lunch and the consumption of such foods as reported by parents at home. The degree of physical activity a child performed during recess was a function of the type of game the child chose to play. Normal playground activities of children are probably more effective in increasing physical activity than the introduction of games unfamiliar to the child that require a large amount of adult supervision and leadership. Most of the research seems to support the conclusion that the involvement of parents in a behavior change program is more ef-

fective than child training alone, especially in children younger than 12 years old.[5,12]

SUMMARY

Normal levels and trends of cardiovascular disease risk factors in childhood have been well documented by numerous epidemiologic surveys. Expected levels of blood pressure, lipids and lipoproteins, and body size can be determined by the child's physician using race- and gender-specific grids. These grids allow for the identification and follow-up of children with high-risk profiles. Evidence of increased left ventricular mass and vascular changes in renal arteries in association with childhood blood pressure level along with atherosclerotic fatty streak and fibrous plaque development in the aorta and coronary arteries shows that children with elevated risk factors are at risk for early target organ damage. These data demonstrate the potential importance of early intervention on the natural history of cardiovascular disease.

Based on our own data from the Bogalusa population, as well as evidence from other epidemiologic investigations in children, the following recommendations can be made, regardless of the risk factor variable under consideration:

1. Cardiovascular disease risk factor variables should be measured carefully and in a serial manner to classify a child as abnormal. Serial measurements serve to reduce the effect of regression to the mean and increase the predictive value of the measurements.

2. The misclassification of normal children into the high-risk category can be avoided by serial and replicate observations. Interventions that have attendant side effects (for example, pharmacologic therapy for high blood pressure) have to be measured against the effectiveness of diet, exercise, and other aspects of primary prevention. Risk factor levels consistently greater than the ninetieth percentile deserve medical attention.

3. Care should be taken prior to using specific grids of normal levels of cardiovascular disease risk factors in children. The measurement techniques employed on individuals should be similar to those used by the epidemiologic study to generate the grids in a reference population.

4. The grids should become part of the child's permanent medical record, as they provide a rapid visual assessment of the cardiovascular disease risk profile over time. High-risk trackers may require more intensive follow-up and will allow for early intervention and an assessment of the efficacy of the intervention program.

In conclusion, cardiovascular disease risk factor screening in childhood is quick, effective, and inexpensive. The potential payoff in prevention of adult cardiovascular disease is enormous and allows the physician to provide more comprehensive care to a pediatric population.[9a]

ACKNOWLEDGMENTS

The Bogalusa Heart Study represents the collaborative efforts of many people whose cooperation is gratefully acknowledged. We especially thank Mrs. Bettye Seal for her outstanding work as Community Coordinator. We also thank the children of Bogalusa and their parents, without whom this study would not be possible.

This research is supported by funds from the National Heart, Lung, and Blood Institute, USPHS, Specialized Center of Research—Arteriosclerosis (SCOR-A) HL15103 and HL02942.

REFERENCES

1. Abraham, S., Carroll, M.D., Najjar, M.F., et al.: Obese and overweight adults in the United States: Data from the National Health Survey, Vital and Health Statistics NCHS. Washington, D.C., Series 11, vol. 230, 1983, p. 1.
2. Aristimuno, G.G., Foster, T.A., Voors, A.W., et al.: Influence of persistent obesity in children on cardiovascular risk factors—The Bogalusa Heart Study. Circulation, 69:895, 1984.
3. Armitage, P., and Rose, G.A.: The variability of measurements of casual blood pressure. I. A laboratory study. Clin. Sci., 30:325, 1966.
4. Armitage, P., and Rose, G.A.: The variability of measurements of casual blood pressure. II. Survey experience. Clin. Sci. 30:337, 1966.
5. Baranowski, T., and Nader, P.R.: Family involvement in health behavior change programs. In Turk, D.C., and Kerno, R.D. (eds.): Health, Illness and Families: A Lifespan Perspective. New York, John Wiley and Sons, 1985.
6. Berenson, G.S., and Epstein, F.H. (Chairmen): Conference on Blood Lipids in Children: Optimal Levels for Early Prevention of Coronary Artery Disease. Workshop Report: Epidemiologic Section, American Health Foundation. Prev. Med., 12:741, 1983.
7. Berenson, G.S., McMahan, C.A., Voors, A.W., et al.: Cardiovascular Risk Factors in Children—The Early Natural History of Atherosclerosis and Essential Hypertension. New York, Oxford University Press, 1980.
8. Berenson, G.S., Voors, A.W., Gard, P., et al.: Clinical and anatomic correlates of cardiovascular disease in children: The Bogalusa Heart Study. In Schettler, F.G., et al. (eds.): Atherosclerosis VI. Proceedings of the Sixth International Symposium on Atherosclerosis. New York, Springer-Verlag, 1982.
9. Berenson, G.S., Cresanta, J.L., and Webber, L.S.: High blood pressure in the young. Annu. Rev. Med., 35:535, 1984.
9a. Berenson, G.S. (ed.): Causation of Cardiovascular Risk Factors in Childhood. New York, Raven Press, 1986.
10. Berenson, G.S., Srinivasan, S.R., Cresanta, J.L., et al.: Dynamic changes of serum lipoproteins in children during adolescence and sexual maturation. Am. J. Epidemiol., 113:157, 1981.
10a. Berenson, G.S., Voors, A.W., Webber, L.S., et al.: A model of intervention for prevention of early essential hypertension in the 1980's. Hypertension, 5:41–55, 1983.
11. Berenson, G.S., Webber, L.S., Srinivasan, S.R., et al.: Black-white contrasts as determinants of cardiovascular risk in childhood: Precursors of coronary artery and primary hypertensive disease. Am. Heart J., 108:672, 1984.
12. Brownell, K.D., Kelman, J.H., and Stunkard, A.J.: Treatment of obese children with and without their mothers: Changes in weight and blood pressure. Pediatrics, 71:515, 1983.
13. Burke, G.L., Webber, L.S., Srinivasan, S.R., et al.: Fasting plasma glucose and insulin levels and their relationship to cardiovascular risk factors in children: The Bogalusa Heart Study. Metabolism, in press.
14. Castelli, W.P.: Epidemiology of coronary heart disease: The Framingham Study. Am. J. Med., 76:4, 1984.
15. Castelli, W.P., Abbott, R.D., and McNamara, P.M.: Summary estimates of cholesterol used to predict coronary heart disease. Circulation, 67:730, 1983.
16. Clarke, W.R., Schrott, H., Leaverton, P.E., et al.: Tracking of blood lipids and blood pressure in children. Circulation, 58:626, 1978.
17. Coates, T.J., Jeffery, R.W., and Slinkard, L.A.: Heart healthy eating and exercise: Introducing and main-

taining changes in health behaviors. Am. J. Public Health, *71*:15, 1981.

18. Coates, T.J., and Thoresen, C.E.: Treating obesity in children and adolescents. A review. Am. J. Public Health, *68*:143, 1978.

19. Cresanta, J.L., Srinivasan, S.R., Foster, T.A., et al.: Serum lipoprotein levels in children: Epidemiologic and clinical implications. J. Chronic Dis., *35*:41, 1982.

20. Cresanta, J.L., Srinivasan, S.R., Foster, T.A., et al.: Distributions of serum lipoproteins in children by repeated measurements. Prev. Med., *12*:554, 1983.

21. Cresanta, J.L., Srinivasan, S.R., Webber, L.S., et al.: Changes of serum lipoprotein cholesterol in children with age and maturation. (Abstract.) Clin. Res., *26*:789A, 1978.

22. Cresanta, J.L., Srinivasan, S.R., Webber, L.S., et al.: Serum lipid and lipoprotein cholesterol grids for cardiovascular risk screening of children. Am. J. Dis. Child., *138*:379, 1984.

23. Culpepper, W.S., Sodt, P.C., Messerli, F.H., et al.: Cardiac status in juvenile borderline hypertension. Ann. Intern. Med., *98*:1, 1983.

24. Enos, W.F., Beyer, J.C., and Holmes, R.H.: Pathogenesis of coronary disease in American soldiers killed in Korea. J.A.M.A., *158*:912, 1955.

25. Five-year findings of the Hypertension Detection and Follow-up Program: Reduction in mortality of persons with high blood pressure, including mild hypertension. J.A.M.A., *242*:2563, 1979.

26. Five-year findings of the Hypertension Detection and Follow-up Program: Mortality by race, sex and age. J.A.M.A., *242*:2572, 1979.

26a.Frank, G.C., Farris, R.P., Ditmarsen, P., et al.: An approach to primary preventive treatment for children with high blood pressure. J. Am. Coll. Nutr., *1*:357–374, 1982.

27. Freedman, D.S., Burke, G.L., Harsha, D.W., et al.: Relationship of changes in obesity to serum lipid and lipoprotein changes in childhood and adolescence. J.A.M.A., *254*:515, 1985.

28. Freedman, D.S., Cresanta, J.L., Srinivasan, S.R., et al.: Longitudinal serum lipoprotein changes in white males during adolescence: The Bogalusa Heart Study. Metabolism, *34*:396, 1985.

29. Freedman, D.S., Shear, C.L., Srinivasan, S.R., et al: Tracking of serum lipids and lipoproteins in children over an eight-year period: Bogalusa Heart Study. Prev. Med., *14*:203, 1985.

30. Garn, S.M.: The origins of obesity. Am. J. Dis. Child., *130*:465, 1976.

31. Garn, S.M.: Continuities and changes in fatness from infancy through adulthood. In Lockhart, J.D. (ed.): Current Problems in Pediatrics. Chicago, Year Book Medical Publishers, 1985.

32. Gordon, T., Castelli, W.P., Hjortland, M.C., et al.; High density lipoprotein as a protective factor against coronary heart disease. Am. J. Med., *62*:707, 1977.

33. Gordon, T., Sorlie, P., and Kannel, W.B.: Problems in the assessment of blood pressure. The Framingham Study. Int. J. Epidemiol., *5*:327, 1976.

34. Harlan, W.R., Oberman, A., Mitchell, R.E., et al.: A 30-year study of blood pressure in a white male cohort. In Onesti, G., Kim, K.E., and Moyer, J.H. (eds.): Hypertension: Mechanisms and Management. New York, Grune and Stratton, 1973, pp. 85–91.

35. Hartz, A., Glesser, E., and Rimm, A.A.: Relative importance of the effect of family environment and heredity on obesity. Ann. Hum. Genet., *41*:185, 1977.

36. Hofman, A.: Epidemiological approach to the etiology of hypertension. J. Hypertension, *2*:323, 1980.

37. Hunter, S.M., Webber, L.S., and Berenson, G.S.: Cigarette smoking and tobacco usage behavior in children and adolescents: The Bogalusa Heart Study. Prev. Med., *9*:701, 1980.

38. Kirkendall, W.M., Feinleib, M., Freis, E.D., et al.: Recommendations for human blood pressure determined by sphygmomanometer: Subcommittee of the AHA Postgraduate Education Committee. Circulation, *62*:1146A, 1980.

39. Kotchen, J.M., and Kotchen, T.A.: Geographic effect on racial blood pressure differences in adolescents. J. Chronic. Dis., *31*:581, 1978.

40. Laird, W.P., and Fixler, D.E.: Left ventricular hypertrophy in adolescents with elevated blood pressure: Assessment by chest roentgenography, electrocardiography, and echocardiography. Pediatrics, *67*:255, 1981.

41. LeBow, M.D.: Child Obesity: A New Frontier of Behavior Therapy. New York, Springer Publishing Co., 1984.

42. Lipid Research Clinics Program: The Lipid Research Clinics Coronary Primary Prevention Trial results. Reduction in incidence of coronary heart disease. J.A.M.A., *251*:351, 1984.

43. Lipid Research Clinics Program: The Lipid Research Clinics Coronary Primary Prevention Trial results. The relationship of reduction in incidence of coronary heart disease to cholesterol lowering. J.A.M.A., *251*:365, 1984.

44. Maxwell, M.H., Waks, A.U., Schroth, P.C., et al.: Error in blood pressure measurement due to incorrect cuff size in obese patients. Lancet, *2*:33, 1982.

45. Mayer, J.: Obesity during childhood. In Winick, M. (ed.): Childhood Obesity. New York, John Wiley and Sons, 1975.

46. McGill, H.C. (ed.): The Geographic Pathology of Atherosclerosis. Baltimore, Williams and Wilkins, 1968.

47. McNamara, J.J., Molot, M.A., Stremple, J.F., et al.: Coronary artery disease in combat casualties in Vietnam. J.A.M.A., *216*:1185, 1971.

48. Miller, W.W.: Familial cardiovascular risk factors: Diagnosis and management in the young. Primary Care, *12*:3–14, 1985.

49. Nader, P.R., Baranowski, T., Vanderpool, N.A., et al.: The family health project: Cardiovascular risk reduction education for children and parents. J. Devel. Behav. Pediatr., *4*:3, 1983.

50. National Heart, Lung and Blood Institute: Report of the Task Force on Blood Pressure Control in Children. Pediatrics, *59(Suppl.)*:797, 1977.

51. National High Blood Pressure Coordinating Committee: The 1984 Report of the Joint National Committee on Detection, Evaluation, and Treatment of High Blood Pressure. NIH Publication No. 84-1088, September, 1984.

52. Newman, W.P., III, Freedman, D.S., Voors, A.W., et al.: Relation of serum lipoproteins and systolic blood pressure to early atherosclerosis. The Bogalusa Heart Study. N. Engl. J. Med., *314*:138, 1986.

53. Pooling Project Research Group: Relationship of blood pressure, serum cholesterol, smoking habit, relative weight and ECG abnormalities to incidence of major coronary events: Final report of the Pooling Project. J. Chronic Dis., *31*:201, 1978.

54. Rose, G.: Standardization of observers in blood pressure measurement. Lancet, *1*:673, 1965.

55. Schieken, R.M., Clarke, W.R., and Lauer, R.M.: Left

ventricular hypertrophy in children with blood pressure in the upper quintile of the distribution. The Muscatine Study. Hypertension, 3:669, 1981.

56. Shear, C.L., Burke, G.L., Freedman, D.S., et al.: The value of childhood blood pressure measurements and family history in predicting future blood pressure status: Results from eight years of follow-up in the Bogalusa Heart Study. Pediatrics, in press.

57. Shear, C.L., Webber, L.S., Freedman, D.S., et al.: The relationship between parental history of vascular disease and cardiovascular disease risk factors in children: The Bogalusa Heart Study. Am. J. Epidemiol., 122:762, 1985.

58. Solberg, L.A., and Strong, J.P.: Risk factors and atherosclerotic lesions: A review of autopsy studies. Arteriosclerosis, 3:187, 1983.

59. Srinivasan, S.R., and Berenson, G.S.: Serum lipoproteins in children and methods for study. In Lewis, L.A., and Opplt, J.J. (eds.): CRC Handbook of Electrophoresis (Lipoproteins). Vol. III. Boca Raton, Florida, CRC Press, 1983, pp. 185–203.

60. Srinivasan, S.R., Webber, L.S., and Berenson, G.S.: Lipid composition and interrelationships of major serum lipoproteins: Observations in children with different lipoprotein profiles—Bogalusa Heart Study. Arteriosclerosis, 2:335, 1982.

61. Srinivasan, S.R., Webber, L.S., and Berenson, G.S.: The relationship between very low density lipoprotein-lipid and measures of carbohydrate metabolism in children with different lipoprotein profiles: Bogalusa Heart Study. Metabolism, 33:760, 1984.

62. Strong, J.P., Johnson, W.D., Oalmann, M.C., et al.: Community pathology of atherosclerosis and coronary heart disease in New Orleans: Relationship of risk factors to atherosclerotic lesions. In Gotto, A.M., Jr., Smith, L.C., and Allen, B. (eds): Atherosclerosis V. New York, Springer-Verlag, 1980, pp. 719–730.

63. Strong, J.P., Oalmann, M.C., Newmann, W.P., III, et al.: Coronary heart disease in young black and white males in New Orleans: Community Pathology Study. Am. Heart J., 108:747, 1984.

64. Tyroler, H.A., Heydens, S., Bartel, A., et al.: Blood pressure and cholesterol as coronary heart risk factors. Arch. Intern. Med., 128:907, 1971.

65. Veterans Administration Cooperative Study Group on Antihypertension Agents: Effects of treatment on morbidity in hypertension: Results in patients with diastolic blood pressure averaging 115 through 129 mm Hg. J.A.M.A., 202:116, 1967.

66. Voors, A.W., Webber, L.S., and Berenson, G.S.: Time course studies of blood pressure in children—The Bogalusa Heart Study. Am. J. Epidemiol., 109:320, 1979.

67. Voors, A.W., Webber, L.S., and Berenson, G.S.: Relationship of blood pressure levels to height and weight in children. J. Cardiovasc. Med., 3:911, 1978.

68. Voors, A.W., Foster, T.A., Frerichs, R.R., et al.: Studies of blood pressures in children, ages 5–14 years, in a total biracial community—The Bogalusa Heart Study. Circulation, 54:319, 1976.

69. Voors, A.W., Webber, L.S., and Berenson, G.S.: A choice of diastolic Korotkoff phases in mercury sphygmomanometry of children. Prev. Med., 8:492, 1979.

70. Webber, L.S., Cresanta, J.L., Croft, J.B., et al.: Transitions from adolescence to young adulthood in terms of cardiovascular risk—The Bogalusa Heart Study. II. Alterations in anthropometric, blood pressure and serum lipoprotein variation. J. Chronic Dis., 39:91, 1986.

71. Webber, L.S., Cresanta, J.L., Voors, A.W., et al.: Tracking of cardiovascular disease risk factor variables in school-age children. J. Chronic Dis., 36:647, 1983.

72. Wilcox, J.: Observer in the measurement of blood pressure. Nurs. Res., 10:4, 1961.

73. Wynder, E.L. (Chairperson): Summary of recommendations of the Conference on Blood Lipids in Children: Optimal levels for early prevention of coronary artery disease. Prev. Med., 12:728, 1983.

74. Ylitalo, V.: Treatment of obese schoolchildren. Acta Paediatr. Scand. (Suppl.), 290:1, 1981.

75. Zahka, K.G., Neill, C.A., Kidd, L., et al.: Cardiac involvement in adolescent hypertension: Echocardiographic determination of myocardial hypertrophy. Hypertension, 3:664, 1981.

Gerald S. Berenson, M.D.
National Research and Demonstration Center—
Arteriosclerosis
Department of Medicine
1542 Tulane Avenue
Louisiana State University Medical Center
New Orleans, Louisiana 70112-2822

Risks for Developing Cardiovascular Risk Factors

Risks for Hyperlipidemia

A. Christine Nestruck, M.Sc., Ph.D.,* and Jean Davignon, M.D.†

Hyperlipidemia is one of the principal factors underlying the risk for cardiovascular disease. Confirmatory evidence from animal studies, clinical case studies, and epidemiologic population studies has clearly established the positive correlation of plasma cholesterol to atherosclerosis and its complications, mainly coronary heart disease (CHD).[50] The predisposition to hyperlipidemia may be purely genetic, for example, the autosomal dominant familial hypercholesterolemia with manifestations displayed very early in life.[34] This is rare, however, and most hyperlipidemias are thought to develop in genetically susceptible individuals in association with other influences.

It has been estimated that the contribution of genetic factors in determining blood cholesterol levels is approximately 50 per cent;[81] environmental factors thus play an almost equal role. Because one of the least understood factors is the duration of exposure to risk, we have chosen to review here some of the genetic factors and some of the relatively long-term environmental factors, such as diet and drug therapies, that are known to increase the risk of hyperlipidemia and likely the predisposition to cardiovascular disease.

HYPERLIPIDEMIA

The cholesterol associated with the low-density lipoproteins (LDL), accounting for 60 to 75 per cent of the plasma levels, is responsible for the powerful direct relationship of plasma cholesterol with coronary heart disease.[42] Furthermore, the cholesterol that accumulates in atheromatous lesions is derived mainly from plasma LDL.[84] Thus, LDL are considered to be the "atherogenic" lipoproteins, and since the early observations of Barr and associates,[4] a vast literature has accumulated on the role of elevated levels of LDL in promoting atherosclerosis.[17,87] High-density lipoproteins (HDL), normally accounting for 20 to 25 per cent of plasma cholesterol, have been shown to be an independent, inverse risk factor for CHD.[66] Not withstanding the obligate role of LDL cholesterol (LDL-C), HDL-associated cholesterol levels (HDL-C) are considered to be protective, that is, "non-atherogenic," and low levels have been linked with increased CHD risk in family studies,[91,98] angiographically defined coronary vessel disease,[67] and pediatric stroke victims.[31]

Hyperlipidemia is defined by elevated levels of the plasma lipids, and the risk for atherosclerosis is associated with the classification types IIa, IIb, III, and perhaps IV, a system of classification based on phenotypic manifestations of increased lipoprotein fractions.[25] The Lipid Research Clinics Program reports plasma lipid and lipoprotein cholesterol distributions of a very large-scale screening of white men and women (both with and without sex hormone usage) aged 20 to 59 years in the United States.[40] Age-related trends for rising triglycerides and cholesterol

*Senior Investigator, Department of Lipid Metabolism and Atherosclerosis Research, Clinical Research Institute of Montreal; Assistant Professor, Department of Medicine, University of Montreal, Montreal, Quebec, Canada

†Director, Department of Lipid Metabolism and Atherosclerosis Research, Clinical Research Institute of Montreal; Chief, Section of Vascular Medicine, Hôtel-Dieu Hospital; Professor, Department of Medicine, University of Montreal, Montreal, Quebec, Canada

with differences between the sexes were clearly demonstrated. The ninety-fifth percentile findings of this study have been suggested as the upper limit of normal (with the fifth percentile being the lower limit for HDL cholesterol).[74]

Today, in the face of our expanding understanding of the very complex metabolism of the plasma lipids, our attention not only is directed to their absolute levels but also is increasingly devoted to the study of lipid distribution among the lipoproteins, anomalies of the lipid moiety, and the role(s) of the apoproteins and their possible defects in directing the properties, functions, and metabolic fates of the lipoproteins.

The "atherogenic" lipoproteins, all containing apolipoprotein B (apo B), include the LDL of familial hypercholesterolemia of normal composition;[34] the LDL of hyperapo-betalipoproteinemia[85] and familial combined hyperlipidemia[41] of abnormal composition,[90] with or without an associated increase in other sterols;[51,77] the cholesterol-rich very-low-density lipoproteins (VLDL) or intermediate-density lipoproteins (IDL) or β-VLDL of type III hyperlipoproteinemia;[9] the lipoprotein Lp(a);[100] and the triglyceride-rich VLDL remnant in familial hypertriglyceridemia.[28] The protective role of the nonatherogenic high-density lipoproteins is not yet well understood,[46] and in humans, there is not yet evidence that interventions that raise HDL cholesterol levels have a beneficial effect on the morbidity and mortality of CHD.[86,99] It has been further suggested that the negative correlation of HDL cholesterol with CHD is a function of the subfraction HDL_2,[67] which adds to the complexity of the interpretation of total HDL cholesterol levels.

NORMOLIPIDEMIC DYSLIPIDEMIAS

It is well established that normolipidemic individuals are not immune to the development of atherosclerosis.[16] Recent emphasis on the apolipoprotein moieties has disclosed several normolipidemic dyslipoproteinemias associated with tissue lipid infiltration: in the case of both apolipoprotein AI absence[78] and apolipoprotein AI–apolipoprotein CIII deficiency,[70] planar xanthomas and premature atherosclerosis were present. On the other hand, plasma apolipoprotein B concentrations were shown to be higher in individuals with CHD than in normal individuals.[3,85] Premature atherosclerosis has also been reported in a hereditary form of hyperapobetalipoproteinemia.[51] Elevated levels of apolipoprotein B may also be a characteristic of fa-

milial combined hypercholesterolemia (multiple phenotype disease) and may be present in 50 per cent of normolipidemic siblings of affected individuals.[41] These findings give credence to the notion that apolipoprotein B itself may have atherogenic properties, whereas apolipoprotein AI may be protective and may have led to the hypothesis that the levels of apolipoprotein B associated with LDL are an independent risk factor for CHD.[69]

NUTRITIONAL ENVIRONMENT

Hyperlipidemia is a significant characteristic of the more affluent Western world. Multifactorial population studies leave little doubt of the powerful role of the environment (predominantly dietary intake of total fat, saturated fats, and calories) in populations of different countries.[45] In the Seven Countries Study,[45] populations with higher levels of cholesterol and LDL cholesterol (and increased atherosclerosis) have saturated fat intakes of 10 per cent or more of calories. The influence of diet is also shown from migration studies of Japanese populations in Japan with those in the United States.[43] In a double-blind study, both mean plasma cholesterol and LDL cholesterol were shown to be elevated in normal American volunteers after cholesterol feeding,[75] confirming earlier studies.[5,62] Further studies of normolipidemic and mildly and severely hypercholesterolemic patients, involving cholesterol feeding or cholesterol restriction, showed increases or decreases in plasma cholesterol, respectively, predominantly affecting the LDL cholesterol fraction. The very important finding here is that the severely hypercholesterolemic patients were much more sensitive to dietary cholesterol levels than the normal subjects.[11] The universality of dietary cholesterol in effecting increases in plasma cholesterol and LDL cholesterol or, when restricted, in effecting decreases has been demonstrated recently in the cross-cultural experiments of Connor and Connor.[10] In these studies, Tarahumara Indians of Mexico, who normally consume a diet poor in fat and very low in cholesterol (when compared with the average American diet), showed marked increases in their normally low plasma cholesterol and LDL cholesterol levels when only the cholesterol content of their usual diet was elevated. Thus, excessive or aberrant eating habits play a role in the risk of developing hyperlipidemia. This is especially important in the genetically susceptible individual; one example is the evidence of tissue lipid infiltration in the form of xanthomas following excessive egg intake.[73]

DRUGS AND HYPERLIPIDEMIA

If drugs adversely affect the lipoprotein profile (predisposing to dyslipoproteinemia and atherosclerosis) and are to be prescribed on a long-term basis, they should be considered as risk factors themselves. Furthermore, pre-existing factors may enhance this effect, for example, as when such drugs are prescribed in an already genetically or ecologically affected individual. In this context, oral contraceptives, antihypertensive therapies, retinoids, and hypolipidemic agents will be considered.

Oral Contraceptives. The use of oral contraceptives was shown very early to predispose to the development of hyperlipidemia.[102] In addition, they predispose to other cardiovascular risk factors that, when combined with smoking, bring about a greatly magnified risk for myocardial infarction.[24,60,83,88] One example of the adverse changes that may be induced by oral contraceptives is shown in Table 1. While taking a norgestrel-containing formulation, a 28-year-old woman with an apo E3/3 phenotype exhibited an elevated LDL cholesterol level, a marked elevation in LDL apolipoprotein B, and a very reduced HDL cholesterol level, especially in HDL$_2$ cholesterol. In view of the studies of Knopp and associates[48] and Wynn and Niththyananthan,[103] these results are not unexpected. What is important here is that both plasma triglyceride and cholesterol measurements did not disclose these adverse changes in lipoprotein cholesterol distribution (see Table 1). Four months after cessation of oral contraceptives, this patient revealed a reversed and normal lipoprotein profile.

Earlier formulations with higher levels of estrogens and progestins had relatively stronger effects on the lipoprotein profile,[30,39] with estrogens promoting elevations and progestins promoting reductions in triglycerides. HDL cholesterol levels were found to fall with increasing dose and potency of progestin and to rise with increasing dose of estrogens.[8] The complexity of the question surrounding the "protective" role of increased HDL cholesterol concentration can be seen in the effect of estrogens. As Stamler has reminded us, estrogen treatment in men surviving a myocardial infarction was associated with a considerable rise in plasma HDL cholesterol but proved ineffective in preventing recurrent infarction and prolonging life.[86] This probable thrombogenic effect of estrogen therapy can also be seen in the increased cardiovascular mortality of male patients being treated with estrogens, despite the reported increase in HDL.[99]

Apart from these known effects of estrogens and progestins, the predisposition to the development of hyperlipidemia and its presumed cardiovascular consequences was elegantly demonstrated in the studies of De Gennes and colleagues.[22] Plasma lipid abnormalities and/or a positive family history of metabolic or cardiovascular disease was found in 74 per cent of first-degree relatives of young women with early vascular disease while taking oral contraceptives. Thus, both the lipoprotein profile of the subject as well as her family history may predict a latent hyperlipoproteinemia.

Antihypertensive Agents. Hypertension is in itself a major risk factor for CHD,[17] and as reviewed by Ames,[1] although the results of eight recently conducted major hypertension treatment trials demonstrated a clear-cut reduction in the incidence of stroke and congestive heart failure through control of hypertension, no such reduction in the morbidity or mortality of CHD could be shown. The breakdown in the link between treatment of hypertension and improvement in CHD may be due to metabolic disturb-

Table 1. *An Example of Changes in Lipoprotein Cholesterol, Plasma Lipids, and Apolipoproteins with an Oral Contraceptive*

MG/DL	ON OC	OFF OC	NORMALS*
Cholesterol	229	228	171 ± 30
Triglycerides	117	58	63 ± 22
VLDL-C	28	7	15 ± 5
LDL-C	172	152	104 ± 29
HDL-C	29	69	52 ± 10
HDL$_2$-C	13	36	24 ± 9
LDL apo B	153	119	83 ± 18
Apo AI	125	140	140 ± 27

*Age-matched women from our clinic, no oral contraceptives; n = 40, values are mean ± S.D.
OC = oral contraceptives (0.25 mg d-norgestrel, 0.05 mg ethinyl estradiol).

ances caused by conventional therapies that predispose to the appearance of other risk factors, including hyperlipidemias or dyslipidemias. Diuretics and adrenergic blocking agents are widely used in the treatment of hypertension, and several studies have examined their effects on plasma lipids and lipoprotein cholesterol.

Diuretic Agents. It is now well established that the thiazide-type diuretic agents raise total cholesterol and LDL cholesterol with variable increases in plasma triglycerides,[2,29,32,37] which, in the case of chlorthalidone, has been shown to be partially countered by concomitant low–saturated fat dietary therapy.[37] HDL cholesterol levels often remain unchanged, but the ratio of total cholesterol to HDL cholesterol increases significantly; according to the results of the Framingham Study, this is considered to be one of the strongest indices of CHD risk.[42]

Adrenergic Inhibitors. Beta-blockers, established drugs for the treatment of hypertension, include those of noncardioselective beta-blockade (for example, propranolol and sotalol), those with cardioselective beta-blockade (for example, metoprolol and atenolol), and those with intrinsic sympathomimetic activity (ISA) (for example, pindolol, and acebutolol). These agents differ not only in their blockade selectivity but also in their effects on lipid levels. Of the noncardioselective beta-blockers, propranolol has been the one studied most often, with consistent findings that plasma triglycerides increase significantly and HDL cholesterol levels decrease significantly, with accompanying subtle and variable changes in cholesterol and LDL cholesterol.[21,53,56] The cardioselective beta-blockers have been shown to have similar but generally less significant effects.[6,21,76] Pindolol, which has intrinsic sympathomimetic activity, has been reported to have no untoward effects on plasma lipids; it increases HDL cholesterol and causes relatively small decreases in LDL cholesterol.[55,65,72] Furthermore, pindolol has been shown to protect against the increase in LDL cholesterol induced by the thiazide-like diuretic clopamide[79] and has therefore been suggested as an effective combined drug treatment.

The alpha$_1$-blocking agent prazosin is generally regarded has having very little effect on plasma lipoprotein cholesterol distribution,[38,49,57] and was shown to counter partially the LDL cholesterol–raising effect but not the HDL cholesterol–lowering effect of propranolol, when given in combination.[55] In view of the many new antihypertensive agents introduced in recent years, the effects of these agents must be evaluated in each individual. Certainly, in young patients who face possibly lifelong drug therapy, the adverse effects on the lipoprotein profile of these patients must be considered. Furthermore, an antiatherogenic diet perhaps should be prescribed in all cases of hypertension treated with beta-blockers and diuretics.

Retinoids. The synthetic retinoids etretinate (the ethyl ester of trimethoxymethylphenyl retinoic acid) and isotretinoin (13-*cis*-retinoic acid) have been shown to be effective in the treatment of several skin diseases with varying side effects, including variable increases in the plasma lipids.[33,44,61,64] Both drugs adversely affect the lipoprotein profile. In a sequential study, isotretinoin was shown to effect an average 20 per cent increase in LDL cholesterol, a parallel rise in total plasma apolipoprotein B levels, and a 12 per cent decrease in HDL cholesterol; similar but smaller changes were found with etretinate.[97] These important and opposite changes nullified a significant change in total plasma cholesterol. In other studies, similar and more pronounced or variable and less marked changes in lipoprotein cholesterol have been found, possibly owing to the confounding factors of different dosages, duration of treatment, sex distribution, and diagnosis.[23,35,64,105] Furthermore, in a study of etretinate by Ellis and associates,[23] a disturbing 32 per cent of patients maintained a 20 per cent increase in plasma cholesterol over baseline as long as 8 weeks after cessation of the drug. Etretinate has been shown to have a biologic half-life of 14 weeks after long-term therapy,[71] which may explain this carry-over effect and introduces an additional confounding factor in clinical cross-over trials. Most importantly, as pointed out by Vahlquist and colleagues,[97] the individual response to retinoid treatment in terms of lipoprotein effects is variable, cannot be predicted, and may not be evident in simple plasma lipid measurements. Therefore, lipoprotein profiling is encouraged with prolonged treatment.

Hypolipidemic Agents. As with all other drug therapies, the differential effects of hypolipidemic agents on plasma lipoprotein cholesterol distribution is of interest not only from the point of view of understanding their mode of action but also in the identification of adverse effects on the lipoprotein profile. The individual variability in response to early drugs such as clofibrate in patients with familial hypercholesterolemia allowed the definition of "responders" and "nonresponders," with the latter being resistant patients having a paradoxic and substantial increase in LDL cholesterol.[14,20] In the Coronary

Drug Project, an overall fall in plasma cholesterol of only 6.5 per cent with clofibrate was associated with a high incidence of cardiovascular complications.[12] In the WHO trial, clofibrate produced a 26 per cent reduction in nonfatal myocardial infarctions but had no significant effect on the incidence of either new infarctions or deaths from CHD. The benefit noted was proportional to cholesterol reduction, which on average was rather small (9 per cent).[12] Both studies failed to take into account the relative proportions of responders and nonresponders. The lack of a marked reduction in average plasma cholesterol indicates that the proportion of resistant patients must have been significant, with the LDL-raising effect offsetting the overall beneficial effect of the drug. Indeed, Lees[52] found a decreased CHD mortality in the responders in the Coronary Drug Project. All of the newer-generation fibrates (gemfibrozil, fenofibrate, ciprofibrate) tested in our clinic have varying proportions of nonresponders, but these appear to be more effective than clofibrate in reducing LDL cholesterol, and generally, the number of nonresponders to these agents is smaller.

Probucol is an effective cholesterol-lowering agent primarily indicated in the treatment of the various forms of hypercholesterolemia. Its effect is mostly on LDL cholesterol, but it lowers HDL cholesterol as well.[54] In view of the protective role ascribed to HDL cholesterol levels, the usefulness of probucol has been a matter of controversy.[15,26] However, renewed interest in this drug as a therapeutic agent stems from studies showing regression of atherosclerosis in hyperlipidemic monkeys[101] and the discovery of a new mechanism for its cholesterol-lowering effect.[68] We have recently reported the results of a partially retrospective study of the combined drug therapy of clofibrate and probucol in which marked reductions in HDL cholesterol were observed in some patients, which, in one case, was associated with regression of xanthelasma and tendon xanthomas.[18] Until the mechanisms and kinetics of the hypolipidemic drugs are established, lipoprotein profiling and cholesterol distribution must be monitored in all patients in order to disclose adverse changes, especially those in LDL cholesterol, which are not revealed by simple plasma lipid measurements.

GENETIC PREDISPOSITION TO HYPERLIPIDEMIA

It has become increasingly apparent that single-gene mutations in apoproteins, lipoproteins, and some of the enzymes involved in lipoprotein metabolism may underlie disorders of hyperlipoproteinemia or hypolipoproteinemia, some of which are very rare, some of which are more common, and some of which predispose to premature atherosclerosis.

Mutations in the LDL Receptor Pathway. Familial hypercholesterolemia is an autosomal dominant disorder characterized by elevated plasma LDL levels, xanthomas, and premature atherosclerosis.[34] The estimated frequency of heterozygotes is 1 in 500 and of homozygotes 1 in 1,000,000.[82] In studies of cultured fibroblasts, Goldstein and Brown[33] originally described three types of receptor defects: "receptor negative" (no detectable binding activity), which was the most common, "receptor defective" (very reduced binding), and "internalization defective" (LDL binding with no transport of the receptor-LDL complex into the cell). These mutations are believed to be the result of mutations at a single genetic locus specifying the LDL receptor.[92] Located on the surface of most body cells, this receptor normally binds LDL and facilitates its uptake and delivery to lysosomes. There, the LDL cholesterol is used in the synthesis of cell membranes, steroid hormones, or bile acids. The decreased rate of removal in familial hypercholesterolemia results in the excess being deposited in other cell types, causing xanthomas and atheromas.[34] To date, there have been no other reported mutations in other lipoprotein receptors.

Apolipoprotein E. Apolipoprotein E is a protein found on the surface of VLDL, IDL, HDL, and chylomicrons. This apoprotein displays a complex isoform pattern that is due to three common alleles coding at a single gene locus and post-translational sialylation.[95,104] The three common alleles, $\epsilon2$, $\epsilon3$, and $\epsilon4$, code for three major isoforms, E2, E3, and E4. The six possible apolipoprotein E phenotypes are found in almost all populations studied at approximately the same frequencies.[80] The homozygous E3/3 phenotype is the most common (approximately 60 per cent), whereas the other homozygous forms are rarer (E2/2—1 to 2 per cent, E4/4—3 to 4 per cent). Evidence has accrued that apolipoprotein E polymorphism may influence the levels of plasma lipids and lipoproteins.[7,19,80,96] By extension, several studies have searched for an influence of the apolipoprotein E gene on the development of atherosclerosis.[13,63,94] Although most bearers of the E2/2 phenotype are normolipidemic, the majority of patients with familial dysbetalipoproteinemia (type III), a disease often associated with progressive

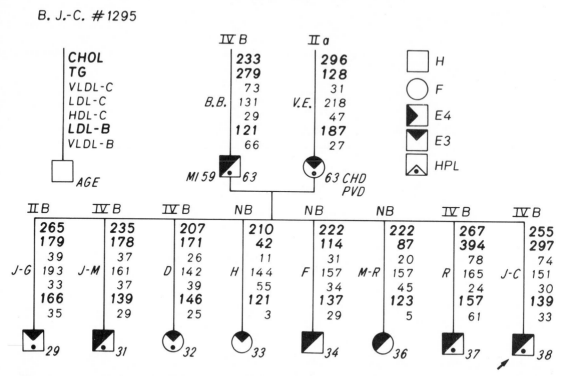

Figure 1. An example of a familial combined hyperlipidemia pedigree (H = male; F = female; E4 and E3 = apo E phenotyping[7]; HPL = hyperlipidemia; B = hyper-apo B; N = normal *lipid* profile; VLDL = very-low-density lipoprotein; LDL = low-density lipoprotein; HDL = high-density lipoprotein; CHOL, C = cholesterol; TG = triglyceride).

atherosclerosis, have the E2/2 phenotype.[93] In type III hyperlipoproteinemia, it is the ligand that is defective. From the elegant studies of Mahley and colleagues,[59] it is known that the E2 isoform differs from the E3 and E4 isoforms by the substitution of cysteine for arginine at position 158 in the amino acid sequence, which results in extremely reduced receptor binding (the apolipoprotein E hepatic receptor or the apolipoprotein B,E receptor of peripheral cells).[9,59] This reduced binding results in the accumulation of remnant particles of both chylomicrons and VLDL, giving the "broad β" pattern on lipoprotein electrophoresis. We have reported an enrichment in the ε2 allele and the E2-bearing phenotypes in an unselected sample of subjects with primary hyperlipidemia, mostly type IV (76 per cent),[19] and more recently, we have reported that this enrichment is associated only with type IV without hyperapobetalipoproteinemia.[58] The common allelic variability at the apolipoprotein E gene locus has a definite influ-

ence on variation in plasma lipids and lipoproteins and thus may contribute to a genetic susceptibility in the development of atherosclerosis.[80] Two other rare forms of apolipoprotein E mutations have recently been reported: apolipoprotein E Bethesda[36] and apolipoprotein E deficiency;[27] both express the features of type III hyperlipoproteinemia.

Hyperapobetalipoproteinemia. People with normal LDL cholesterol levels but elevated levels of LDL apolipoprotein B are at increased risk for developing atherosclerosis (hyperapolipoprotein B).[85] A second disorder, familial combined hyperlipidemia, shares the characteristic of a diminished LDL cholesterol–to–LDL apolipoprotein B ratio.[41,47] Familial combined hyperlipidemia is also defined by multiple hyperlipidemic phenotypes within the same family. Recently, it has been suggested that a common feature of both familial combined hyperlipidemia and normolipidemic hyperapolipoprotein B is overproduction of apolipoprotein B.[47] Furthermore, the denser and smaller LDL particles of patients with hyperapolipoprotein B, with and without hyperlipidemia, were recently shown to have reduced immunoreactivity in some of the apolipoprotein B antigenic determinants, which may possibly be related to their affinity for the apolipoprotein B,E receptor.[89] Although the genetic factors underlying these two (and not necessarily different) disorders are not yet understood, the important factor is the finding of elevated levels of LDL apolipoprotein B as a predictive risk factor. An example of a family positive for familial combined hyperlipidemia, as revealed by both multiple hyperlipidemia phenotypes and hyperapolipoprotein B within the same family, is shown in Figure 1. Here, the only clue in the three normolipidemic offspring is the presence of elevated LDL apolipoprotein B. Followed over time, these pure hyperapolipoprotein B individuals may show an abnormal increase in lipoprotein cholesterol levels and/or triglycerides. Indeed, 1 year after the initial family screening, the subject identified as "NB (F, male, age 34)" now displays a type IV phenotype with hyperapolipoprotein B.

CONCLUSION

In summary, the risk for developing the risk factor hyperlipidemia rests on both genetic and environmental factors and their interplay. Until the discrete and likely numerous genetic factors are better understood, the primary role of LDL (its cholesterol or apoprotein B components) must be considered, especially if elevated by diet and/or drugs and/or smoking. The accurate assessment of HDL-associated cholesterol must also be considered, especially when reductions accompany elevation in LDL. Finally, "normolipidemia" does not preclude premature atherosclerosis; the cryptic clues of potential dyslipidemias, hyperapobetalipoproteinemia, and a positive family history for early coronary vascular disease are all predisposing risk factors.

REFERENCES

1. Ames, R.P.: Negative effects of diuretic drugs on metabolic risk factors for coronary heart disease: Possible alternative drug therapies. Am. J. Cardiol., *51*:632, 1983.
2. Ames, R.P., and Hill, P.: Increase in serum lipids during treatment of hypertension with chlorthalidone. Lancet, *1*:721, 1976.
3. Avogaro, P., Bittolo Bon, G., Cazzalato, G., et al.: Plasma levels of apolipoprotein AI and apolipoprotein B in human atherosclerosis. Artery, *4*:384, 1978.
4. Barr, D.P., Russ, E.M., and Eder, H.A.: Protein-lipid relationships in human plasma. II. In atherosclerosis and related conditions. Am. J. Med., *11*:480, 1951.
5. Beveridge, J.M.R., Connel, W.B., Mayer, G.A., et al.: The response of man to dietary cholesterol. J. Nutr., *71*:61, 1960.
6. Bielmann, P., Leduc, G., and Davignon, J.: Beta-bloquants sélectif (métroprolol) vs non-sélectif (propranolol): Effets comparés sur la composition des lipoportéines plasmatiques et la pression sanguine. Union Med. Can., *109*:1734, 1980.
7. Bouthillier, D., Sing, C.F., and Davignon, J.: Apolipoprotein E phenotyping with a single gel method: Application to the study of informative matings. J. Lipid Res., *24*:1060, 1983.
8. Bradley, D.D., Winger, D.J., Petitti, D.B., et al.: Serum high-density-lipoprotein cholesterol in women using oral contraceptives, estrogens and progestins. N. Engl. J. Med., *299*:17, 1978.
9. Brown, M.S., Goldstein, J.L., and Fredrickson, D.S.: Familial type 3 hyperlipoproteinemia (dysbetalipoproteinemia). *In* Stanbury, J.B., et al. (eds.): Metabolic Basis of Inherited Disease. Edition 5. New York, McGraw-Hill, 1983.
10. Connor, S.L., and Connor, W.E.: The interaction of genetic and nutritional factors in hyperlipidemia. *In* Valazquez, A., and Bourges, H. (eds.): Genetic Factors in Nutrition. New York, Academic Press, 1984.
11. Connor, W.E., and Connor, S.L.: The dietary treatment of hyperlipidemia. Med. Clin. North Am., *66*:485–518, 1982.
12. Coronary Drug Project Research Group: Clofibrate and niacin in coronary heart disease. J.A.M.A. *231*:360, 1975.
13. Cumming, A.M., and Robertson, F.W.: Polymorphism at the apoprotein E locus in relation to risk of coronary disease. Clin. Genet., *25*:310, 1984.
14. Davignon, J., Aubry, F., Noël, C., et al.: Heterogeneity of familial hyperlipoproteinemia type II on the basis of fasting plasma triglyceride/cholesterol ratio and plasma cholesterol response to chlorophenoyisobutyrate. Rev. Can. Biol., *30*:307, 1971.
15. Davignon, J., and Bouthillier, D.: Probucol and familial hypercholesterolemia. Can. Med. Assoc. J., *126*:1024, 1982.
16. Davignon, J., Bouthillier, D., Dufour, R., et al.: Xanthomes et athérosclérose en présence de lipides plasmatiques normaux. Ann. Med. Interne, *134*:483, 1983.
17. Davignon, J., Dufour, R., and Cantin, M.: Current views on the etiology and pathogenesis of atherosclerosis. *In* Genest, J., Koiw, E., and Küchel, O., (eds.): Hypertension: Physiopathology and Treatment. Edition 2. New York, McGraw-Hill, 1983.
18. Davignon, J., Nestruck, A.C., Alaupovic, P., et al.: Severe hypoalphalipoproteinemia induced by a combination of probucol and clofibrate. *In* Symposium on Lipoprotein Deficiency Syndromes. New York, Plenum Press, in press.
19. Davignon, J., Sing, C.F., Lussier-Cacan, S., et al.: Xanthelasma, latent dyslipoproteinemia and atherosclerosis: Contribution of apo E polymorphism. *In* De Gennes, J.L., Polonovsky, J.J., and Paoletti, R. (eds.): Latent Dyslipoproteinemia and Atherosclerosis. New York, Raven Press, 1984.
20. Davignon, J., Sniderman, A., Cayen, M.N., et al.: Sensitivity and resistance to the cholesterol-lowering effect of clofibrate—pharmacokinetic studies, plasma apolipoprotein B levels and therapeutic im-

plications. *In* Fumagalli, R., Kritchevsky, D., and Paoletti, R. (eds.): Drugs Affecting Lipid Metabolism. Amsterdam and New York, Elsevier–North Holland, 1980.

21. Day, J.L., Metcalfe, J., and Simpson, C.N.: Adrenergic mechanisms in control of plasma lipid concentrations. Br. Med. J., *284*:1145, 1982.

22. De Gennes, J.L., Turpin, G., and Truffert, J.: Vascular disease and oral contraceptives: Familial hyperlipoproteinemia as a predisposing factor. Diabete Metab., *2*:81, 1976.

23. Ellis, C.N., Swanson, N.A., Grekin, R.C., et al.: Etretinate therapy causes increases in lipid levels in patients with psoriasis. Arch. Dermatol., *118*:559, 1982.

24. Frederiksen, H., and Ravenholt, R.T.: Thromboembolism, oral contraceptives and cigarettes. Public Health Rep., *85*:197, 1970.

25. Frederickson, D.S., Levy, R.I., and Lees, R.S.: Fat transport in lipoproteins—an integrated approach to mechanisms and disorders. N. Engl. J. Med., *276*:32, 94, 148, 215, 273, 1967.

26. Gagné, C., Lupien, P.J., Brun, M., et al.: Probucol and high density lipoprotein cholesterol. Can. Med. Assoc. J., *123*:356, 1980.

27. Ghiselli, G., Schaefer, E.J., Gascon, P., et al.: Type III hyperlipoproteinemia associated with apolipoprotein E deficiency. Science, *214*:1239, 1981.

28. Gianturco, S.H., Gotto, A.M., Hwang, S.L.C., et al.: Apolipoprotein E mediates uptake of Sf100–400 hypertriglyceridemic very low density lipoproteins by the low density lipoprotein receptor pathway in normal human fibroblasts. J. Biol. Chem., *258*:4526, 1983.

29. Gluck, Z., Weidmann, P., Mordasini, R., et al.: Increased serum low density lipoprotein cholesterol in men treated short-term with the diuretic chlorthalidone. Metabolism, *29*:240, 1980.

30. Glueck, C.J., Scheel, D., Fishback, J., et al.: Progestagens, anabolic androgenic compounds, estrogens: Effects on lipids and post-heparin lipolytic enzymes. Lipids, *7*:110, 1972.

31. Glueck, C.J., Daniels, S.R., Bates, S., et al.: Pediatric victims of unexplained stroke and their families: Familial lipid and lipoprotein abnormalities. Pediatrics, *69*:308, 1982.

32. Goldman, A.I., Steele, B.W., Schnaper, H.W., et al.: Serum lipoprotein levels during chlorthalidone therapy. J.A.M.A. *224*:1691, 1980.

33. Goldstein, J.L., and Brown, M.S.: The low density lipoprotein pathway and its relation to atherosclerosis. Annu. Rev. Biochem., *46*:897, 1977.

34. Goldstein, J.L., and Brown, M.S.: Familial hypercholesterolemia. *In* Stanbury, J.B., et al. (eds.): Metabolic Basis of Inherited Diseases. Edition 5. New York, McGraw-Hill, 1983.

35. Gollnick, H., Tsambaos, D., and Orfanos, C.E.: Risk factors promote elevations of serum lipids in acne patients under oral 13-*cis*-retinoic acid (isotretinoin). Arch. Dermatol. Res., *271*:189, 1981.

36. Gregg, R.E., Ghiselli, G., and Brewer, B., Jr.: Apolipoprotein E-Bethesda: A new variant of apolipoprotein E associated with type III hyperlipoproteinemia. J. Clin. Endocrinol. Metabl., *57*:969, 1983.

37. Grimm, R.H., Jr., Leon, A.S., Hunninghake, D.B., et al.: Effects of thiazide diuretics on plasma lipids and lipoproteins in mildly hypertensive men. Ann. Intern. Med., *94*:7, 1981.

38. Harvard, C.W.H., Khokhar, A.M., and Flax, J.S.: Open assessment of the effect of prazosin on plasma lipids. J. Cardiovasc. Pharmacol, *4*(Suppl. 2):239, 1982.

39. Hazzard, W.R., Spiger, J.M., Bagdade, J.D., et al.: Studies on the mechanism of increased plasma triglyceride levels induced by oral contraceptives. N. Engl. J. Med., *280*:471, 1969.

40. Heiss, G., Tamir, I., Davis, C.E., et al.: Lipoprotein cholesterol distributions in selected North American populations. The Lipid Research Clinics Program Prevalence Study. Circulation, *61*:302, 1980.

41. Hershon, K., Brunzell, J., Albers, J., et al.: Hyperapo-B-emia with variable lipid phenotype (familial combined hyperlipidemia). Circulation, *64*:103, 1981.

42. Kannel, W.B., Castelli, W.P., and Gordon, T.: Cholesterol in the prediction of atherosclerotic disease. Ann. Intern. Med., *90*:85, 1979.

43. Kato, H., Tillotson, J., Nichamon, M., et al.: Epidemiologic studies of coronary heart disease and stroke in Japanese men living in Japan, Hawaii and California. Am. J. Epidemiol., *97*:372, 1973.

44. Katz, R.A., Jogensen, H., and Nigra, T.P.: Elevation of serum triglyceride levels from oral isotretinoin in disorders of keratinization. Arch. Dermatol., *116*:1396, 1980.

45. Keys, A. (ed.): Coronary heart disease in seven countries. Circulation, *41*(Suppl. 1):11, 1970.

46. Kinnunen, P.K.: High-density lipoprotein may not be antiatherogenic after all. Lancet, *2*:34, 1979.

47. Kissebah, A.H., Alfarsi, .S., and Evans, D.J.: Low density lipoprotein metabolism in familial combined hyperlipidemia. Mechanism of the multiple lipoprotein phenotypic expression. Arteriosclerosis, *4*:614, 1984.

48. Knopp, R.H., Walden, C.E., Wahl, P.M., et al.: Effects of oral contraceptives on lipoprotein triglyceride and cholesterol: Relationship to estrogen and progestin potency. Am. J. Obstet. Gynecol., *142*:(Suppl.):725, 1982.

49. Kokubu, T., Itoh, I., Kurita, H., et al.: Effect of prazosin on serum lipids. J. Cardiovasc. Pharmacol., *4*(Suppl. 2):228, 1982.

50. Kuller, L.H.: Epidemiology of cardiovascular diseases: Current perspectives. Am. J. Epidemiol., *104*:425, 1976.

51. Kwiterovich, P.O., Jr., Bachorik, P.S., Smith, H.H., et al.: Hyperapobetalipoproteinaemia in two families with xanthomas and phytosterolaemia. Lancet, *1*:466, 1981.

52. Lees, R.S.: Clofibrate and atherosclerosis. N. Engl. J. Med., *300*:491, 1979.

53. Lehtonen, A., and Viikari, J.: Long-term effect of sotalol on plasma lipids. Clin. Sci., *57*(Suppl.):405, 1979.

54. LeLorier, J., Dubreuil-Quidoz, S., Lussier-Cacan, S., et al.: Diet and probucol in lowering cholesterol concentrations. Arch. Intern. Med., *137*:1429, 1977.

55. Leren, P., Foss, O.P., Helgeland, A., et al.: Effects of pindolol and hydrochlorothiazide on blood lipids: The Olso Study. Clin. Trials J., *18*:254, 1981.

56. Leren, P., Helgeland, A., Holme, I., et al.: Effect of propranolol and prazosin on blood lipids: The Oslo Study. Lancet, *2*:4, 1980.

57. Lithell, H., Waern, U., and Vessby, B.: Effect of prazosin on lipoprotein metabolism in premenopausal, hypertensive women. J. Cardiovasc. Pharmacol., *4*(Suppl. 2):242, 1982.

58. Lussier-Cacan, S., Bouthillier, D., and Davignon, J.: Apo E allele frequency in primary endogenous hy-

pertriglyceridemia (type IV) with and without hyperapobetalipoproteinemia. Arteriosclerosis, 5:639, 1985.

59. Mahley, R.W., Innerarity, T.L., Stanley, C., et al.: Plasma lipoproteins: Apolipoprotein structure and function. J. Lipid Res., 25:1277, 1984.

60. Mann, J.I., Vessey, M.P., Thorogood, M., et al.: Myocardial infarction in young women with special reference to oral contraceptive practice. Br. Med. J., 2:241, 1975.

61. Marsden, J.R., Trinick, T.R., and Laker, M.F.: Effects of isotretinoin on serum lipids and lipoproteins, liver and thyroid function. Clin. Chim. Acta, 143:243, 1984.

62. Mattson, F.H., Erickson, B.A., and Klingman, A.M.: Effect of dietary cholesterol on serum cholesterol in man. Am. J. Clin. Nutr., 25:589, 1972.

63. Menzel, H.J., Kladetsky, R.G., and Assmann, G.: Apolipoprotein E polymorphism and coronary artery disease. Arteriosclerosis, 3:310, 1983.

64. Michaëlsson, G., Bergqvist, A., and Whalquist, A.: The influence of "Tigason" (R010–9359) on the serum lipoproteins in man. Br. J. Dermatol., 107:591, 1982.

65. Miettinen, T.A., Vanhanen, H., Huttunen, J.K., et al.: HDL cholesterol and β-adrenoceptor blocking agents in a 5-year multifactorial primary prevention trial. Br. J. Clin. Pharmacol., 13(Suppl. 2):431, 1982.

66. Miller, G.J., and Miller, N.E.: Plasma high density lipoprotein concentration and development of ischemic heart disease. Lancet, 1:16, 1975.

67. Miller, N.E., Hammett, F., Saltissi, S., et al.: Relation of angiographically defined coronary artery disease to plasma lipoprotein subfractions and apolipoprotein. Br. MEd. J., 282:1741, 1981.

68. Naruszewicz, M., Carew, T.E., Pittman, R.C., et al.: A novel mechanism by which probucol lowers low density lipoprotein levels demonstrated in the LDL receptor-deficient rabbit. J. Lipid Res., 25:1206, 1984.

69. Noma, A., Yokosura, T., and Kitamura, K.: Plasma lipids and apolipoproteins as discriminators for presence and severity of angiogrpahically defined coronary artery disease. Atherosclerosis, 49:1, 1983.

70. Norum, R.A., Lakier, J.B., Goldstein, S., et al.: Familial deficiency of apolipoproteins AI and CIII and precocious coronary artery disease. N. Engl. J. Med., 306:1513, 1982.

71. Paravicini, U., Stockel, K., MacNamara, P.J., et al.: On metabolism and pharmacokinetics of an aromatic retinoid. Ann. N.Y. Acad. Sci., 359:54, 1981.

72. Pasotti, C., Capra, A., Fiorella, G., et al.: Effects of pindolol and metoprolol on plasma lipids and lipoproteins. Br. J. Clin. Pharmacol., 13(Suppl. 2):435, 1982.

73. Rhomberg, H.P., and Braunsteiner, H.: Excessive egg consumption, xanthomatosis and hypercholesterolemia. Br. Med. J., 1:1188, 1976.

74. Rifkind, B.M., and Segal, D.: Lipid Research Clinics Program: Reference values for hyperlipidemia and hypolipidemia. J.A.M.A., 250:1869, 1983.

75. Roberts, S.L., McMurry, M.P., and Connor, W.E.: Does egg feeding (i.e., dietary cholesterol) affect plasma cholesterol levels in humans? The results of a double-blind study. Am. J. Clin. Nutr., 34:2092, 1981.

76. Rössner, S., and Weiner, L.: Atenolol and metoprolol: Comparison of effects. Eur. J. Clin. Pharmcol., 24:573, 1983.

77. Salen, G., Shefer, S., and Berginer, V.M.: Familial diseases with storage of sterols other than cholesterol: Cerebrotendinous xanthomatosis and sitosterolemia with xanthomatosis. In Stanbury, J.B., et al. (eds.): Metabolic Basis of Inherited Diseases. Edition 5. New York, McGraw-Hill, 1983.

78. Schaefer, E.J., Heaton, W.H., Wetzel, M.G., et al.: Plasma apolipoprotein AI absence associated with a marked reduction of high density lipoproteins and premature coronary artery disease. Arteriosclerosis, 2:16, 1982.

79. Schiffl, H., Weidmann, P., Mordasini, R., et al.: Reversal of diuretic-induced increases in serum low density lipoprotein cholestrol by the betablocker pindolol. Metabolism, 31:411, 1982.

80. Sing, C.F., and Davignon, J.: Role of the apolipoprotein E polymorphism in determining normal plasma lipid and lipoprotein variation. Am. J. Hum. Genet., 37:268, 1985.

81. Sing, C.F., and Orr, J.D.: Analysis of genetic and environmental sources of variation in serum cholestrol in Tecumseh, Michigan. IV. Separation of polygene from common environmental effects. Am. J. Hum. Genet., 30:491, 1978.

82. Slack, J.: Inheritance of familial hypercholesterolemia. Atherosclerosis Rev., 5:35, 1979.

83. Slone, D., Shapiro, S., Rosenburg, L., et al.: Relation of cigarette smoking to myocardial infarction in young women. N. Engl. J. Med., 298:1273, 1978.

84. Smith, E.B., and Slater, R.S.: Relationship between low density lipoprotein in aortic intima and serum lipid levels. Lancet, 1:463, 1972.

85. Sniderman, A.D., Shapiro, S., Marpole, D., et al.: Association of coronary atherosclerosis with hyperapobetalipoproteinemia (increased protein but normal cholesterol levels in human plasma low density [β] lipoproteins). Proc. Natl. Acad. Sci. USA, 77:604, 1980.

86. Stamler, J.: Dietary and serum lipids in the multifactorial etiolgoy of atherosclerosis. Arch. Surg., 113:21, 1978.

87. Steinberg, D.: Lipoprotein and atherosclerosis. Arteriosclerosis, 3:283, 1983.

88. Stolley, P.D.: Drugs, thromboembolism and myocardial infarction. In Bristow, M. (ed.): Drug-induced Heart Disease. Amsterdam, Elsevier, 1980.

89. Teng, B., Sniderman, A., Krauss, R.M., et al.: Modulation of apolipoprotein B antigenic determinants in human low density lipoprotein subclasses. J. Biol. Chem., 260:5067, 1985.

90. Teng, B., Thompson, G.R., Sniderman, A., et al.: Composition and distribution of low density lipoprotein fraction in hyperapobetalipoproteinemia, normolipidemia and familial hypercholesterolemia. Proc. Natl. Acad. Sci. USA, 80:6662, 1983.

91. Third, J.L.H.C., Montag, J., Flynn, M., et al.: Primary and familial hypoalphalipoproteinemia. Metabolism, 33:136, 1984.

92. Tolleshaug, H., Hobgood, K.K., Brown, M.S., et al.: The LDL receptor locus in familial hypercholesterolemia: Multiple mutations disrupt transport and processing of a membrane receptor. Cell, 32:941, 1983.

93. Utermann, G.: Role in lipoprotein metabolism and pathophysiology of hyperlipoproteinemia type III. La Ricerca Clin. Lab., 12:23, 1982.

94. Utermann, G., Hardewig, A., and Zimmer, F.: Apolipoprotein E phenotypes in patients with myocardial infarction. Hum. Genet., 65:237, 1984.

95. Utermann, G., Hees, M., and Steinmetz, A.: Polymorphism of apolipoprotein E and occurrence of dysbetalipoproteinemia in man. Nture, *269*:604, 1977.

96. Utermann, G., Kindermann, I., and Kaffarnik, H.: Apolipoprotein E phenotypes and hyperlipidemia. Hum. Genet., *65*:232, 1984.

97. Vahlquist, C., Michaëlsson, G., Vhalquist, A., et al.: A sequential comparison of etretinate (Tigason) and isotretinoin (Roaccutane) with special regard to their effects on serum lipoproteins. Br. J. Dermatol., *112*:69, 1985.

98. Vergani, C., and Bettale, G.: Familial hypo-alpha-lipoproteinemia, Clin. Chim. Acta, *114*:45, 1981.

99. Wallentin, L., and Varenhorst, E.: Changes of plasma lipid metabolism in males during estrogen treatment for prostatic carcinoma. J. Clin. Endocrinol. Metab., *47*:596, 1975.

100. Walton, K.W., Hitchens, J., Magnani, H.N., et al.: A study of methods of identification and estimation of Lp(a) lipoprotein and of its significance in health, hyperlipidemia and atherosclerosis. Atherosclerosis, *20*:323, 1974.

101. Wissler, R.W., and Vesselinovitch, D.: Combined effects of cholestyramine and probucol on regression of atherosclerosis in rhesus monkey aortas. Appl. Pathol., *1*:89, 1983.

102. Wynn, V., Doge, J.W.H., and Mills, G.L.: Some effects of oral contraceptives on serum lipid and lipoprotein levels. Lancet, *2*:720, 1966.

103. Wynn, V., and Niththyananthan, R.: The effect of progestins in combined oral contraceptives on serum lipids with special reference to high-density lipoproteins. Am. J. Obstet. Gynecol., *142*:(Suppl.):766, 1982.

104. Zannis, V.I., and Breslow, J.L.: Human very low density lipoprotein apolipoprotein E isoprotein polymorphism is explained by genetic variation and post-translational modification. Biochemistry, *20*:1033, 1981.

105. Zech, L.A., Gross, E.G., Peck, G.L., et al.: Changes in plasma cholesterol and triglyceride levels after treatment with oral isotretinoin. Arch. Dermatol., *119*:987, 1983.

Department of Lipid Metabolism and
Atherosclerosis Research
Clinical Research Institute of Montreal
110 Pine Avenue, West
Montreal, Quebec, Canada
H2W 1R7

Risks for Arterial Hypertension

Roland E. Schmieder, M.D.,* Franz H. Messerli, M.D.,†
and Heinz Ruddel, M.D.‡

In the United States, approximately 35 million people have what is conventionally called established essential hypertension (blood pressure of 160/95 mm Hg or higher) or are using antihypertensive medication. Another 25 million are estimated to have so called "borderline hypertension" (systolic blood pressure of 140 to 160 mm Hg or diastolic blood pressure of 90 to 95 mm Hg).[60,62]

During the past decade, cardiovascular mortality and morbidity in the United States have been declining, at least to some extent as the result of the reduction of various risk factors.[84,95] Risk factor reduction has therefore become an increasingly important goal in medicine. Primary prevention should occur early in life, because the Bogalusa Heart Study[66] found that even in childhood, vascular changes in the arteries were closely related to pressure levels and serum lipoproteins. However, an even more important goal, reducing pre-existing risk factors, would be achieved by preventing the development of cardiovascular risk factors de novo. Borderline hypertension deserves special attention, as it often progresses to established hypertension, as demonstrated more than 40 years ago.[42]

The prevalence of borderline hypertension in westernized populations ranges from 10 to 20 per cent, depending on the definition used. Indeed, individuals with borderline or transient hypertension are at approximately two to five times greater risk of developing established hypertension than comparative normotensive sub-

jects (Fig. 1).[34,42] Furthermore, persons with borderline hypertension develop cardiovascular disease at a rate twice that in the general population.[34] Because borderline hypertension does not always progress to established hypertension, it is crucial to identify those individuals whose hypertensive cardiovascular disease progresses and to distinguish them from those with transient blood pressure elevation.

In this discussion, the most important risk factors that may predict the transition from borderline to established hypertension are reviewed. Although several biochemical, physiologic, and behavioral abnormalities have been noted in the early stages of hypertension,[34,35] these might be consequences or manifestations rather than precursors of established hypertension. Thus, this discussion is restricted to those pathophysiologic changes that have been investigated for their value as predictors of established hypertension.

DEFINITION

In 1978 borderline hypertension was arbitrarily defined by the World Health Organization as blood pressure equal to or greater than 140/90 mm Hg but less than 160/95 mm Hg.[97] Yet more commonly, a patient is diagnosed as a borderline hypertensive if several pressure values are somewhere above as well as below 140/90 mm Hg.[55] Such patients are usually recog-

*Section on Hypertensive Diseases, Department of Internal Medicine, Ochsner Clinic and Alton Ochsner Medical Foundation, New Orleans, Louisiana
†Section on Hypertensive Diseases, Department of Internal Medicine, Ochsner Clinic and Alton Ochsner Medical Foundation, New Orleans, Louisiana
‡Medizinische Universitatsklinik, Bonn-Venusberg, Federal Republic of Germany

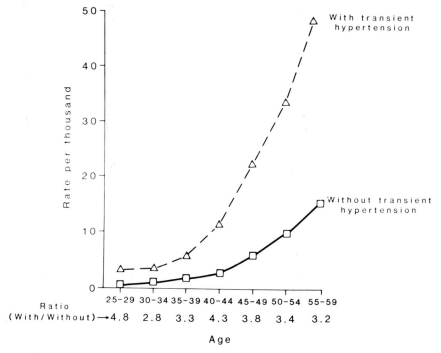

Figure 1. Prevalence of sustained hypertension in later life in normotensive subjects and patients who initially had transient (borderline) hypertension. Each cohort was followed for 5 years. (*From* Julius, S., and Ester, M.: Autonomic nervous cardiovascular regulation in borderline hypertension. Am. J. Cardiol., *36*:685–696, 1975; with permission.)

nized as hypertensive when they are less than 40 years old, although some seem to exhibit a borderline blood pressure pattern throughout their lives. Based on the risk of death related to hypertension in a two-stage screening, the Working Group on Risk and High Blood Pressure divided subjects on their first occasion of measurement into groups with minimal risk (diastolic blood pressure less than 80 mm Hg), intermediate risk (diastolic blood pressure greater than or equal to 80 mm Hg and less than 90 mm Hg), and high risk (diastolic blood pressure greater than or equal to 90 mm Hg) for hypertension. In the rescreening of the latter group, the subjects were characterized by intermediate risk (diastolic blood pressure less than 90 mm Hg) or confirmed risk (diastolic blood pressure of 90 mm Hg or greater) for high blood pressure.[96]

CONGENITAL FACTORS

Genetic Factors. Essential hypertension, by and large, is an inherited disorder. Familial aggregation of elevated blood pressure was found among first-degree relatives in adults and also between young children or newborns and their mothers.[98] Twin studies in monozygotic and bizygotic twins have established the degree to which heredity and environment determine the blood pressure pattern.[19] In contrast, no significant correlation has been noted between blood pressure in adopted children and in their adoptive parents.[19,36] The pressure levels of natural children were more closely correlated with their parents' levels than were the pressure levels of adopted children with their parents' levels.[36]

Most studies favor the hypothesis of polygenic inheritance of essential hypertension, but the detailed nature of heredity is still disputed.[98] Our knowledge of the genetic etiology of pathophysiologic hypertension is fragmentary. Hemodynamic responses to the performance of mental arithmetic problems were enhanced in children with a family history of hypertension when compared with children without such a family hsitory.[18] In a follow-up of more than 3 years, children who responded to mental arithmetic exercises with elevated blood pressure later developed higher blood pressure values than the control group.[17]

Several biochemical markers reflect the hereditary etiology of established hypertension. Patients with a positive family history often have a characteristic variation in the electrophoretic pattern of plasma proteins.[59] Urinary concentration of kallikrein also has been reported to correlate significantly with familial aggregation of blood pressure.[100] In addition, recent studies have revealed that the cell membrane transport of cations is altered in essential hypertension. For instance, the ratio of net sodium/potassium fluxes in red cells is reduced in patients with essential hypertension and the sodium/potassium ATPase activity is higher in offspring of hypertensive parents compared with offspring of normotensive subjects.[5,14,26,27,71,99]

Age. In Western populations, arterial pressure increases throughout life. In the United States, approximately 40 per cent of white people and more than 50 per cent of black people over age 65 have hypertension (blood pressure of 160/95 mm Hg or greater) or isolated systolic hypertension (systolic blood pressure greater than 160 mm Hg and diastolic blood pressure less than 95 mm Hg).[29,67] Both systolic blood pressure and diastolic blood pressure are equally important predictors of stroke and coronary heart disease.[73] In contrast, in populations that do not add salt to food, blood pressure does not increase during the life span (Fig. 2).[47,80]

Race. Essential hypertension is more prevalent and vascular disease more severe in blacks than in whites.[11,16,22,37] Even when the prevalence of hypertension was controlled for socioeconomic variables, the mortality risk remained greater among black than white hypertensive subjects.[32,63] Moreover, black men with borderline or mild hypertension progressed more frequently to moderate or even severe hypertension than their matched white counterparts. The reason for the increased prevalence of hypertension in black patients remains unknown. Most recently, we demonstrated that at any level of arterial pressure, renal blood flow was lower and renal vascular resistance higher in black patients than in white patients.[24] For a given level of arterial pressure, black patients also had a higher left ventricular mass.[32]

ENVIRONMENTAL FACTORS

Obesity. The association between obesity and hypertension is well documented.[6,25] Obesity increases the prevalence of hypertension (three to eight times).[76] A maximum of 30 per cent of hypertension in a given population could be attributed to overweight.[49] Body weight, body mass index, skin fold thickness, and circumferences of arm, chest, waist, and hips are all strongly correlated with arterial pressure.[86,87] Closer examination, however, disclosed that this holds true only for the characteristics of lean body mass, body build, and upper-body fat pattern, whereas absolute fat mass, central fat pattern, and fat cell characteristics do not necessarily predict increases in mean arterial pressure.[4,79,92] Nevertheless, evidence that weight loss reduces blood pressure has been well established.[6,74,76]

Obese patients are characterized by an expanded intravascular volume, expanded central blood volume, which leads to an increase in stroke volume, increased cardiac output, and increased cardiac workload caused by increasing venous return.[54] Thus, the increase in blood volume and cardiac output could conceivably be the cause of elevated arterial pressure. However, regardless of pressure elevation, these factors will eventually produce left ventricular dilatation and hypertrophy (eccentric hypertrophy)[56] in obesity hypertension. The fact that resting plasma catecholamines tend to be elevated in obese patients and decrease with weight reduction could indicate that in obesity, activity of the sympathetic nervous system increases.[74] However, other pathophysiologic abnormalities regarding sodium balance, insulin, carbohydrate metabolism, and the renin-angiotensin-aldosterone system in obesity hypertension have also been documented.[76]

Salt Intake. As early as 1904, arterial hypertension was linked to excessive dietary salt intake.[1] Since then, numerous studies on this subject have been published, but results remain controversial.[23,46,72,80] In a cross-cultural analysis, a strong relationship between salt intake and the prevalence of hypertension was observed.[46,47] The modifying impact of sodium intake on the increasing prevalence of hypertension with age was also noted.[47] When people migrate from areas with low sodium intake (3 gm or less per day) to communities where the daily salt intake is high (7 to 8 gm or more), their blood pressure increases proportionally.[72] These data, however, should not be overestimated, because possible confounding influences such as social change and altered overall nutritional state were not ruled out in this study. Levels of calcium, potassium, and magnesium in the diet might be equally important.[45,47] In therapeutic trials, including well-controlled double-blind studies, sodium restriction caused a decrease in blood pressure.[33,47] However, this decline in arterial pressure was

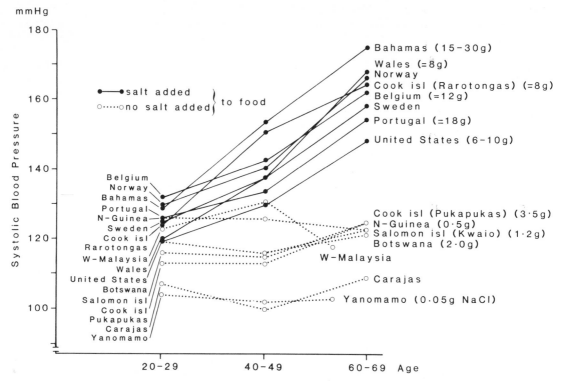

Figure 2.   Comparative international data on salt intake and blood levels at varying data. (*From* MacGregor, G.A.: Sodium is more important than calcium in essential hypertension. Hypertension, 7:628–637, 1985; with permission.)

not noted in each individual. Thus, many authors now believe that it is reasonable to assume that there are "salt-sensitive" and "salt-resistant" subjects.[38,44,81] Salt-sensitive subjects retain more sodium when exposed to a high-salt diet, and arterial pressure rises considerably more than in salt-resistant subjects.[38] Moreover, salt-sensitive subjects are characterized by enhanced sensitivity to circulating norepinephrine levels and more often exhibit a positive family history of essential hypertension.[81,82]

Alcohol, Caffeine, and Tobacco. The association between alcohol abuse and elevated arterial pressure has been established by various epidemiologic studies.[2,10,39,91] In a report of 83,947 subjects, consumption of 60 mg per day of alcohol caused an increase in arterial pressure averaging 10.9/4.5 mm Hg in men and 5.4/2.1 mm Hg in women.[39] Conversely, withdrawal of alcohol was followed by a decrease in arterial pressure after a few days. Hypertensive patients who stop drinking can often reduce or discontinue antihypertensive treatment.[2,30] Most studies show a linear correlation between alcohol consumption and level of arterial pressure (Fig. 3).[2] A maximum of 11 per cent of hypertension in men and only 1 per cent in women could be

attributed to alcohol consumption. These percentages were slightly reduced when age and body mass index were taken into account.[49]

Caffeine intake also produces an increase in arterial pressure; however, the effect is transient and rather small. The difference between non–coffee drinkers and those with the highest level of coffee consumption averaged 2.5/0.8 mm Hg.[40] Tobacco consumption is not an established risk factor for blood pressure elevation.[40] Recently, however, it has been implied that excessive tobacco chewing has a pressor effect leading to hypokalemia, similar to licorice abuse. A variety of chemical agents (drugs, foods, poisons) have been shown to elevate arterial pressure.[53] However, the increase in pressure is usually mild and transient. Only a few agents are known to provoke malignant hypertension.[7,53]

Oral Contraceptives. Premenopausal women have a lower prevalence of essential hypertension and its risk factors than men of the same age, probably because of the influence of estrogen.[61,90] However, if these women take oral contraceptives, arterial pressure increases and transient hypertension, often severe or even malignant, can be induced.[8,28,69,85] Young women

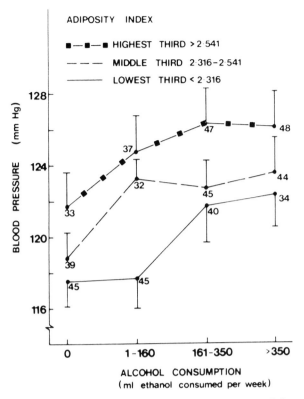

Figure 3.   Mean systolic blood pressure (x ± SEM) of men with known drinking habits according to body mass index (gm/cm). Effect of alcohol on systolic pressure is independent of obesity (F = 4.04 3 df p < 0.007). Effect of obesity on systolic pressure is independent of alcohol (F = 8.143 2 df p < 0.01). (*From* Arkwright, P.D., et al.: Effects of alcohol use and other aspects of lifestyle on blood pressure levels and prevalence of hypertension in a working population. Circulation, 66:60–66, 1982; with permission.)

with a positive family history of high blood pressure are at a particularly high risk of developing established hypertension with oral contraceptives.[20] However, no correlation has been found between the duration of contraceptive intake and the development of arterial hypertension.[20] Although the estrogen component is related to transient hypertension, the dose of estrogen is not related to blood pressure elevation.[51] In an epidemiologic study of 14,000 women, the prevalence of essential hypertension was 1.76 times higher in those who were taking oral contraceptives than in those who were not. However, because women taking oral contraceptives are more often examined by their physicians, the likelihood of discovering hypertension is greater in this cohort. If this factor is taken into account, the relative risk of arterial hypertension in women taking oral contraceptives is reduced from 1.76 to 1.29 compared with those without treatment.[20]

Stress and Socioeconomic Factors. Stress, noise, and socioeconomic factors may contribute to blood pressure elevation. Air traffic controllers working in a stressful environment (busy airports) developed a high incidence of arterial hypertension.[75] By comparing residents living near roads with heavy traffic with those who lived near light traffic, it was found that the average blood pressure of residents in the noisy district was higher; the longer they lived in the noisy area, the higher was the percentage of antihypertensive therapy.[64] In a preliminary follow-up study, noise was found to be one factor among various common stressors that determined blood pressure levels after 3 years.[64,65] In addition, the effect on blood pressure of the physical and mental demands of occupation, as well as of category of social class, was discovered in 1959.[15] However, the degree to which these environmental factors determine pathogenesis of blood pressure elevation still remains unclear.

DIAGNOSTIC CLUES FOR FUTURE HYPERTENSION

Tachycardia. In the Framingham Study, an increase in heart rate correlated with an increase in arterial pressure, particularly in men.[36] A fast heart rate seems to predispose one to the development of hypertension later in life.[41,68,88] Even normotensive subjects with a fast resting heart rate are at twice the risk of developing hypertension as those who have a normal resting heart rate.[43] Thus, tachycardia is clearly a risk factor for the development of hypertension.

Average Blood Pressure Level. Based on the close relationship between physical activity and subjectively reported emotional arousal to each blood pressure value, monitoring of ambulatory blood pressure seems to be a more appropriate assessment of "true" blood pressure.[52,77] The prediction of risk factors that might lead to hypertension was more successful when blood pressure was monitored over 24 hours than when it was monitored casually.[12,83]

Blood Pressure Variability. Several findings indicate that exaggerated blood pressure elevations that occur during daily life may ultimately lead to the development of sustained hypertension and to morphologic changes in arterial walls.[21] Experimentally, an increase in blood pressure lability will accelerate vascular wall protein synthesis in a manner similar to that seen in the arterial wall in hypertension.[48] Although blood pressure variability may be increased in patients with essential hypertension, when compared with normotensive subjects, variation coefficients (corrected for the absolute magnitude of blood pressure elevation) are usually normal.[50] Thus, at present, there is no strong evidence that increased blood pressure variability predicts future hypertension.

Blood Pressure Response to Dynamic Exercise. Exercise treadmill or bicycle testing does not always reveal an increased blood pressure response in hypertensive or prehypertensive patients.[9,70] However, it seems that the hypertensive response puts a patient at risk for developing subsequent hypertension that is between two and four times higher than in patients with a normotensive response.[13,93] Young healthy men who were normotensive at rest but who showed an exaggerated blood pressure response to bicycling (systolic blood pressure greater than 200 mm Hg and/or diastolic blood pressure increase greater than 10/90 mm Hg) had a distinct risk of developing hypertension after follow-up of almost 6 years.[13] Although the data are not entirely conclusive, we believe that exercise testing may be useful in predicting hypertension in prehypertensive subjects.

Blood Pressure Response to Mental Arithmetic. Patients with mild established essential hypertension (World Health Organization,

Stage 1) exhibited a greater increase in blood pressure or heart rate response when performing mental arithmetic tasks than a normotensive control group.[78] Even in children with a positive family history of hypertension, an enhanced hemodynamic response to mental challenge was noted.[18] After follow-up of 41 months, normotensive adolescents with an increase in blood pressure when performing mental arithmetic problems more frequently developed arterial hypertension.[17] However, this group was also characterized by a strong family history of hypertension, higher resting heart rate, and slightly higher initial resting blood pressure. Thus, these results are not entirely conclusive.

Response to Cold Pressure Tests. Almost 50 years ago, it was proposed that the development of high blood pressure in response to an external cold pressure stimulus could perhaps predict future hypertension.[31,58] The cold pressure test is predominantly an adrenergic stimulus requiring only a few minutes of testing and is easy to perform. However, its usefulness in the prediction of subsequent established hypertension is contested. In a recent long-term follow-up of patients of the Mayo Clinic, arterial hypertension occurred in 71 per cent of the hyperreactors and in only 19 per cent of the normal reactors.[94] These results are, however, subject to some criticism, because the follow-up rate in this study was only about 50 per cent.

MULTIFACTOR STUDIES

Several trials have been conducted to weigh these risk factors according to their predictive value. However, the results remain controversial. When baseline blood pressure, age, resting heart rate, relative weight, hematocrit, 1-hour postprandial blood sugar, and cholesterol were considered, more than half of the patients who developed hypertension were found to score in the highest quintile of these risk factors.[58] In contrast, the Australian Therapeutic Trial studying age, sex, family history, cigarette smoking, and serum cholesterol did not improve its prediction of hypertension after a 3-year follow-up in the placebo group.[3] In a recent attempt, baseline blood pressure, parental history of stroke or hypertension, smoking, and interior weight gain were found to be the most significant predictors distinguishing future hypertensive subjects from normotensive subjects.[89]

Table 1. *Predictors for Future Hypertension*

Congenital Risk Factors
  Family history of hypertension
  Age
  Race

Environmental Risk Factors
  Obesity
  Salt intake
  Alcohol, caffeine (?)
  Oral contraceptives
  Noise
  Socioeconomic status
  Other chemical agents

Prognostic Clues
  Resting tachycardia
  Ambulatory blood pressure monitoring
  Response to dynamic exercise
  Response to mental stress (?)
  Response to cold pressure test (?)

CONCLUSIONS

In a given population of patients with borderline hypertension, the incidence of de novo established essential hypertension averages 2 per cent per year. Clearly, primary prevention has to focus on identifying individuals who are at highest risk and delaying or reversing further elevation of arterial pressure levels (Table 1). A review of the literature indicates that several environmental and congenital factors can be identified as risk factors for the development of hypertension, including family history of essential hypertension, age, race, obesity, alcohol consumption, salt intake, hormonal status, and some stress factors. Some behavioral patterns and personality traits appear to be associated with borderline hypertension, but evidence that these factors determine the transition from borderline to established hypertension in later life has not yet been demonstrated. Of all approaches to predict the development of hypertension, measurements of resting heart rate and responses to dynamic exercise have some predictive value. Moreover, ambulatory monitoring of blood pressure might allow us to differentiate patients with transiently elevated blood pressure from those with more sustained hypertension.

REFERENCES

1. Ambard, L., and Beaujard, E.: Causes de l'hypertension arterielle. Arch. Intern. Med., *1*:520, 1904.
2. Arkwright, P.D., Beilin, L.J., Rouse, I., et al.: Effect of alcohol use and other aspects of lifestyle on blood pressure levels and prevalence of hypertension in a working population. Circulation, *66*:60–66, 1982.
3. Australian Therapeutic Trial in Mild Hypertension: Untreated mild hypertension. Am. J. Cardiol., *36*:685–696, 1975.
4. Berglund, G., Ljungman, S., Hartfort, M., et al.: Type of obesity and blood pressure. Hypertension, *4*:692–696, 1982.
5. Canessa, M., Adragna, N., Soloman, H.S., et al.: Increased sodium-lithium countertransport in red cells of patients with essential hypertension. N. Engl. J. Med., *302*:772–776, 1980.
6. Chaing, B.N., Perlman, L.V., and Epstein, F.H.: Overweight and hypertension: A review. Circulation, *39*:403–421, 1969.
7. Crane, M.G.: Iatrogenic hypertension. *In* Genest, J., Kuchel, O., Hamet, P., et al. (eds): Hypertension: Physiopathology and Treatment. New York, McGraw-Hill Book Company, 1983, pp. 976–988.
8. Crane, M.G., Harris, J.J., et al.: Hypertension, oral contraceptive agents, and conjugated estrogens. Ann. Intern. Med., *74*:13–21, 1971.
9. Criqui, M.H., Haskell, W.L., Heiss, et al.: Predictors of systolic blood pressure response to treadmill exercise: The Lipid Research Clinics Program Prevalence Study. Circulation, *68*:225–233, 1983.
10. Criqui, M.H., Wallace, R.B., Mishkey, M., et al.: Alcohol consumption and blood pressure: The Lipid Research Clinics Prevalence Study. Hypertension, *3*:557–565, 1981.
11. Cruickshand, J.K., and Beevers, D.G.: Epidemiology of hypertension: Blood pressure in blacks and whites. Clin. Sci., *62*:1–6, 1982.
12. Devereux, R.B., Pickering, T.G., Harshfield, G.A., et al.: Left ventricular hypertension in patients with hypertension: Importance of blood pressure response to regularly recurring stress. Circulation, *68*:470–476, 1983.
13. Dlin, R.A., Hanne, N., Silverberg, D.S., et al.: Follow-up of normotensive men with exaggerated blood pressure response to exercise. Am. Heart J., *106*:316–320, 1983.
14. Doyle, A.E., and Frazier, J.R.E.: Essential hypertension and inheritance of vascular reactivity. Lancet, *2*:509–511, 1961.
15. Edwards, F., McKeown, T., and Whitfield, A.G.W.: Arterial pressure in men over sixty. Clin. Sci., *18*:289–300, 1959.
16. Entwisle, G., Apostolides, A.Y., Hebel, J.R., et al.: Target organ damage in black hypertensives. Circulation, *55*:729–796, 1977.
17. Falkner, B., Kushner, H., Onesti, G., et al.: Cardiovascular characteristics in adolescents who develop essential hypertension. Hypertension, *3*:521–527, 1981.
18. Falkner, B., Onesti, G., and Angelakos, E.T.: Hemodynamic response to mental stress in normal adolescents with varying degree of genetic risk for essential hypertension. *In* Yamori, Y., Lovenberg, W., and Freis, E. (eds.): Prophylactic Approach to Hypertensive Diseases. New York, Raven Press, 1979, pp. 149–156.
19. Feinleib, H., Garrison, R., Borhani, N., et al.: Studies of hypertension in twins. *In* Paul, O. (ed.): Epidemiology and Control of Hypertension. New York, and Stuttgart, Stratton Intercontinental Medical Books, 1975, pp. 3–17.
20. Fisch, J.R., Freedman, S.H., and Wyatt, A.V.: Oral contraceptives, pregnancy and blood pressure. J.A.M.A., *222*:1507–1510, 1972.

21. Folkow, B.: Physiological aspects of primary hypertension.. Physiol. Rev., *62*:327–329, 1980.

22. Freis, E.D.: Age, race, sex and other indices of risk in hypertension. Am. J. Med., *55*:275–280, 1973.

23. Freis, E.D.: Salt volume and the prevention of hypertension. Circulation, *53*:589–595, 1976.

24. Frohlich, E.D., Messerli, F.H., Dunn, F.G., et al.: Greater renal vascular involvement in the black patient with essential hypertension: A comparison of systemic and renal dynamics in black and white patients. Miner. Electrolyte Metab., *10*:173–177, 1984.

25. Frohlich, E.D., Messerli, F.H., Reisin, E., et al.: The problem of obesity and hypertension. Hypertension, 5(Suppl. III):71–78, 1983.

26. Garay, R.P., Elghozi, J.L., Dagher, G., et al.: Laboratory distinction between essential and secondary hypertension by measurement of erythrocyte cation fluxes. N. Engl. J. Med., *302*:769–771, 1980.

27. Garay, R.P., and Meyer, P.: A new test showing abnormal net Na^+, K^+ fluxes in erythrocytes of essential hypertensive patients. Lancet., *1*:349–353, 1979.

28. Harris, P.W.R.: Malignant hypertension associated with oral contraceptives. Lancet, 2:466–467, 1969.

29. Health, and Nutritional Examination Study (HANES), 1971–1974: Blood pressure levels of persons 60–74, U.S. National Center for Health Statistics, Department of Health, Education and Welfare. Vital and Health Statistic Series II, No. 203, 1977.

30. Henningsen, N.C.: Hypertension, levels of serum gamma glutamyl transpeptidase and degree of blood pressure control in middle-aged males. Acta Med. Scand., *207*:245–251, 1980.

31. Hines, E.A., and Brown, G.E.: The cold pressor test for measuring the reactibility of the blood pressure: Data concerning 571 normal and hypertensive subjects. Am. Heart J., *11*:1–9, 1936.

32. Hypertension Detection and Follow-up Program Cooperative Group: Race, education and prevalence of hypertension. Am. J. Epidemiol., *106*:351–361, 1977.

33. Joossens, J.V.: Dietary salt restriction: The case in favor. The Therapeutics of Hypertension. London, Royal Society of Medicine (International Congress and Symposium Series; No. 26) 1980, pp. 243–250.

34. Julius, S.: Borderline hypertension; clinical and pathophysiologic significance. Adv. Intern. Med. Pediatr., *41*:51–84, 1978.

35. Julius, S., and Esler, M.: Autonomic nervous cardiovascular regulation in borderline hypertension. Am. J. Cardiol., *36*:685–696, 1975.

36. Kannel, W.B.: Host and environmental determinants of hypertension. Perspective from the Framingham Study. *In* Kesteloot, H., and Joossens, F.V. (eds.): Epidemiology of Arterial Blood Pressure. The Hague, Boston, and London, Martinus Nijhoff Publishers, 1980, Edition 2. pp. 266–295.

37. Kaplan, N.M.: Clinical Hypertension. Edition 2. Baltimore, Williams and Wilkins, 1978.

38. Kawasaki, T., Delea, C.S., and Bartter, F.C.: The effect of high-sodium and low-sodium intakes on blood pressure and other related variables in human subjects with idiopathic hypertension. Am. J. Med., *64*:193–198, 1978.

39. Klatsky, A.L., Friedman, G.D., Siegelaub, A., et al.: Alcohol consumption and blood pressure. N. Engl. J. Med., *296*:1194–1200, 1977.

40. Lang, T., Degoulet, P., and Aime, F.: Relation between coffee drinking and blood pressure: Analysis of 6,321 subjects in the Paris region. Am. J. Cardiol., *52*:1238–1242, 1983.

41. Langewitz, W., von Eiff, A.W., and Goglin, E.: Reliability and validity of ambulatory blood pressure recording in children.·J. Clin. Exp. Hypertension, A7:217–225, 1985.

42. Levy, R.L., Hillmann, C.C., Stroud, W.D., et al.: Transient hypertension. J.A.M.A., *126*:829–833, 1944.

43. Levy, R.L., White, P.D., Stroud, W.D., et al.: Transient tachycardia: Prognostic significance alone and in association with transient hypertension. J.A.M.A., *129*:585–588, 1945.

44. Longworth, D.K., Drayer, J.I.M., and Weber, M.A.: Divergent blood pressure responses during short-term sodium restriction in hypertension. Clin. Pharmacol. Ther., *27*:544–546, 1980.

45. MacCarron, D.A.: Is calcium more important than sodium in the pathogenesis of essential hypertension? Hypertension, 7:607–627, 1985.

46. MacFate-Smith, W.: Epidemiology of hypertension. Med. Clin. North Am., *61*:467–486, 1977.

47. MacGregor, G.A.: Sodium is more important than calcium in essential hypertension. Hypertension, 7:628–637, 1985.

48. MacLean, A.G., Bevan, R.D., and Hume, W.R.: Rapid onset of vascular wall protein synthesis with increase in lability of blood pressure in rabbits. Clin. Sci., 59:327–329, 1980.

49. MacMahon, S.W., Blacket, R.B., and MacDonald, G.J.: Obesity, alcohol consumption and blood pressure in Australian men and women. The National Heart Foundation of Australia Risk Factor Prevalence Study. J. Hypertension, 2:85–91, 1984.

50. Mancia, G., and Zanchett, A.: Blood pressure variability and the assessment of blood pressure: Implications for epidemiologic research and for treatment. *In* Gross, F., and Strasser, T. (eds.): Mild Hypertension. Recent Advances. New York, Raven Press, 1983, pp. 251–262.

51. Meir, R.J., Wilson, E.S.B., and Cruikshank, J.K.: Effects on blood pressure of low-dose estrogen and progestagen only oral contraceptives. (Abstract.) Ricera Scientifica et Educazione Permante, *33*(Suppl.):479, 1983.

52. Messerli, F.H.: Continuous noninvasive automatic blood pressure recording. Postgrad. Med., 75:115–124, 1984.

53. Messerli, F.H.: High blood pressure. A side effect of drugs, poisons, and food. Arch. Intern. Med., *139*:682–687, 1979.

54. Messerli, F.H., Christie, B., DeCarvalho, J.G.P., et al.: Obesity and essential hypertension. Arch. Intern. Med., *141*:81–85, 1981.

55. Messerli, F.H., DeCarvalho, J.G.P., Christie, B., et al.: Systemic and regional hemodynamics in low, normal and high cardiac output borderline hypertension. Circulation, 58:441–448, 1978.

56. Messerli, F.H., Sungaard-Riise, B.A., Reisin, E.D., et al.: Dimorphic cardiac adaptation to obesity and arterial hypertension. Ann. Intern. Med., 99:757–761, 1983.

57. Messerli, F.H., Sundgaard-Riise, B.A., Reisin, E., et al.: Disparate cardiovascular effect of obesity and arterial hypertension. Am. J. Med., 74:808–812, 1983.

58. Murakami, E., Hiwada, K., and Kokubu, T.: Pathophysiological characteristics of labile hypertensive

patients determined by the cold pressor test. Jpn. Circ. J., *44*:438–442, 1980.

59. Nardi, R., Carreta, R., Sawa, H., et al.: Characteristic variation in electrophoretic pattern of plasma proteins in essential hypertension. Lancet, 2:182–183, 1980.

60. National Center for Health Statistics: Hypertension in adults 25–74 years of age, United States 1971–75. Hyattsville, Maryland, DHHS publication No. (PHS) 81-1671, Vital and Health Statistics Series II, No. 221, April 1981.

61. National Health Survey: Hypertension and hypertensive heart disease in adults, U.S. 1960–1962, Washington, D.C., U.S. Department of Health, Education and Welfare. Vital and Health Statistics Series II, No. 13, U.S. Government Printing Office, 1966.

62. National High Blood Pressure Education Program Coordinating Committee: New Hypertension Prevalence Data and Recommended Public Statements. Bethesda, Maryland, National Heart, Lung and Blood Institute, February 1978.

63. Neser, W.B., Tyroler, H.A., and Cassel, J.C.: Social disorganization and stroke mortality in the black population of North Carolina. Am. J. Epidemiol., *93*:166–175, 1971.

64. Neus, H., von Eiff, A.W., Ruddel, H., et al.: Traffic noise and hypertension. The Bonn traffic noise study. Proceedings of the Fourth International Congress on Noise as a Public Health Problem. Milano, Centro Ricerche e Studi Amplifon, 1983, pp. 693–698.

65. Neus, H., Ruddel, H., Schute, W., et al.: The long-term effect of noise on blood pressure. J. Hypertension, *1*(Suppl. 2):251–253, 1983.

66. Newman, W.P., Freedmann, D.S., Voors, A.W., et al.: Serum lipoproteins and systolic blood pressure are related to atherosclerosis in early life: The Bogalusa Heart Study. N. Engl. J. Med., *314*:138–149, 1986.

67. Osfeld, A.M.: Elderly hypertensive patient: Epidemiologic review. N.Y. State J. Med., *78*:1125–1129, 1978.

68. Pfaffenberger, R.S., Thorne, M.C., and Wing, A.L.: Chronic disease in former college students—VIII. Characteristics in youth predisposing to hypertension in later years. Am. J. Epidemiol., *88*:25–32, 1968.

69. Pfeffer, R.I.: Estrogen use, hypertension and stroke in postmenopausal women. J. Chronic Dis., *31*:389–398, 1978.

70. Pickering, T.G., Harshfield, G.A., Kleinert, H.D., et al.: Blood pressure during normal daily activities, sleep and exercise: comparison of values in normal and hypertensive subjects. J.A.M.A., *247*:992–996, 1982.

71. Postnov, Y.V., Orlov, S.N., Schevchenko, A.S., et al.: Altered sodium permeability, calcium binding and NA-K-ATPase activity in the red blood cell membrane in essential hypertension. Pflugers Arch., *371*:263–269, 1977.

72. Prior, I.A.M., Evans, J.G., Harvey, H.B.P., et al.: Sodium intake and blood pressure in two Polynesian populations. N. Engl. J. Med., *279*:515–520, 1968.

73. Rabbin, S.W., Mathemson, R.A.G., and Tate, R.B.: Predicting and risk of ischemic heart disease and cerebrovascular disease from systolic and diastolic blood pressure. Ann. Intern. Med., *88*:342–345, 1978.

74. Reisin, E., Frohlich, E.D., Messerli, F.H., et al.: Cardiovascular changes after weight reduction in obesity hypertension. Ann. Intern. Med., *98*:315–319, 1983.

75. Rose, R.M., Jenkins, C.D., and Hurst, M.W.: Air traffic controller health damage study. In Levin, M.A. (ed.): Report to the FAA. Contract DOT-FA73WA-3211, August 1978.

76. Rosenfeld, J., and Shohat, J.: Obesity and hypertension. In Gross, F., and Strasser, T. (eds.): Mild Hypertension: Recent Advances. New York, Raven Press, 1983, pp. 197–208.

77. Schmieder, R., Ruddell, H., Laugwitz, W., et al.: The influence of monotherapy with oxprenolol and nitrendipine on ambulatory blood pressure in hypertensives. Clin. Exp. Hypertension, A7:445–454, 1985.

78. Schulte, W., Neus, H., and von Eiff, A.W.: Blutdruckreaktivitat unter emotionalem Stress bei unkomplizierten Formen des Hochdrucks. Klin, Wochenschr., *59*:1243–1249, 1981.

79. Siervogel, R.M., Rodie, A.F., Chumlea, W.C., et al.: Blood pressure, body composition and fat tissue cellularity in adults. Hypertension, *4*:382–386, 1982.

80. Simpson, F.O.: Salt and hypertension: A skeptical review of the evidence. Clin. Sci., *57*(Suppl. 5):463–482, 1979.

81. Skrabal, F., Aubock, J., and Hortnagl, H.: Low sodium/high potassium diet for prevention of hypertension: Probable mechanisms of action. Láncet, 2:895–900, 1981.

82. Skrabal, F., Herholz, H., et al.: Neues Konzept fur die Entstehung der essentiellen Hypertonie. Dtsch. Med. Wochenschr., *108*:1122–1126, 1983.

83. Sokolow, M., Werdegar, D., and Kain, H.K.: Relationship between the level of blood pressure measured casually and by portable recorders and severity of complications in essential hypertension. Circulation, *34*:279–298, 1966.

84. Stamler, J.: The marked decline in coronary heart disease mortality rates in the United States 1968–1981: Summary of findings and possible explanations. Cardiology, *72*:11–22, 1985.

85. Stern, M.P., Brown, B.W., Haskell, W.L., et al.: Cardiovascular risk and use of estrogen-progestagen combinations. J.A.M.A., *235*:811–815, 1976.

86. Svardsudd, K., Wedel, H., and Wilhelmsen, L.: Factors associated with the initial blood pressure level and with the subsequent blood pressure increase in a longitudinal population study: The study of men born in 1913. Eur. Heart. J., *1*:345–354, 1980.

87. Svardsudd, K., and Wilhelmsen, L.: Change of blood pressure in relation to other variables and to development of hypertensive disease indices in a longitudinal population study: The study of men born in 1913. Eur. Heart J., *1*:355–360, 1980.

88. Thomas, C.B., and Duszynski, K.R.: Blood pressure levels in young adulthood as predictors of hypertension and the fate of the cold pressor test. The Johns Hopkins Medical Journal, *151*:93–100, 1982.

89. Thomas, J., Semenya, K.A., Neser, W.B., et al.: Risk factors and the incidence of hypertension in black physicians: The Meharry Cohort Study. Am. Heart. J., *110*:637–645, 1985.

90. von Eiff, A.W., Plotz, E.F., and Beck, K.J.: The effect of estrogens and progestins on blood pressure regulation of normotensive women. Am. J. Obstet. Gynecol., *109*:887–892, 1971.

91. Wallace, R.B., Lynch, C.S., Pomrehn, P.R., et al.: Alcohol and hypertension: epidemiologic and ex-

perimental considerations. The Lipid Research Clinics Program. Circulation, *64*(Suppl. 3):41–47, 1981.

92. Weinsier, R.L., Birch, N.R., Bernstein, R.S., et al.: The relative contribution of body fat and fat pattern to blood pressure level. Hypertension, 7:578–585, 1985.

93. Wilson, N.V., and Meyer, B.M.: Early prediction of hypertension using exercise blood pressure. Prev. Med., *10*:62–68, 1981.

94. Wood, D.L., Sheps, S.G., Elveback, L.R., et al.: A cold pressor test as a predictor of hypertension. Hypertension, 6:301–306, 1984.

95. Working Group on Arteriosclerosis of the National Heart, Lung and Blood Institute: Decline in Coronary Heart Disease Mortality, 1968–1978. Vol. 2. Bethesda, Maryland, National Institutes of Health (DHHS publication No. (NIH) 82-2035), 1981, pp. 157–158.

96. Working Group on Risk and High Blood Pressure: An epidemiological approach to describing risk associated with blood pressure levels. Hypertension, 7:641–651, 1985.

97. World Health Organization Expert Committee: Arterial hypertension, WHO Technical Report Service, 1978, p. 628.

98. Yamori, Y.: The genetics of essential hypertension. *In* Gross, F., and Strasser, T. (eds.): Mild Hypertension: Recent Advances. New York, Raven Press, 1983, pp. 187–196.

99. Yamori, Y., Nara, Y., Hoerie, R., et al.: Abnormal membrane characteristics of erythrocytes in rat models and men with predisposition to stroke. Clin. Exp. Hypertension, 2:1009, 1980.

100. Zinner, S.H., Margolius, H.S., and Rosen, B.: Familial aggregation of urinary kallikrein concentration in childhood: Relation to blood pressure, race and urinary electrolytes. Am. J. Epidemiol., *104*:124, 1976.

Franz H. Messerli, M.D.
Ochsner Clinic
1514 Jefferson Highway
New Orleans, Louisiana 70121

Risks for Glucose Intolerance

Leslie J. Klaff, M.D., Ph.D.,* and Jerry P. Palmer, M.D.†

Premature vascular disease is one of the most common and serious complications of diabetes. Most studies demonstrate that the prevalence of cardiovascular disease is increased among diabetics compared with nondiabetics. Although there appears to be a relationship between plasma glucose levels and the prevalence of diabetic microvascular disease, the relationship between glucose and macrovascular disease is not nearly as well defined.

Although the risk of developing cardiovascular disease is high in diabetics, not all diabetics are at equal risk. Many other variables, including genetic factors, geographic factors, sex, age, and the presence of other risk factors, interact with glucose intolerance as a risk factor for the development of cardiovascular disease. In this article, we shall review the epidemiologic data dealing with the increased risk of cardiovascular disease associated with glucose intolerance and some of the possible mechanisms that may account for this increased risk.

POPULATION PREVALENCE STUDIES

A large body of literature has accumulated that confirms that cardiovascular disease is the major cause of death and morbidity in diabetics. One of the earliest studies was performed at the Joslin Clinic in 1964.[4] This study included 2364 patients with diabetes and reported that about 75 per cent died of vascular causes. When the mortality data from Caucasians in New England were used for comparison, death due to vascular disease was two to four times more common in this diabetic clinic population.

The Framingham Study was the first large community-based prospective study in which diabetics were compared with nondiabetics from the same population group.[7,10,21–23] This study found that the mortality from sudden death, cardiac infarctions, and cerebrovascular disease was significantly higher in diabetics.[7] Furthermore, the average annual incidence of cardiovascular events was increased in the diabetics[21] (Table 1).

Prospective studies have now been performed among such divergent groups and communities as men of Japanese descent living in Hawaii[50]; urban and rural Puerto Ricans[3]; British male civil servants[6]; and in Bedford, England.[26] The results of these studies are essentially the same as those of the Framingham Study, namely that the age-adjusted incidence of cardiovascular events and the death rate from cardiovascular causes are between 1.5- and 4-fold higher in diabetics than in nondiabetics. Retrospective studies in diabetic clinic patients in Warsaw, Poland,[27] and in a population-based study in Rochester, Minnesota,[30] also confirm these results.

Prevalence studies showing a higher prevalence of cardiovascular disease in diabetics than in nondiabetics have also been performed in many communities throughout the world, including Finland,[47] Japan,[11,16] the Pacific Islands,[51] Arizona (among the Pima Indians),[15] and Tecumseh, Michigan.[31,32]

One of the factors contributing toward the increased mortality rate from cardiovascular disease may relate to the finding that diabetics are

*Assistant Professor, Division of Metabolism, Endocrinology, and Nutrition, Department of Medicine, University of Washington School of Medicine, Seattle, Washington

†Associate Professor, Division of Metabolism, Endocrinology, and Nutrition, Department of Medicine, University of Washington School of Medicine, Seattle, Washington

68   Leslie J. Klaff and Jerry P. Palmer

Table 1. Average Annual Age-Adjusted Incidence per 1000 Specified Cardiovascular Events*

CARDIOVASCULAR EVENT	MEN Diabetic	MEN Nondiabetic	WOMEN Diabetic	WOMEN Nondiabetic
Cardiovascular disease	39.1	19.1	27.2	10.2
Cardiovascular disease death	17.4	8.5	17.0	3.6
Congestive heart failure	7.6	3.5	11.4	2.2
Intermittent claudication	12.6	3.3	8.4	1.3
Atherothrombotic brain infarction	4.7	1.9	6.2	1.7
Coronary heart disease	24.8	14.9	17.8	6.9

*Framingham cohort, including men and women aged 45 to 74 years.
From Kannel, W.B., and McGee, D.L.: Diabetes and cardiovascular disease: The Framingham Study. J.A.M.A., 241:2035–2038, 1979; with permission.

more likely to die in the acute stage of myocardial infarction than nondiabetics. In comparing diabetics and nondiabetics admitted to coronary care units, Soler and coworkers reported an overall mortality rate of 35.3 per cent in diabetics and 18.0 per cent in nondiabetics.[45] This excess mortality did not occur in the diet-treated patients. Rytter and associates reported that the mortality rate after admission for acute myocardial infarcts was 42 per cent for diabetics and 20 per cent for nondiabetics.[41] In the non–insulin-dependent diabetics, insulin treatment was associated with a reduced mortality rate compared with treatment with oral agents. The mortality rate was higher in patients with poor metabolic control, and diabetics were more prone to develop cardiogenic shock and conduction disorders than nondiabetics. In slight contrast, however, Harrower and Clarke reported an overall mortality rate from acute myocardial infarction of 24 per cent in diabetics, which was only slightly higher than that in nondiabetics.[12] This was not influenced by prior treatment but was influenced by prior metabolic control, with poorly controlled patients having a significantly higher mortality rate than the well-controlled patients.

One factor that may adversely influence survival may be the presence of diabetic cardiopathy. In the Framingham Study, it was noted that congestive cardiac failure occurred more frequently in diabetics[22] (see Table 1). This increased frequency could not be explained by overt coronary artery disease or other risk factors and may have been due, in part, to this entity.

SEX

The relative impact of impaired glucose tolerance as a risk factor for vascular disease is substantially greater for women than for men. In the Framingham Study, the excess of coronary artery disease in diabetic women was particularly striking, with the cardiovascular mortality in diabetic women being equal to that in diabetic men (see Table 1).[10,21,22] This increased risk has now been confirmed in several other studies both in the United States[1] and in Britain,[20,44] although it has not been noted in two European studies.[27,34]

In the Framingham Study, it was found that after adjustment for differences in the other cardiovascular risk factors in the two sexes, the relative impact of diabetes on coronary heart disease, peripheral arterial disease, and stroke is the same in each sex. However, for cardiovascular mortality and for cardiac failure, the impact remained greater in women even after adjustment for coexisting risk factors. Similarly, in a Finnish study, the increased risk of electrocardiographic abnormalities was similar (about 3.3 times higher in diabetics than in the nondiabetic controls of both sexes), but the frequency of definite electrocardiographic evidence of myocardial infarction was 4.4 times higher in diabetic women compared with 1.7 times higher in diabetic men.[47] Rytter and colleagues did not find that men with non–insulin-dependent diabetes had a significantly higher risk of acute myocardial infarctions, but the risk in women was approximately doubled.[41]

The reason for this apparent increased susceptibility of diabetic women to cardiovascular mortality is not clear. Walden and associates found that diabetes caused consistently greater adverse effects on lipoprotein triglycerides and cholesterol concentrations in women than in men.[49] However, these effects were relatively modest, and we must postulate other additional factors to account for the greater propensity for atherosclerotic disease in diabetic women.

GENETIC AND GEOGRAPHIC FACTORS

The frequency and severity of cardiovascular disease in populations vary widely among different geographic and ethnic groups. Within most groups, arterial disease is more common in individuals with diabetes than in those without diabetes. However, differences in cardiovascular mortality and morbidity among ethnic groups, populations, and individuals are not explained satisfactorily by the variation of risk factors alone. For example, in the WHO study of vascular disease and diabetes, it was noted that diabetics from Japan and Hong Kong, despite being older, being among the heaviest cigarette smokers, and having relatively high blood pressures, had lower frequencies of symptoms of major arterial disease and electrocardiographic signs than the European and American groups.[24] In contrast, the frequency of microangiopathy (nephropathy and retinopathy) did not differ significantly among the 14 centers studied.[25] The International Atherosclerosis Project, which quantitated arterial wall changes on autopsy material from diabetics and nondiabetics in 19 centers, made the observation that although arteries of diabetics showed more disease than those of nondiabetics in all centers, the prevalence of atherosclerosis varied considerably from center to center and showed distinct parallelism with overall prevalence variations in the national ethnic groups.[39] It would appear, therefore, that the frequency of macrovascular disease in the diabetic population is related to the frequency of macrovascular disease in the nondiabetic population. For example, in Japan, where the mortality due to ischemic heart disease is very low, coronary heart disease appeared to be the cause of death, based on postmortem examinations, in only 6 per cent of a large series of diabetics.[11] Most current figures from Europe and the United States would exceed 40 per cent. In South Africa, both coronary heart disease and peripheral vascular disease occurred less frequently in black diabetics than in nondiabetics of other ethnic groups, although microvascular disease occurred with equal frequency in all groups.[43] The Pima Indians, with their very high frequency of diabetes, have only half the frequency of coronary heart disease compared with the Caucasian population of Tecumseh.[15]

SEVERITY OF GLUCOSE INTOLERANCE

So far, the relationship between clinically evident diabetes and cardiovascular morbidity and mortality has been considered. In 1979, the National Diabetes Data Group made a distinction between the entities of diabetes and impaired glucose tolerance.[29] Diabetes is characterized by raised fasting blood sugar (greater than 140 mg per dl) and/or severe and prolonged postprandial hyperglycemia (greater than 200 mg per dl). Impaired glucose tolerance is diagnosed when the fasting blood sugar is normal or slightly raised (less than 140 mg per dl) and the postprandial blood glucose is intermediate between diabetic and normal range (140 to 200 mg per dl). Persons with impaired glucose tolerance but not diabetes have only a slightly increased risk of developing microvascular complications. However, several studies have indicated that persons with impaired glucose tolerance are at risk of developing macrovascular disease and have approximately double the risk of coronary heart disease mortality compared with normal individuals.

In the Bedford study,[26] Keen and associates reported that at baseline, the prevalence of arterial disease in borderline diabetics (patients with impaired glucose tolerance) was intermediate between those of the diabetics and the normal individuals. Similarly, the age-corrected mortality rates over 10 years of follow-up in these patients were intermediate between those of diabetics and nondiabetic controls.[20] Twenty-two of 249 borderline diabetics became diabetic in the first 5 years of follow-up. Of these, 22.7 per cent died a cardiovascular death, as compared with 9.9 per cent of those who did not progress to diabetes within the first 5 years. Although this comparison did not reach statistical significance, it suggested a particularly adverse cardiovascular effect of deteriorating glucose tolerance. Similar observations were made by Sartor and coworkers.[42] In their prospective study of patients with impaired glucose tolerance, 31.4 per cent of those with deteriorating glucose tolerance died during follow-up, compared with 15.2 per cent of those who did not show deterioration.

In the Whitehall study among British male civil servants,[6] 18,403 persons were ranked according to their blood glucose level 2 hours after a 50-gm glucose load. Analysis of 1077 deaths that had occurred after 7.5 years showed an abrupt doubling of the coronary heart disease mortality rate in those persons falling above the ninety-fifth percentile for glucose levels. The cutoff point determining the ninety-fifth percentile corresponded to a blood glucose of only 96 mg per dl. The mortality rate among these persons was similar to that of a group who, at screening, were found to have frank diabetes.

In the Honolulu Heart Program,[50] a prospective study of Japanese men born in the years 1900 to 1919 and examined in 1965 to 1968, age-adjusted coronary heart disease mortality rates over 9 years of follow-up were not significantly different between men with previously diagnosed diabetes and men with post–glucose load hyperglycemia (above the ninetieth percentile for the cohort). Both groups had mortality rates from coronary heart disease twofold to threefold greater than men with blood glucose below the ninetieth percentile. In the Finnish Policemen Study, Pyorala[37] found that the risk of coronary artery disease did not relate to fasting blood glucose but to the 1-hour blood glucose and integrated values after a glucose load. Persons with only mildly impaired glucose tolerance had increased risk of coronary heart disease. Likewise, in the Puerto Rican Heart Program an abnormal glucose tolerance test was found to be an independent risk factor for death from coronary heart disease in urban men.[3] As in the Whitehall Study and Helsinki Study, fasting blood glucose levels alone were not an important predictor of mortality from coronary heart disease. Thus, it would appear that impaired glucose tolerance is associated with an increased risk of cardiovascular disease and that this increased risk occurs at fairly low levels of hyperglycemia.

DURATION OF GLUCOSE INTOLERANCE

It is well documented that the microvascular complications of diabetes are closely related to the duration of diabetes.[36] In contrast, a relationship between the duration of diabetes or hyperglycemia and cardiovascular disease has not been demonstrated. Two studies have compared diabetic patients who were first diagnosed by a screening program with an age-matched group of known diabetics who had been diagnosed previously by other means. Because the former group were not known to be diabetic prior to the screening program, it is reasonable to assume that their duration of hyperglycemia would be shorter than that of the known diabetics. In both studies, after follow-up for 10 years (Erfurt [German Democratic Republic] Study)[33] and 5 years (Israeli Ischemic Heart Disease Survey),[13] the mortality and morbidity rates from cardiovascular disease were similar in both groups. In the Whitehall Study, age-adjusted coronary heart disease mortality rates in known diabetics with an average duration of nearly 10 years were not significantly different from those in the group with impaired glucose tolerance.[6] In the diabetic men, there was no significant relationship between duration of glucose intolerance and mortality from coronary heart disease.

THE EFFECTS OF OTHER RISK FACTORS

Diabetics not only have a higher risk for cardiovascular disease but also have a higher frequency of other cardiovascular risk factors. The following question therefore arises: Is hyperglycemia a truly independent risk factor for cardiovascular disease? Data on this question are conflicting. The Framingham Study found that associated risk factors could not explain the high incidence of cardiovascular disease in those known to have diabetes.[22] However, of all the major risk factors, diabetes had the smallest attributable risk of cardiovascular disease among men. On the other hand, among women, the attributable risk factor associated with diabetes was substantial; it exceeded the risk for cigarette smoking and was surpassed only by hypertension.

Several other studies have reported the predictive value of putative risk factors in diabetic subjects with specific reference to coronary heart disease. In the Whitehall Study, hyperglycemia was an independent risk factor for coronary heart disease,[6] and in the Honolulu Study, both the serum glucose level and the type of treatment for diabetes were significantly predictive of mortality from coronary heart disease.[5] Similarly, in the Puerto Rican Heart Health Program, abnormal glucose tolerance remained an independent risk factor for coronary heart disease in men after controlling for smoking, systolic blood pressure, cholesterol, and relative weight.[3] In contrast, in the Evans County (United States) Study, 4.5-year coronary heart disease mortality rates, when standardized for age, systolic blood pressure, serum cholesterol and triglyceride levels, body weight, and cigarette smoking, were not increased in diabetic men but were increased in diabetic women.[14] However, the total number of deaths was small, and any conclusion should be tentative. In the Bedford 10-year follow-up study, after adjusting for three putative risk factors, namely systolic blood pressure, obesity, and cigarette smoking, risk of cardiovascular mortality was still greater in diabetics and borderline diabetics than in normal individuals but was statistically significant only in female "borderline diabetics."[20] Small numbers may have prevented these risk ratios in the other groups from reaching statistical significance, but if so, it confirms that the increased risk of diabetes and hyperglycemia in men after adjustment for other risk factors is small, whereas in women, the risk is greater.

GLUCOSE INTOLERANCE: RISK FACTOR OR ASSOCIATION?

Jarret has questioned whether impaired glucose tolerance is a true risk factor for coronary heart disease.[18] Several factors would favor the concept that impaired glucose tolerance is not a risk factor but an association. First, there is the lack of association between the duration of glucose intolerance and the development of coronary heart disease.[13,33] Second, several studies have demonstrated that other cardiovascular risk factors are present before the onset of glucose intolerance. The Israeli Ischemic Heart Disease Study demonstrated that hypertension and peripheral vascular disease occurred more frequently in men with normal glucose tolerance at the time of the study who subsequently became diabetic.[28] In the DuPont Company Study, retrospective analysis of medical records also showed hypertension to be more common in people subsequently diagnosed as diabetic,[35] and in the Framingham Study, subjects with diabetes had higher lipid values and a higher frequency of hypertension before the diagnosis of diabetes.[7] Comparison of people with impaired glucose tolerance and age-matched control subjects has shown higher average blood pressure[19] and higher cholesterol levels.[32,50] Thus, Jarret has argued that a certain metabolic milieu may predispose to both coronary artery disease and impaired glucose tolerance. He suggests that arteriosclerosis and diabetes may share a number of antecedents and that the balance between them may determine the clinical outcome. Thus, one factor that may sway the balance in the direction of diabetes is obesity. The common antecedents, namely the association between levels of blood pressure, blood glucose, and plasma lipids, have been demonstrated in the young as well as in adults,[5,46,48] and for both serum cholesterol and blood pressure, there is an increase in level with increasing age.[7,8] Thus, the newly diagnosed middle-aged diabetic patient may have many years of exposure to factors that promote atherogenesis, and the final decompensation of blood glucose with resultant clinical diabetes may not add to the risk of coronary heart disease. Although this is an interesting concept, it does not explain the findings in the studies cited previously in which glucose intolerance was found to be an independent risk factor. Furthermore, the predominance in women is not explained.

PATHOGENESIS OF MACROVASCULAR DISEASE ASSOCIATED WITH DIABETES

As indicated previously, much of the increased risk of morbidity and mortality due to cardiovascular disease in diabetics may be ascribed to the increased prevalence of other putative risk factors in these patients. These risk factors include hypertension, abnormal lipid levels, including low high-density lipoprotein (HDL) cholesterol and high very-low-density lipoprotein (VLDL) levels, and obesity, which are discussed in other articles. There are, however, several unique factors that occur in diabetes that may contribute to the high prevalence of vascular disease in diabetics.

Hematologic Disturbances. According to one popular theory, injury to the endothelium may be the primary lesion in the development of atherosclerosis.[40] Depending on host responses, this may be reversed or may be followed by platelet deposition at the site of injury. Platelets aggregate and release vasoconstrictor and proaggregatory arachidonic acid metabolites, as well as platelet-derived growth factors. These, in turn, may stimulate smooth muscle cell proliferation, and circulating lipoproteins deliver cholesterol to the site of the injury. This process may progress to the complete atherosclerotic lesion and arterial thrombotic occlusion. Several lines of evidence indicate a state of hypercoagulability and abnormal endothelial function as well as enhanced platelet aggregability in diabetics that could theoretically enhance this process.

Endothelial Function in Diabetes Mellitus. Several factors produced by the endothelium have been studied and found to be abnormal in diabetes. The glycoprotein Von Willebrand factor, which is present in plasma as part of the Factor VIII complex, is increased in diabetes.[17] Prostacyclin, which is a potent vasodilator and antagonist of platelet aggregation and adherence of platelets to the vessel wall, is produced at lower levels in diabetics, and plasminogen activator, an enzyme in the fibrinolytic system, is also reduced in diabetes.[2] These abnormalities may indicate that the endothelium, the site of the primary lesion in atherosclerosis, is abnormal in diabetes. Furthermore, these abnormalities may relate to the increased tendency toward arterial thrombosis seen in many diabetic patients.

Platelet Function in Diabetes Mellitus. Altered platelet function in vitro has been observed in many studies involving both human subjects with diabetes and diabetic animals. Platelet adhesiveness has been found to be increased in diabetes, and platelets from diabetic subjects have an increased sensitivity to aggregating agents such as ADP, adrenalin, collagen, arachidonic acid, and thrombin.[2] Plasma concentrations of platelet factor 4 and beta-thromboglobulin, which are released by aggregating platelets, are increased in diabetes and may indicate increased in vivo aggregation.[38] Furthermore, studies have demonstrated that some diabetic patients have decreased platelet survival, again possibly indicating in vivo aggregation. Platelet aggregation may release factors that enhance endothelial permeability and mitogens that stimulate smooth muscle cell proliferation.

Effect of Insulin. Considerable controversy exists regarding the role of insulin, and evidence for both a protecting and a promoting influence of insulin on the development of atherosclerosis has been presented in experimental situations. In superphysiologic doses, insulin has been shown to stimulate arterial smooth muscle cell proliferation, to enhance the synthesis of cholesterol and other lipids, and to inhibit lipolysis in the arterial wall. In a study from Finland in nondiabetic men, hyperinsulinemia was incriminated as a risk factor of coronary disease.[37] Peripheral hyperinsulinemia is common both in type I diabetes, as a result of insulin treatment, and in type II diabetes, as a result of insulin resistance. However, whether hyperinsulinemia is a factor in the accelerated atherosclerosis of diabetes is not known. Further elucidation is also required on the effects of other growth factors that may be mitogenic for vascular endothelium and may be abnormal in diabetes.

IMPLICATIONS FOR TREATMENT

We have discussed evidence that impaired glucose tolerance may be a risk factor for the development of cardiovascular disease. In men, there is evidence that it is a fairly weak independent risk factor, whereas in women, the risk is greater. The risk appears to occur at low levels of glucose intolerance and, unlike microvascular disease, does not appear to relate to a threshold level of significant glycemia. The implications for treatment are therefore unclear. If the risk factor is hyperglycemia, what levels of blood sugar should we aim for? How can this best be achieved? Possibly the degree of normalization of hyperglycemia that may prevent or retard retinopathy and nephropathy will be ineffective for cardiovascular disease. If hyperinsulinism is a risk factor for atherosclerosis, should oral hypoglycemic agents that stimulate insulin secretion be used? At this time, answers to these questions are unclear, and the approach with the most common sense to prevent cardiovascular disease would be the early detection and treatment of other risk factors and the prevention of obesity.

REFERENCES

1. Barrett-Connor, E., and Wingard, D.: Sex differential in ischemic heart disease in diabetes: A prospective population-based study. *In* Alberti, K.G.M.M., Ogada, T., Aluoch, J.A., et al. (eds.): Abstracts of the 11th Congress of the International Diabetes Federation (1982), Excerpta Medica International Congress Series 577, Amsterdam, Excerpta Medica, 1982, p. 65.
2. Colwell, J.A., Winocour, P.D., Lopes-Virella, M., et al.: New concepts about the pathogenesis of atherosclerosis in diabetes mellitus. Am. J. Med., 75(Suppl. 5b):67–80, 1983.
3. Cruz-Vidal, M., Garcia-Palmieri, M.R., Costas, R., et al.: Abnormal blood glucose and coronary heart disease: The Puerto Rico Heart Health Program. Diabetes Care, 6:556–561, 1983.
4. Entmacher, P.S., Root, H.F., and Marks, H.H.: Longevity of diabetic patients in recent years. Diabetes, 13:373–382, 1964.
5. Florey, C.duV., Uppal, S., and Lowy, C.: Relation between blood pressure, weight and plasma sugar and serum insulin levels in school children aged 9–12 years in Westland, Holland. Br. Med., J., 1:1368–1371, 1976.
6. Fuller, J.H., Shipley, M.J., Rose, G., et al.: Coronary heart disease risk and impaired glucose tolerance: The Whitehall Study. Lancet, 1:1373–1376, 1980.
7. Garcia, M.J., McNamara, P.M., Gordon, T., et al.: Morbidity and mortality in diabetes in the Framingham Study: Sixteen year follow-up. Diabetes, 23:105–111, 1974.
8. Gillum, R.F., Taylor, H.L., Brozek, J., et al.: Blood lipids in young men followed 32 years. J. Chronic Dis., 35:635–641, 1982.
9. Gillum, R.F., Taylor, H.L., Brozek, J., et al.: Indices of obesity and blood pressure in young men followed 32 years. J. Chronic Dis., 35:211–219, 1982.
10. Gordon, T., Castelli, W.P., Hjortland, M.C., et al.: Diabetes, blood lipids and the role of obesity in coronary heart disease risk for women: The Framingham Study. Ann. Intern. Med., 87:393–397, 1977.
11. Goto, Y., Sako, S.I., and Masuda, M.: Causes of death in 3151 diabetic autopsy cases. Tohoku J. Exp. Med., 112:339–353, 1974.
12. Harrower, A.D.B., and Clarke, B.F.: Experience of coronary care in diabetes. Br. Med. J., 1:126–128, 1976.
13. Herman, J.B., Medalie, J.H., and Goldbourt, U.: Differences in cardiovascular morbidity and mortality between previously known and newly diagnosed adult diabetics. Diabetologia, 13:229–234, 1977.

14. Heyden, S., Heiss, G., Bartel, A.G., et al.: Sex differences in coronary mortality among diabetics in Evans County, Georgia. J. Chronic Dis., *33*:265–273, 1980.

15. Ingelfinger, J.A., Bennet, P.H., Liebow, I.M., et al.: Coronary artery disease in the Pima Indians: Electrocardiographic findings and post-mortem evidence of myocardial infarction in a population with a high prevalence of diabetes mellitus. Diabetes, *25*:561–565, 1976.

16. Ishihara, M., Yukimura, Y., Yamada, T., et al.: Diabetic complications and their relationships to risk factors in a Japanese population. Diabetes Care, *7*:533–538, 1984.

17. Jaffe, E.A.: Endothelial cells and the biology of factor VIII. N. Engl. J. Med., *296*:377–383, 1977.

18. Jarret, R.J.: Type II (non-insulin dependent) diabetes mellitus and coronary heart disease—chicken, egg or neither. Diabetologia, *26*:99–102, 1984.

19. Jarret, R.J., Keen, H., McCartney, M., et al.: Glucose tolerance and blood pressure in two population samples: Their relation to diabetes mellitus and hypertension. Int. J. Epidemiol., *7*:15–24, 1978.

20. Jarret, R.J., McCartney, P., and Keen, H.: The Bedford Survey: Ten year mortality rates in newly diagnosed diabetics, borderline diabetics and normoglycemic controls and risk indices for coronary heart disease in borderline diabetics. Diabetologia, *22*:79–84, 1982.

21. Kannel, W.B., and McGee, D.L.: Diabetes and cardiovascular disease. The Framingham Study. J.A.M.A., *241*:2035–2038, 1979.

22. Kannel, W.B., and McGee, D.L.: Diabetes and cardiovascular risk factors: The Framingham Study. Circulation, *59*:8–13, 1979.

23. Kannel, W.B., and McGee, D.L.: Diabetes and glucose tolerance as risk factors for cardiovascular disease: The Framingham Study. Diabetes Care, *2*:120–126, 1979.

24. Keen, H., and Jarret, R.J.: the WHO multi-national study of vascular disease in diabetes: 2. Macrovascular disease prevalence. Diabetes Care, *2*:187–195, 1979.

25. Keen, H., and Jarret, R.J.: The WHO multi-national study of vascular disease in diabetes: 3. Microvascular disease. Diabetes Care, *2*:196–201, 1979.

26. Keen, H., Rose, G., Pyke, D.A., et al.: Blood sugar and arterial disease. Lancet, *2*:505–508, 1965.

27. Krolewski, A.S., Czyzyk, A., Janeczko, D., et al.: Mortality from cardiovascular diseases among diabetics. Diabetologia, *13*:345–350, 1977.

28. Medalie, J.H., Papier, C.M., and Goldbourt, U.: Major factors in the development of diabetes mellitus in 10,000 men. Arch. Intern. Med., *135*:811–817, 1975.

29. National Diabetes Data Group: Classification and diagnosis of diabetes mellitus and other categories of glucose intolerance. Diabetes, *28*:1039–1057, 1979.

30. Ochi, J.W., Melton, L.J., Palumbo, P.J., et al.: A population-based study of diabetes mortality. Diabetes Care, *8*:224–229, 1985.

31. Ostrander, L.D., Francis, T., Hayner, N.S., et al.: The relationship of cardiovascular disease to hyperglycemia. Ann. Intern. Med., *62*:1188–1198, 1965.

32. Ostrander, L.D., Lamphiear, D.E., Black, W.E., et al.: Physiological variables and diabetic status: Findings in Tecumseh, Michigan. Arch. Intern. Med., *140*:1215–1219, 1980.

33. Panzram, G., and Ruttman, B.: Prognose des diabetes mellitus nach fruhdiagnose durch glucosurie-screening. Schweiz. Med. Wochenschr., *108*:221–225, 1978.

34. Panzram, G., and Zabel-Langhennig. R.: Prognosis of diabetes mellitus in a geographically defined population. Diabetologia, *20*:587–591, 1981.

35. Pell, S., and D'Alonzo, C.A.: Some aspects of hypertension in diabetes mellitus. J.A.M.A., *202*:104–110, 1967.

36. Pirart, J.: Diabetes mellitus and its degenerative complications: A prospective study of 4400 patients observed between 1947 and 1973. Diabetes Care, *1*:168–198, 252–263, 1978.

37. Pyorala, K.: Relationship of glucose tolerance and plasma insulin to the incidence of coronary heart disease: Results from two population studies in Finland. Diabetes Care, *2*:131–141, 1979.

38. Rak, K., Beck, P., Udvardy, M., et al.: Plasma levels of beta thromboglobulin and factor VIII–related antigen in diabetic children and adults. Throm. Res., *29*:155–162, 1983.

39. Robertson, W.B., and Strong, J.P.: Atherosclerosis in persons with hypertension and diabetes mellitus. Lab. Invest., *18*:538–551, 1968.

40. Ross, R., and Glomsett, J.A.: The pathogenesis of atherosclerosis. N. Engl. J. Med., *295*:369–377, 420–425, 1976.

41. Rytter, L., Troelsen, S., and Beck-Nielsen, H.: Prevalence and mortality of acute myocardial infarction in patients with diabetes. Diabetes Care, *8*:230–234, 1985.

42. Sartor, G., Schersten, B., Carlstrom, S., et al.: Ten year follow up of subjects with impaired glucose tolerance. Prevention of diabetes by tolbutamide and diet regulation. Diabetes, *29*:41–49, 1980.

43. Seftel, H.C., Joffe, B.I., and Goldberg, R.B.: Vascular disease in diabetes in Africans. *In* Keen, H., Pickup, J.C., and Talwalker, C.V. (eds.): Epidemiology of Diabetes and Its Vascular Complications. London, International Diabetes Federation, 1978, p. 77.

44. Shenfield, G.M., Elton, R.A., Bhalla, I.P., et al.: Diabetic mortality in Edinburgh. Diabete Metab., *5*:149–158, 1979.

45. Soler, N.G., Pentecost, B.L., Bennet, M.A., et al.: Coronary care for myocardial infarction in diabetes. Lancet, *1*:475–478, 1974.

46. Tzagournis, M., Chiles, R., Ryan, J.M., et al.: Interrelationships of hyperinsulinism and hypertriglyceridemia in young patients with coronary heart disease. Circulation, *38*:1156–1163, 1968.

47. Uusitupa, M., Siitonen, O., Aro, A., et al.: Prevalence of coronary heart disease, left ventricular failure and hypertension in middle-aged newly diagnosed type II (non-insulin-dependent) diabetic subjects. Diabetologia, *28*:22–27, 1985.

48. Voors, A.W., Radhakrishnamurphy, B., and Srinavasan, S.E.: Plasma glucose level related to blood pressure in 272 children ages 7–15 years sampled from a total biracial population. Am. J. Epidemiol., *113*:347–356, 1981.

49. Walden, C.E., Knopp, R.H., Wahl, P.W., et al.: Sex differences in the effect of diabetes mellitus on lipoprotein triglyceride and cholesterol concentrations. N. Engl. J. Med., *311*:953–959, 1984.

50. Yano, K., Kagan, A., McGee, D., et al.: Glucose intolerance and nine year mortality in Japanese men in Hawaii. Am. J. Med., *72*:71–80, 1982.

51. Zimmet, P.: Epidemiology of diabetes and its macrovascular manifestations in Pacific populations: The medical effects of social progress. Diabetes Care, *2*:144–153, 1979.

Diabetes Research Center, Quarters 8/9
Pacific Medical Center
1200 12th Avenue South
Seattle, Washington 98144

Risks for Obesity

Celso Amodeo, M.D.,* and Franz H. Messerli, M.D.†

A number of factors associated with increased probability for developing cardiovascular and cerebrovascular disease have been identified. Thus, a survey by Hopkins and Williams in 1981[23] revealed no less than 246 coronary risk factors. Among these, high blood pressure,[3,26,29] hyperlipidemia,[14,32,57] glucose intolerance,[18,30,65,70] left ventricular hypertrophy,[28,33,44] and obesity[25,43,62] were considered major risk factors.

The concept of obesity per se as an independent risk factor is controversial.[67] However, the association of obesity with other important risk factors has been demonstrated extensively.[20,25,55,58] The purpose of this article is to discuss the influence of obesity on some of the major risk factors for cardiovascular disease.

OBESITY AND GLUCOSE INTOLERANCE

The most profound metabolic alteration in obesity is peripheral resistance to the action of insulin on glucose utilization, which seems to be a direct function of increased fat cell size.[7] Studies show evidence of impaired insulin action on adiposity, most likely resulting from decreased numbers of insulin receptors.[13,16]

As a result of peripheral resistance to insulin action, the beta cells of the pancreas are stimulated to produce insulin. High blood levels of insulin may be observed in obesity.[7] Bar and associates[4] observed that circulating levels of insulin affect the receptors on cell surfaces. In addition, muscle metabolism probably has an

important role in obesity insulin resistance, as Bjortorp and colleagues[9] reported that physical training decreases hyperinsulinemia in obesity without changing adipose cellularity. Thus, increased peripheral resistance to insulin associated with an exhaustion of the beta cells of the pancreatic islets, in those subjects who are genetically susceptible, impairs glucose utilization, leading to glucose intolerance. Therefore, the appearance of diabetes mellitus may be related to the degree and duration of obesity.[71]

OBESITY AND HYPERLIPIDEMIA

Hyperlipidemia is a disturbance of lipid transport that results from abnormalities in the synthesis or metabolization of plasma lipoproteins.[11] Some hyperlipidemias result from primary defects in lipoprotein metabolism, whereas others may be a result of metabolic system disorders, such as thyroid hormone deficiency or insulin deficiency.

Hypertriglyceridemia and hypercholesterolemia are important risk factors for atherosclerosis and, consequently, for cerebrovascular and cardiovascular disease.[14,57,72] Obesity may increase triglyceride levels partly as a result of associated hyperinsulinism.[7] There is evidence that triglyceride levels are positively related to weight gain[2] and to circulating insulin levels in adults.[8] In general, hyperinsulinemia and hypertriglyceridemia are reversible with weight reduction.[48]

Association between obesity and hypercholesterolemia is not as evident as that between

---

*Section on Hypertensive Diseases, Department of Internal Medicine, Ochsner Clinic and Alton Ochsner Medical Foundation, New Orleans, Louisiana

†Section on Hypertensive Diseases, Department of Internal Medicine, Ochsner Clinic and Alton Ochsner Medical Foundation, New Orleans, Louisiana

obesity and hypertriglyceridemia, but a relationship does exist.[47] This connection may be related to the increased propensity of obese subjects to develop gallstones.

OBESITY AND HYPERESTROGENEMIA

Common hormonal abnormalities observed in obesity are an increase in estrogen levels, a decrease in serum testosterone (but with a normal level of free testosterone), and an increase in the estrogen-to-testosterone ratio.[36,61]

Epidemiologic studies[34,59] show that women have reduced incidence of coronary heart disease when compared with men at similar age. This difference tends to disappear in women after menopause. The fact that women lose protection against cardiovascular disease after menopause led to the idea that the sexual difference in incidence of cardiovascular disease was related to estrogen levels. Indeed, reduction of coronary attack rates was observed in women receiving estrogen therapy.[12] However, other hormones also differ in plasma concentration before and after menopause. In premenopausal women, there is a high plasma concentration of progesterone that is significantly reduced after menopause. Progesterone has also been shown to have antiestrogen effects.[24] Thus, postmenopausal women might be more vulnerable to cardiovascular disease not because of a loss of estrogen protection but, in fact, because of a decrease in plasma levels of progesterone.

Increasing evidence supporting the concept of hyperestrogenemia as a risk factor for cardiovascular disease has been published.[22,52] High estrogen levels and an increased estradiol-to-testosterone ratio are associated with hypercholesterolemia,[41,60] hypertension,[51] and diabetes.[53] Other studies show that administration of estrogen may lead to myocardial infarction[66] and may increase other risk factors.[49] Studying young men after myocardial infarction, Phillips observed increased mean serum concentrations of estradiol and estrone.[54] He also observed that the ratio of serum concentrations of estradiol to testosterone was closely related to abnormal glucose tolerance and lipid metabolism.

How estrogen works in this context remains speculative, and the higher incidence of thrombophlebitis and pulmonary embolism in the estrogen-treated group observed in The Coronary Drug Project[66] suggests that an alteration of the clotting mechanism may be involved.

OBESITY AND HYPERTENSION

Epidemiologic studies of blood pressure in populations have shown significant correlation between blood pressure and body mass and between hypertension and obesity.[15,20,64] Weight gain during adult life is an important risk factor for the development of hypertension.[31] In the Framingham Study the risk of developing hypertension was proportional to weight gain. Patients who weighed 20 per cent more than their ideal weight had an eight times greater risk for hypertension than patients who weighed 10 per cent less than their ideal weight. The exact mechanism through which obesity predisposes a person to increased risk for hypertension remains unclear, although it has been suggested that obese subjects have a higher intake of calories and salt.[17] However, the association between obesity and hypertension is observed even in groups in which habitual sodium intake is low.[50] Reisin and colleagues observed that weight loss without restriction of sodium intake was associated with a drop in blood pressure.[56,56a] Even in patients who maintained a "normal" salt intake, a hypocaloric diet produced a fall in arterial pressure that was similar to the pressure of subjects on a low-salt diet.[42a]

Another possible explanation could be hormonal status. As discussed previously, obesity is related to glucose insulin defects, hyperestrogenemia, and an increased estrogen-to-testosterone ratio. Hypertension has been precipitated in women by the administration of estrogen[19] and is associated with glucose intolerance.[53] Therefore, hyperestrogenism and insulin resistance could have the same role in the increased risk for hypertension observed in obese patients. Studies are needed to determine how estrogen produces high blood pressure, but unquestionably, more than one system plays a role in the development of hypertension by estrogen. Studies have shown that renin substrate is increased during pregnancy and during estrogenic therapy.[39] The excess in substrate to renin increases the rate of generation of angiotensin II, a potent vasoconstrictor. In addition, estrogen probably has a mineralocorticoid effect by direct action on renal tubular cells, therefore causing sodium retention.[27] Hence, obesity may increase the risk for hypertension, at least to some extent, through hormonal modification.

Although a strong correlation has been demonstrated between obesity and hypertension, the hypothesis that obesity increases the risk for cardiovascular disease in hypertensive patients remains controversial. Some studies show that obese hypertensive patients are at greater risk for cardiovascular disease and have higher mortality rates than nonobese hypertensive patients.[15,42] However, for many years, this concept has been refuted. In 1946, Bechgaard[6] reported results showing that in a 25-year follow-up of 1000 hypertensive patients, those who weighed 20 kg more than their ideal weight did not have worse prognoses in terms of cardiovascular mortality rates. Sokolow and Perloff observed that hypertensive patients who were obese had better prognoses than nonobese hypertensive patients.[63] Similarly, Barrett-Connor and Khaw recently published a 9-year follow-up of 1727 men 50 to 79 years of age that suggested that in the presence of hypertension, obesity does not increase the risk for cardiovascular disease and appears to be protective.[5]

DIFFERENT TYPES OF OBESITY

Based on clinical observations, two well-defined types of obesity are described.[7] One is called lifelong obesity and is characterized by a typical history of obesity since early childhood with some important gain in weight during puberty and often, in women, a history of constant increase in weight with each successive pregnancy. These patients have difficulty losing weight and, in general, after successful weight reduction, tend to return to pretreatment levels of weight. In this pattern of obesity, hyperplasia of fat cells appears to be more pronounced than a cellular hypertrophy.

The other clinical type is adult-onset obesity, which is characterized by weight gain beginning in adulthood. This is frequently associated with environmental factors and a sedentary lifestyle. In this clinical type, in contrast to lifelong obesity, there is predominant adipose cell hypertrophy with only minimal increase in cell number, but fat cell hyperplasia may become evident when accentuated levels of overweight are achieved.

Whether or not these two clinical types of obesity have similar effects on the major risk factor for cardiovascular disease remains unclear. There are studies suggesting that adult-onset obesity (hypertrophic obesity) seems to be more closely associated with hypertension in the various metabolic complications than does lifelong obesity (hyperplastic obesity).[10,31]

Disparate sexual distribution of the adipose tissue also seems to influence cardiovascular risk. Men have adipose cell deposits predominantly in the abdominal region (male-pattern obesity or upper-body obesity), whereas women's body fat cell deposits are prevalent on the buttocks and legs (female-pattern obesity or lower-body obesity).[37] A study from Vague[69] showed a difference between the prevalence of cardiovascular risk factors in subjects with male-pattern obesity and those with female-pattern obesity. Krotkiewski and associates[37] reported that men and women with male-pattern obesity exhibited more profound disturbances of lipid and carbohydrate metabolism. Furthermore, Larsson and colleagues reported a prospective study indicating that abdominal adipose tissue distribution associated with serum cholesterol concentration and blood pressure may be used as a predictor of cardiovascular disease.[40]

An attractive pathophysiologic mechanism for the association between abdominal obesity and cardiovascular risk factor is the interesting manipulation of free fatty acid by the abdominal adipose cells. Intra-abdominal adipocytes empty their free fatty acids directly into the portal vein, exposing the liver to high concentrations of free fatty acids.[40] The concentration of free fatty acid might decrease the liver uptake of insulin, which is more likely to result in an increased plasma level of this hormone. As pointed out previously, hyperinsulinemia may affect the receptors on cell surfaces and produce glucose intolerance.[13,16] In addition, a high portal concentration of free fatty acid causes increased triglyceride plasma levels. This mechanism, however, is not observed with the gluteal and femoral adipocytes, which appear to be more sensitive to corticosteroids and estrogen.[38]

OBESITY AND LEFT VENTRICULAR HYPERTROPHY

Left ventricular hypertrophy has been demonstrated to be an important risk factor for cardiovascular disease.[28,33,44] The prevalence of left ventricular hypertrophy in obese patients is higher than that observed in lean subjects.[45] A recent study by Messerli and coworkers[45] suggests a possible pathophysiologic mechanism through which obesity increases the risk for left ventricular hypertrophy. In this comparison with lean subjects, obese patients had high cardiac output, stroke volume, plasma volume, and left ventricular mass measured by M-mode echocardiography, despite similar blood pressure levels. The elevated cardiac output was produced mainly by a high stroke volume, because heart rate remained unchanged. High stroke volume associated with expanded total blood volume leads to an increase in the preload to the left ventricle, which reacts with dilatation. As a result, an increase in ventricular wall tension (stress) is observed. The left ventricle adapts to this state by increasing muscle mass. Therefore, left ventricular adaptation to obesity consists of eccentric hypertrophy, regardless of arterial pressure. Moreover, eccentric left ventricular hypertrophy as a consequence of longstanding obesity is a major risk factor for sudden death and other types of cardiovascular morbidity and mortality.[42b] Holter monitoring documents that obese patients with eccentric left ventricular hypertrophy seem to have increased ectopy when compared with those without left ventricular hypertrophy.[42b–42d]

REFERENCES

1. Abraham, G.E., Hopper, K., Tulchinsky, D., et al.: Simultaneous measurement of plasma progesterone, 17-hydroxyprogesterone and estradiol-17 B by radioimmunoassay. Anal. Letters, 4:325, 1971.
2. Albrink, M.J., et al.: Weight gain and serum triglycerides in normal men. N. Engl. J. Med., 266:484, 1962.
3. American Heart Association, Steering Committee of Medical and Community Program: Risk factors and coronary disease: A statement for physicians. Circulation, 62:445A, 1980.
4. Bar, R.S., et al.: Fluctuations in the affinity and concentration of insulin receptors on circulating monocytes of obese patients. J. Clin. Invest., 58:1123, 1976.
5. Barrett-Connor, E., and Khaw, K.T.: Is hypertension more benign when associated with obesity? Circulation, 72:53–60, 1985.
6. Bechgaard, P.: Arterial hypertension; a followup study of one thousand hypertonics. Acta Med. Scand., 172(Suppl.):3, 1946.
7. Bierman, E.L., and Hirsch, J.: Obesity. *In* Williams, R.H. (ed.): Textbook of Endocrinology. Edition 6. Philadelphia, W.B. Saunders Company, 1981, pp. 907–921.
8. Bierman, E.L., et al.: Hypertriglyceridemia and glucose intolerance in man. *In* Jeaurrnaud, B., and Hepp, D. (eds.): Adipose Tissue, Regulation and Metabolic Functions. New York, Academic Press, 1970.
9. Bjorntorp, P., et al.: Physical training in human hyperplastic obesity. IV. Effects on the hormonal status. Metabolism, 26:319, 1977.
10. Bray, G.A.: Obesity: Definition, diagnosis and disadvantages. Med. J. Aust., 142:52–58, 1985.
11. Brown, M.S., and Goldstein, J.L.: The hyperlipoproteinemias and other disorders of lipid metabolism. *In* Petersdorf, R.G., et al. (eds.): Principles of Internal Medicine. Edition 10. New York, McGraw-Hill, 1983, pp. 547–559.
12. Bush, T.L., Cowan, L.D., Barrett-Connor, E., et al.: Estrogen use and all cause mortality. Preliminary results from the Lipid Research Clinics Program Follow-up Study. J.A.M.A., 249:903, 1983.
13. Butterfield, W.J.H., et al.: Peripheral metabolism of glucose and free fatty acids during oral glucose tolerance tests. Metabolism, 14:851, 1965.
14. Castelli, W.P., Doyle, J.T., Gordon, T., et al.: HDL cholesterol and other lipids in coronary heart disease. The Cooperative Lipoprotein Phenotyping Study. Circulation, 55:767, 1977.
15. Chiang, B.N., Rerlman, L.V., and Epstein, F.H.: Overweight and hypertension. Circulation, 39:403, 1969.
16. Czech, M.P., et al.: Biochemical basis of fat cell and insulin resistance in obese rodents and man. Metabolism, 26:1057, 1977.
17. Dahl, L.K., Silver, L., and Christie, R.W.: The role of salt in the fall of blood pressure accompanying obesity. N. Engl. J. Med., 258:1186–1194, 1958.
18. Epstein, F.H.: Hyperglycemia. A risk factor in coronary disease. Circulation, 36:606, 1967.
19. Fisch, I.R., Freedman, S.H., and Myatt, A.V.: Oral contraceptives, pregnancy and blood pressure. J.A.M.A., 222:1507–1510, 1972.
20. Gordon, T., and Kannel, W.B.: Obesity and cardiovascular disease: The Framingham Study. Clin. Endocrinol. Metab., 5:367, 1976.
21. Gordon, T., Garcia-Palmieri, M.R., Kagan, A., et al.: Differences in coronary heart disease in Framingham, Honolulu and Puerto Rico. J. Chronic Dis., 27:329, 1974.
22. Gordon, T., Kannel, W.B., Hjortland, M.C., et al.: Menopause and coronary heart disease. The Framingham Study. Ann. Intern. Med., 89:157, 1978.
23. Hopkins, P.N., and Williams, R.R.: A survey of 246 suggested coronary risk factors. Atherosclerosis, 40:1–52, 1981.
24. Hsueh, A.J.W., Peck, E.J., Jr., and Clark, J.H.: Control of estrogen receptor levels by progesterone. Endocrinology, 98:438, 1976.
25. Hubert, H.G., Feinleib, M., McNamara, P.M., et al.: Obesity as an independent risk factor for cardiovascular disease: A 26-year follow-up of participants in the Framingham Heart Study. Circulation, 67:968, 1983.
26. Hypertension Detection and Follow-up Program Cooperative Group: The hypertension detection and follow-up program: A progress report. Circ. Res., 40(Suppl. I):I–106, 1977.
27. Johnson, J.A., Davis, J.O., Brown, P.R., et al.: Effects of estradiol on sodium and potassium in adrenalectomized dogs. Am. J. Physiol., 223:194–197, 1972.
28. Kannel, W.B.: Some lesions in cardiovascular epidemiology from Framingham. Am. J. Cardiol., 37:269–282, 1976.
29. Kannel, W.B.: Role of blood pressure in cardiovascular disease: The Framingham Study. Angiology, 26:1, 1975.
30. Kannel, W.B., and McGee, D.L.: Diabetes and glucose tolerance as risk factors for cardiovascular disease: The Framingham Study. Diabetes Care, 2:120, 1979.
31. Kannel, W.B., Brand, N., Skinner, J.J., et al.: The relation of adiposity to blood pressure and development of hypertension. Ann. Intern. Med., 67:48–59, 1967.
32. Kannel, W.B., Castelli, W.P., and Gordon, T.: Cholesterol in the prediction of atherosclerotic disease. New perspectives based on the Framingham Study. Ann. Intern. Med., 90:85, 1979.
33. Kannel, W.B., Gordon, T., Castelli, W.P., et al.: Electrocardiographic left ventricular hypertrophy and risk of coronary heart disease. Ann. Intern. Med., 72:813–822, 1970.
34. Kannel, W.B., Hjortland, M.C., McNamara, P.M., et

al.: Menopause and risk of cardiovascular disease: The Framingham Study. Ann. Intern. Med., 85:447, 1976.

35. Keys, A.: A Multivariate Analysis of Seven Countries: Death and Coronary Heart Disease. Cambridge, Massachusetts, Harvard University Press, 1980.

36. Kley, H.K., Edelmann, P., and Kruskemper, H.L.: Relationship of plasma sex hormones to different parameters of obesity in male subjects. Metabolism, 29:1041–1045, 1980.

37. Krotkiewski, M., Bjorntorp, P., Sjostrom, L., et al.: Impact of obesity on metabolism in men and women: Importance of regional adipose tissue distribution. J. Clin. Invest., 72:1150–1162, 1983.

38. Krotkiewski, M., Sjostrom, L., Bjorntorp, P., et al.: Regional adipose tissue cellularity in relation to metabolism in young and middle-aged women. Metab. Clin. Exp., 24:703–710, 1975.

39. Laragh, J.H., Sealy, J.E., Ledingham, J.J.G., et al.: Oral contraceptives: Renin, aldosterone, and high blood pressure. J.A.M.A., 201:918–922, 1967.

40. Larsson, B., Svardsudd, K., Wellin, L., et al.: Abdominal adipose tissue distribution, obesity and risk of cardiovascular disease and death: 13-year follow-up of participants in the study of men born in 1913. Br. Med. J., 288:1401–1404, 1984.

41. Laskarzewski, P.M., Morrison, J.A., Gutai, J., et al.: High and low density lipoprotein cholesterols in adolescent boys: Relationships with endogenous testosterone, estradiol and Quetelet index. Metabolism, 32:262–271, 1983.

42. Lew, E.A.: Blood pressure and mortality-life insurance experience. *In* Stamler, J., Stamler, R., and Pullman, T.N. (eds.): The Epidemiology of Hypertension. New York, Grune and Stratton, 1976, p. 392.

42a. Maxwell, M.H., Kushiro, T., Dornfield, L.P., et al.: Blood pressure changes in obese hypertensive subjects during rapid weight loss: Comparison of restricted vs. unchanged salt intake. Arch. Intern. Med., 144:1581–1584, 1984.

42b. Messerli, F.H., Venturo, H.O., Elizardi, D.J., et al.: Hypertension and sudden death: Increased ventricular ectopic activity in left ventricular hypertrophy. Am. J. Med., 77:18–22, 1984.

42c. Messerli, F.H., Venturo, H.O., and Synder, D.W.: Eccentric left ventricular hypertrophy—a determinant of increased ventricular ectopy in obesity. (Abstract.) J. Am. Coll. Cardiol., in press.

42d. Messerli, F.H.: Cardiomyopathy of obesity—a not-so-Victorian disease. N. Engl. J. Med., in press.

43. Messerli, F.H.: Cardiovascular effects of obesity and hypertension. Lancet, 1:1165–1168, 1982.

44. Messerli, F.H.: Clinical determinants and consequences of left ventricular hypertrophy. Am. J. Med., 75:51–57, 1983.

45. Messerli, F.H., Sundgaard-Riise, K., Reisin, E., et al.: Dimorphic cardiac adaptation to obesity and arterial hypertension. Ann. Intern. Med., 99:757–761, 1983.

46. Miller, N.E.: The evidence for the antiatherogenicity of HDL in man. (Symposium on HDL structure, functions analysis, clinical, epidemiological and metabolic aspects of HDL.) Lipids, 13:914–919, 1978.

47. Montoye, H.J., Epstein, F.H., and Kjelsberg, M.O.: Relationship between serum cholesterol and body fatness. An epidemiologic study. Am. J. Clin. Nutr., 18:397, 1966.

48. Olefsky, J., et al.: Effects of weight reduction on obesity: Studies of lipid and carbohydrate metabolism in normal and hyperlipoproteinemic subjects. J. Clin. Invest., 53:64, 1974.

49. Ostrander, L.D., Lamphiear, D.E., Block, W.D., et al.: Oral contraceptives and physiological variables. J.A.M.A., 244:677–679, 1980.

50. Page, L.B., Damon, A., and Moellering, R.C., Jr.: Antecedents of cardiovascular disease in six Solomon Islands societies. Circulation, 49:1132–1147, 1974.

51. Phillips, G.B.: Hyperestrogenemia, diet and disorders of Western Societies. Am. J. Med., 78:363–366, 1985.

52. Phillips, G.B.: Sex hormones, risk factors and cardiovascular disease. Am. J. Med., 65:7–11, 1978.

53. Phillips, G.B.: Evidence for hyperestrogenemia as the link between diabetes mellitus and myocardial infarction. Am. J. Med., 76:1041–1048, 1984.

54. Phillips, G.B.: Evidence for hyperestrogenemia as a risk factor for myocardial infarction in men. Lancet, 2:14–18, 1976.

55. Pooling Project Research Group: Relationship of blood pressure, relative weight and ECG abnormalities to incidence of major coronary events: Final report. J. Chronic Dis., 31:201–306, 1978.

56. Reisin, E., Abel, R., Modan, M., et al.: Effect of weight loss without salt restriction on the reduction of blood pressure in overweight patients. N. Engl. J. Med., 298:1–6, 1978.

56a. Reisin, E., Frohlich, E.D., Messerli, F.H., et al.: Cardiovascular changes after weight reduction in obesity hypertension. Ann. Intern. Med., 98:315–319, 1983.

57. Rhoads, G.G., Gulbrandsen, C.L., and Kagan, A.: Serum lipoproteins and coronary heart disease in a population study of Hawaii-Japanese men. N. Engl. J. Med., 294:293, 1976.

58. Rimm, A.A., and White, P.L.: Obesity: Its risks and hazards. *In* Bray, G.A. (ed.): Obesity in America. Washington, D.C., U.S. Department Health, Education and Welfare, NIH Publication No. 79-359, 1979.

59. Robinson, R.W., Higano, N., and Cohen, W.D.: Increased incidence of coronary heart disease in women castrated prior to the menopause. Arch. Intern. Med., 104:908, 1959.

60. Rosenthal, M.B., Barnard, J., Rose, D.P., et al.: Effects of high complex carbohydrate, low fat, low cholesterol diet on levels of serum lipids and estradiol., Am. J. Med., 78:23–27, 1985.

61. Schneider, G., Kirschner, M.A., Berkowitz, R., et al.: Increased estrogen production in obese man. J. Clin. Endocrinol. Metab., 48:633–638, 1979.

62. Society of Actuaries and Association of Life Insurance Medical Directors: Build Study 1979. Chicago, Recording and Statistical Corporation, 1980.

63. Sokolow, M., and Perloff, D.: The prognosis of essential hypertension treated conservatively. Circulation, 23:697, 1961.

64. Stamler, R., Stamler, J., Riedlinger, W.F., et al.: Weight and blood pressure: Findings in hypertension screening of 1 million Americans. J.A.M.A., 240:1607, 1978.

65. Stout, R.W.: Blood glucose and atherosclerosis. Atherosclerosis, 1:227, 1981.

66. The Coronary Drug Project: Initial findings leading to modifications of its research protocol. J.A.M.A., 214:1303–1313, 1970.

67. Truett, J., Cornfield, J., and Kannel, W.: A multivariate analysis of the risk of coronary heart disease in Framingham. J. Chronic Dis., 20:511, 1967.

68. Tuck, M.L., Sawers, J., Dornfeld, L., et al.: The effect of weight reduction on blood pressure, plasma renin activity and plasma aldosterone levels in obese patients. N. Engl. J. Med., 304:930–933, 1981.

69. Vague, J.: The degree of masculine differentiation of obesities, a factor determining predisposition to diabetes, atherosclerosis, gout and uric calculus disease. Am. J. Clin. Nutr., 4:20–34, 1956.

70. Wahlqvist, M.L., Rilg, I.R., Myers, K.A., et al.: Diabetes and macrovascular disease: Risk factors for atherogenesis. Hum. Nutr. Clin. Nutr., 38:175–184, 1984.

71. West, K.M.: Epidemiology of Diabetes and its Vascular Lesions. New York, Elsevier–North Holland Press, 1978.

72. Yaari, S., Eren-Zshar, S., Goldhourt, V., et al.: Associations of serum high density lipoprotein and total cholesterol with total cardiovascular and cancer mortality in a 7-year prospective study of 10,000 men. Lancet, 1:1011, 1981.

Franz H. Messerli, M.D.
Ochsner Clinic
1514 Jefferson Highway
New Orleans, Louisiana 70121

Risk for Cardiac Involvement in Essential Hypertension

Kenneth G. Zahka, M.D. *

Owing in large part to advances in echocardiography, our knowledge of cardiovascular structure and function in hypertension has expanded dramatically over the last decade. Left ventricular hypertrophy has been observed consistently in a proportion of individuals with essential hypertension, in some cases regardless of the duration or severity of the disease. This has prompted extensive investigation of the development and pathogenesis of ventricular hypertrophy in essential hypertension. Included in these studies are the relationship of the blood pressure to hypertrophy, the association of hypertrophy with long-term morbidity, systolic and diastolic function of the hypertrophied left ventricle, and the effect of lowering of the blood pressure on hypertrophy.

DEFINITION OF HYPERTROPHY

At the cellular level, myocardial hypertrophy is an increase in the diameter of the individual muscle cells with a concomitant increase in the number of contractile units. In the hypertrophied intact heart, there is a thickening of the ventricular wall and an increase in the total ventricular muscle mass. Hyperplasia, an increase in the number of muscle cells, is not encountered outside of the perinatal period,[89] and this does not contribute to the thickening of the ventricular wall in essential hypertension. Myocardial fibrosis or infiltration may mimic hypertrophy by increasing wall thickness without any alteration in the size of the muscle cells.

By this definition, hypertrophy is a dynamic process that occurs with normal growth as well as in pathologic states. *Physiologic* hypertrophy occurs as the heart grows to meet the cardiovascular demands of the developing animal. The growth is proportional to the increase in cardiac output and arterial blood pressure.[85,89] The muscle mass thus must be related to the size of the individual patient and possibly to the degree of physical activity independent of the blood pressure. Left ventricular posterior wall thickness increases with body surface area,[39] degree of obesity,[46] and physical activity.[32] *Pathologic* hypertrophy is an increase in wall thickness and muscle mass out of proportion to body size or physical activity.[85] In a particular patient, the diagnosis of left ventricular hypertrophy depends on normalization for body size and cognizance of physical conditioning.

CAN HYPERTROPHY BE MEASURED CLINICALLY?

Several noninvasive tests, including electrocardiography, echocardiography, computed tomography (CT), and magnetic resonance imaging (MRI), may be used to assess left ventricular mass. Of these, only the electrocardiogram and echocardiogram have been studied extensively in hypertensive patients. Electrocardiographic criteria most frequently cited are the Romhilt-Estes point system[58] and the Sokolow-Lyon voltage criteria.[75] These initial studies showed only a fair correlation with autopsy left ventricular mass.[3,44,69] Although changes in the electrocardiogram have been noted during the course of

*Assistant Professor of Pediatrics, Division of Pediatric Cardiology, The Johns Hopkins University School of Medicine, Baltimore, Maryland

the disease, the electrocardiogram alone has not been a consistently powerful tool for the diagnosis and follow-up of left ventricular hypertrophy.[20,25,35]

Several echocardiographic indices of left ventricular hypertrophy have been evaluated, including posterior wall and ventricular septal thickness,[83] cross-sectional muscle area,[65] left ventricular mass,[13,83] and the radius-to-thickness ratio.[28] The radius-to-thickness ratio is a measure of relative wall thickness, the inverse of which, the thickness-to-radius ratio, has also been advocated by some authors. The three-dimensional correlate of the thickness-to-radius ratio is the mass-to-volume ratio.

Troy and associates[83] showed a high correlation of posterior wall thickness by echocardiography (r = 0.89) and calculated left ventricular mass by echocardiography (r = 0.88) with angiographically derived values. Devereux and Reichek later showed an excellent correlation (r = 0.96) between M-mode echocardiographic calculated ventricular mass and left ventricular mass at autopsy[13] (Fig. 1). Although it has not been as critically studied, the cross-sectional muscle area, either calculated from M-mode echocardiogram measurements or measured directly from two-dimensional images,[38] should also accurately reflect left ventricular hypertrophy, because it uses similar methodology to the mass calculations. The radius-to-thickness ratio can be determined accurately by M-mode echocardiography[28] and is decreased by hypertrophy of the left ventricle. Conversely, the thickness-to-radius ratio and the mass-to-volume ratio are increased by left ventricular hypertrophy.

Direct comparisons of echocardiography and electrocardiography have demonstrated consistently the improved sensitivity of the echocardiogram for the diagnosis and quantitation of left ventricular hypertrophy.[16,30,55] Reichek and Devereux evaluated the sensitivity of the M-mode echocardiogram and the electrocardiogram in predicting the left ventricular mass determined at autopsy.[55] They found that the echocardiographic diagnosis of left ventricular hypertrophy was both sensitive (93 per cent) and specific (95 per cent) and that the correlation with autopsy left ventricular mass was excellent (r = 0.95). In contrast, the electrocardiogram was an insensitive (50 per cent) but specific (95 per cent) means of diagnosing left ventricular hypertrophy.

Despite the excellent correlation between the echocardiographic determination of left ventricular mass and the mass measured at autopsy, there are several additional issues that must be addressed before these data can be used for the evaluation of an individual patient or to expand our knowledge of the pathogenesis of essential hypertension. The measurements of left ventricular wall thickness and mass must be reproducible on several occasions over a period of time. Schlant and colleagues[68] have demonstrated excellent consistency between different observers and repeat measurements by the same observer. Tarazi and Fouad[80] showed in a group of 11 normotensive subjects that the posterior wall and septal thickness and the calculated left ventricular mass could be measured with less than a 5 per cent variation on three occasions over a 6-month interval.

Indexing the posterior wall thickness, ventricular septal thickness, cross-sectional muscle area, and muscle mass to body surface area is the most common normalization method. It is most appropriate for left ventricular mass because mass is linearly related to body surface area.[39] Although the relationship of septal and posterior wall thickness to body surface area is nonlinear,[39] over the relatively narrow range of

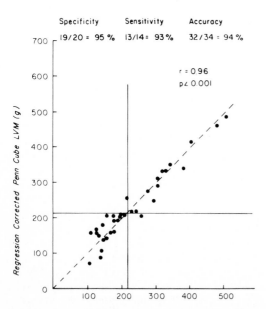

Figure 1. Regression-corrected left ventricular mass using the Penn convention correlates well with anatomic left ventricular weight. (*From* Reichek, N., and Devereux, R.B.: Left ventricular hypertrophy: Relationship of anatomic, echocardiographic and electrocardiographic findings. Circulation, 63:1391–1398, 1981; with permission.)

body size encountered from adolescence to adulthood, this should not introduce a marked error. The radius-to-thickness ratio is independent of body size and thus does not require normalization.

Over the past several years, most investigators have adopted the recommendations of the American Society of Echocardiography,[63] using the leading edge method for measurement of wall thickness and ventricular dimensions. Although calculations of left ventricular mass from measurements using other conventions may provide somewhat better correlation with autopsy mass, this method should be followed for the sake of uniformity.[10] Two-dimensional echocardiography has been useful to guide localization of the M-mode beam between the mitral valve papillary muscles after obtaining a true cross-sectional image. With improved imaging, it has become practical to measure cross-sectional muscle area in two planes and to calculate left ventricular mass based on these cross-sectional areas.[57]

LEFT VENTRICULAR HYPERTROPHY IN ESSENTIAL HYPERTENSION

Left ventricular hypertrophy has been documented in adolescents[7,31,42,67,88] and young adults[4,19,40,59,61,66] early in the course of their disease as well as in adults[19] with well-established hypertension. Savage and coworkers[66] found that 60 per cent of a group of adults, including those in the third decade, with a mean blood pressure of 144/94 mm Hg had increased left ventricular mass (Fig. 2). Similarly, Schlant and associates[68] documented increased posterior wall thickness in a group of 83 hypertensive adults with mild to moderate hypertension (diastolic blood pressure of 90 to 115 mm Hg). In young hypertensive adults with left atrial abnormality on the electrocardiogram, Dunn and colleagues[19] demonstrated increased posterior wall and septal thickness. In our study of hypertensive adolescents, we documented a 40 per cent increase in left ventricular mass and significant thickening of the posterior wall and ventricular septum.[88] Schieken and coworkers[67] also showed that left ventricular mass, when corrected for body size, was increased in children whose blood pressures were in the upper quintile of the distribution. Although there is considerable overlap in the left ventricular mass index between patients with essential hypertension and normal subjects, 40 to 50 per cent of hypertensive patients (mean blood pressure of

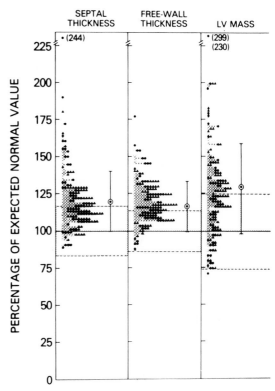

Figure 2. Distribution of echocardiographic ventricular septal thickness, posterior wall thickness, and left ventricular mass in 234 hypertensive subjects. Each value is plotted as a percentage of the predicted value determined from normal data. *Shaded areas* represent the 95 per cent prediction interval derived from normal data. (*From* Savage, D.D., et al.: Echocardiographic assessment of cardiac anatomy and function in hypertensive subjects. Circulation, 59:623–632, 1979; with permission.)

147/94 mm Hg)[10] will have left ventricular hypertrophy. These studies clearly demonstrated early myocardial involvement in the hypertensive process, which previously had not been clinically apparent.

Pathogenesis

Data from both human and animal studies suggest several mechanisms for left ventricular hypertrophy in essential hypertension. Increased afterload is certainly a major factor in the pathogenesis of ventricular hypertrophy. However, early studies in the spontaneously hypertensive rat[8,9,71,87] indicated that left ventricular hypertrophy was present prior to the development of or in spite of prevention of hypertension. Thus, many clinical studies have evaluated the additional role of the sympathetic nervous system and the renin-angiotensin system as well as a variety of indices of left ventricular afterload.

Increased Afterload

Confirmation of increased afterload in the pathogenesis of left ventricular hypertrophy in essential hypertension has been hampered to some extent by the difficulty in defining and quantitating afterload in clinical settings. Systolic, diastolic, or mean blood pressures have shown either a weak or no correlation with left ventricular mass. Devereux and associates[15] showed significant but weak ($r < 0.35$) correlation between mean, systolic, and diastolic blood pressure and left ventricular mass index and no correlation with the thickness-to-radius ratio. The thickness-to-radius ratio correlated best ($r = 0.52$, $p < 0.001$) with the peripheral vascular resistance. Similarly, Ren and associates[57] showed no correlation with casual systolic blood pressure and left ventricular mass. The study of Bouthier and colleagues[2] is one of the few that found a high correlation ($r = 0.71$, p. < 0.001) between systolic blood pressure and the left ventricular mass–to–volume ratio. They suggested that the improved correlation documented in their study was due to the particular suitability of the mass-to-volume ratio in patients with chronically elevated afterload and to their use of serial rather than occasional blood pressure measurements.

One possible reason for the weak relationship between blood pressure and hypertrophy is that the casual blood pressure does not accurately reflect the average load placed on the left ventricle. To test this hypothesis, Ren and colleagues[57] also evaluated the relationship of treadmill exercise maximum systolic blood pressure and left ventricular mass index determined by two-dimensional echocardiography. They found that the correlation of exercise systolic blood pressure with left ventricular mass index was better than that of the resting systolic pressure ($r = 0.58$ versus $r = 0.16$) (Fig. 3). Nathwani and coworkers[50] showed that although the correlation between casual blood pressures and left ventricular mass index was poor, the correlation between systolic blood pressure at submaximal exercise was good ($r = 0.68$, $p < 0.01$). In moderately hypertensive individuals, left ventricular mass appears to be related to diastolic blood pressure during isometric exercise.[37]

Twenty-four–hour ambulatory blood pressure recording may better characterize the average load placed on the left ventricle. Rowlands and associates[60] performed continuous ambulatory intra-arterial monitoring on 50 hospitalized patients with moderately elevated casual blood pressures (162/102 mm Hg) and found that the mean systolic blood pressure over 24 hours correlated best with posterior wall thickness ($r = 0.52$) and left ventricular mass index ($r = 0.60$). Although still significant, the correlations with casual systolic blood pressure ($r = 0.38$, 0.45) and mean diastolic blood pressure over 24 hours ($r = 0.37$, 0.35) were weaker. In their study using noninvasive ambulatory monitoring, Devereux and colleagues[12] found that only ambulatory recordings of blood pressure while the patients were at work (Figs. 4 and 5) correlated with the left ventricular mass index, leading them to conclude that the blood pressure response to recurrent stress was related to the development of left ventricular hypertrophy.

Some investigators have proposed left ventricular systolic wall stress as a more complete assessment of left ventricular afterload than systolic or mean arterial blood pressure.[6,77,81] Increased wall stress is also an important stimulus for hypertrophy.[33] The tension (T), or force developed within the ventricular wall, is related inversely to the radius (r) of the ventricle and directly to the wall thickness (h) and ventricular pressure (P) as expressed by the law of LaPlace with $T = Pr/2h$. Instantaneous systolic wall stress can be calculated from simultaneous measurement of intra-arterial pressure and echocardiographic ventricular diameter and wall thickness at multiple points throughout systole.[33] Wall stress changes throughout the cardiac cycle; it is lowest in early diastole and reaches a peak in early systole before the peak ventricular pressure is reached (Fig. 6).[33] Several studies have calculated peak systolic wall stress based on noninvasive systolic pressure and the diastolic ventricular diameter and wall thickness or end-systolic stress from systolic pressure and end-ejection ventricular diameter and wall thickness.[44] Although these are only an approximation of either average wall stress throughout the cardiac cycle or actual peak wall stress based on simultaneous pressure and dimension data, they do offer a clinically feasible estimate of wall stress.

In general, essential hypertension produces concentric hypertrophy with no significant change or a slight decrease in left ventricular systolic volume and thickening of the ventricular posterior wall and septum. Wall thickening would be expected to offset the increased intracavitary pressure, thus normalizing wall stress. Based on these concepts, the slope of a plot of wall stress versus left ventricular mass or wall

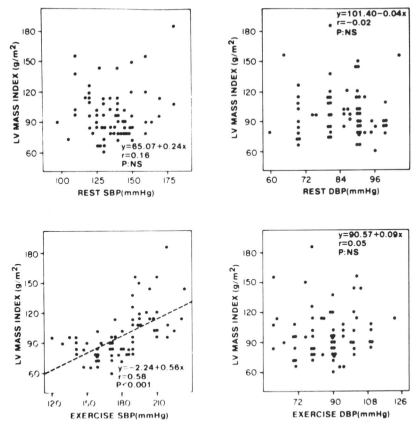

Figure 3. Left ventricular mass index in hypertensive subjects (n = 67) in relation to systolic blood pressure (SBP) at rest, diastolic blood pressure (DBP) at rest, exercise systolic blood pressure, and exercise diastolic blood pressure. Only exercise systolic blood pressure correlates with left ventricular mass index. (*From* Ren, J., et al.: Exercise systolic blood pressure: A powerful determinant of increased left ventricular mass in patients with hypertension. J. Am. Coll. Cardiol., 5:1224–1231, 1985; with permission.)

thickness should be zero. If, on the other hand, the elevation of the afterload is acute and compensatory hypertrophy had not occurred to normalize wall stress or there are other mechanisms governing wall stress in essential hypertension, an increase in wall stress would be expected.

Abi-Samra and coworkers[1] calculated peak and end-systolic wall stress in a group of 37 untreated patients with hypertension and found that both were increased by nearly 20 per cent. The relationship between left ventricular mass index and peak systolic wall stress was weak (r = −0.30) but statistically significant (p < 0.05), suggesting that there were patients in whom the increased wall stress was not offset by compensatory wall thickening or was associated with ventricular dilatation. Bouthier and associates[2] studied 20 patients with a mean blood pressure of 169/104 mm Hg and demonstrated an increased left ventricular mass index and a 33 per cent increase in end-systolic wall stress. Wikstrand[86] noted that hypertension associated with high cardiac output was associated with an increased peak systolic stress compared with hypertensive patients with elevated peripheral resistance and the same level of end-systolic stress. In their study of 27 patients with essential hypertension prior to instituting therapy, Reichek and colleagues[56] showed that estimated end-systolic left ventricular wall stress was normal. Because none of their patients had been receiving antihypertensive medications, the estimates of wall stress were made during a steady-state period. In contrast, in the patients in the other studies, medication had been discontinued for as little as 2 weeks. Although hypertrophy has been documented to occur rapidly, especially in experimental animals,[89] it is possible that following the cessation of therapy, the increase in arterial blood pressure occurred more rapidly than the ventricular wall thickening. These patients may not have been in a steady state and would not necessarily have had sufficient time to normalize wall stress completely.

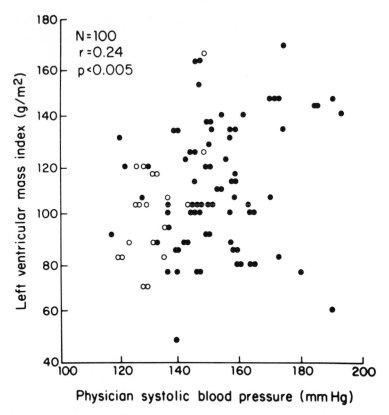

Figure 4. A weak relationship is observed between clinical (physician) measurements of systolic blood pressure and left ventricular mass index. *Open circles* = normal subjects; *closed circles* = hypertensive subjects. (*From* Devereux, R.B., et al.: Left ventricular hypertrophy in patients with hypertension: Importance of blood pressure response to regularly recurring stress. Circulation, 68:470–476, 1983; with permission.)

Our inability to measure wall stress directly and its variability throughout the cardiac cycle complicate the application of the principle of afterload as it is defined in isolated muscle studies to the intact ventricle. If afterload is defined as the external opposition to ventricular outflow rather than a property of the muscle, the rigorous description of the properties of the vascular bed provided by the measurement of arterial impedance should provide a better understanding of the afterload of the left ventricle in essential hypertension.[6,49,51] The measurement of aortic impedance permits separation of the contribution of the pulsatile and the steady-state components of blood flow to the total work of the ventricle. The former is affected primarily by the diameter and distensibility of the aorta and the reflection of waves back from the periphery. The latter is determined by the diameter and number of the small resistance arterioles. The application of the principles of aortic impedance has been limited by the need for simultaneous recording of high-fidelity aortic pressure and flow waveforms, which then must be subjected to lengthy analysis.

In their study of aortic impedance in 12 hypertensive patients, Merillon and associates[45] demonstrated an increase in both the mean and pulsatile components of left ventricular power, suggesting that in addition to the peripheral vascular resistance, the properties of the aorta produced alterations in the pulsatile blood flow that further increased ventricular afterload. The ratio of the pulsatile to mean power was increased in the hypertensive patients, indicating that the blood flow was less efficient, with a greater proportion of energy required to move blood in a pulsatile fashion. The characteristics of the impedance spectrum also indicated that pulse wave velocity and reflected waves in the aorta were increased because of a combination of an increase in aortic diameter, a decrease in aortic distensibility, and increased peripheral vascular resistance. This contribution of the pulsatile nature of blood flow to the total left ventricular afterload may explain in part some of the inconsistencies encountered in the studies of the relationship of left ventricular hypertrophy to blood pressure or wall stress.

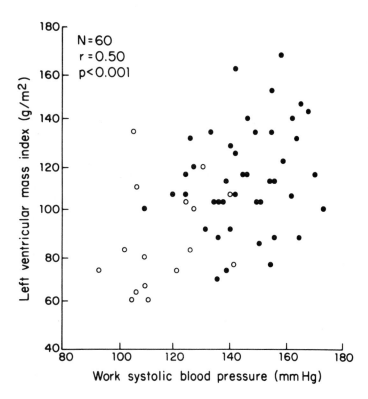

Figure 5. A closer relationship exists between automatic recorder measurements of systolic blood pressure at work and left ventricular mass index. *Open circles* = normal subjects; *closed circles* = hypertensive subjects. (*From* Devereux, R.B., et al.: Left ventricular hypertrophy in patients with hypertension: Importance of blood pressure response to regularly recurring stress. Circulation, *68*:470–476, 1983; with permission.)

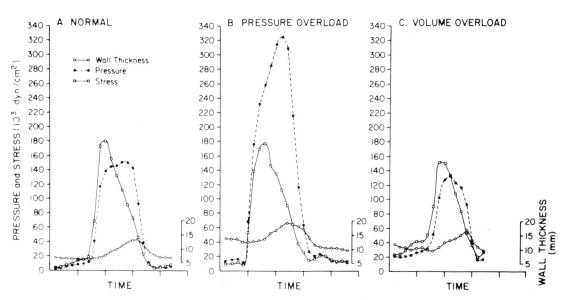

Figure 6. Comparison of changes in left ventricular pressure (*solid dots*), wall thickness (*open dots*), and meridional stress (*open squares*) throughout the cardiac cycle for representative normal (A), pressure-overloaded (B), and volume-overloaded (C) left ventricles. Measurements are plotted at 40-msec intervals. In the pressure-overloaded ventricle (B), the markedly elevated systolic pressure is exactly counterbalanced by increased wall thickness, with the result that the wall stress remains normal. (*From* Grossman, W., et al.: Wall stress in the normal and hypertrophied human left ventricle. J. Clin. Invest., *56*:56–64, 1975; with permission.)

Decreased arterial distensibility and increased pulse wave velocity in essential hypertension have been consistent findings by a variety of techniques in addition to arterial impedance.[47] Arterial distensibility is related to systolic blood pressure.[54] Using a bidirectional pulsed Doppler system, Bouthier and colleagues[2] analyzed brachioradial pulse wave velocity and compliance in essential hypertension and found a direct correlation between brachioradial pulse wave velocity and the left ventricular mass–to–volume ratio. Similarly, brachial artery compliance was inversely related to the mass–to–volume ratio. This study and those of Merillon and coworkers suggest that the development of left ventricular hypertrophy in essential hypertension is strongly influenced by ventricular afterload.

The Adrenergic Nervous System

Catecholamines have been implicated in the pathogenesis of experimental and clinical myocardial hypertrophy.[26,27,82] Catecholamines induce hypertrophy in cultured myocytes,[73] and norepinephrine stores are increased in the hypertrophied rat heart.[21] The data regarding the role of the adrenergic nervous system in essential hypertension are less compelling. Beta-blockade in the spontaneously hypertensive rat does not prevent the development of left ventricular hypertrophy or reverse established left ventricular hypertrophy, despite lowering of blood pressure.[84] Similarly, immunosympathectomy of the spontaneously hypertensive rat does not prevent the development of hypertrophy.[9] In support of the role of the sympathetic nervous system, Sen and associates[70] found that in the spontaneously hypertensive rat, blocking the sympathetic nervous system with methyldopa lowered both blood pressure and ventricular mass, whereas hydralazine, which leaves the sympathetic nervous system intact, decreased only the blood pressure.

Inferences regarding the role of catecholamines in left ventricular hypertrophy in man have been drawn primarily from the regression of hypertrophy following pharmacologic treatment of hypertension. Fouad and colleagues[22] have shown that the addition of methyldopa decreased left ventricular mass without a significant improvement in the blood pressure control achieved by diuretic alone. In patients with mean arterial blood pressure greater than 100 mm Hg, Hartford and coworkers[37] demonstrated a significant correlation between 24-hour urinary norepinephrine excretion and left ventric-

ular mass, but no correlation with plasma norepinephrine concentration. Analysis of patients with mean blood pressure below 100 mm Hg showed no pattern of catecholamine concentration or excretion. Corea and associates[5] found that septal thickness was related to plasma norepinephrine concentration, and posterior wall thickness correlated weakly with mean blood pressure. Left ventricular mass index was not related to blood pressure or to plasma catecholamines. Treatment with atenolol decreased blood pressure and left ventricular mass index significantly but resulted in no significant change in plasma catecholamines. This suggests that although the sympathetic nervous system may be responsible in part for the 5 to 10 per cent incidence of mild asymmetric septal hypertrophy in patients with essential hypertension,[4,19,66,68] it probably does not play a major role in the pathogenesis of left ventricular hypertrophy in essential hypertension.

The Renin-Angiotensin System

Speculation regarding the direct role of angiotensin in the pathogenesis of left ventricular hypertrophy arises in part from the observation that treatment of the spontaneously hypertensive rat with hydralazine or minoxidil increases the plasma renin levels without changing left ventricular hypertrophy and that other drugs that lower the blood pressure and decrease left ventricular muscle mass also inhibit the renin-angiotensin system.[70,71] Clinical studies, however, have shown no relationship between plasma renin concentration and indices of left ventricular hypertrophy.[5,14,37] Although these findings do not support the role of angiotensin in the pathogenesis of essential hypertension, Devereux and coworkers[14] do note that their high-renin hypertension patients were younger than the low- and normal-renin group, suggesting that they may have developed hypertrophy more rapidly.

Blood Viscosity

Essential hypertension is associated with mild yet significant elevations of the hematocrit, hemoglobin, and whole blood viscosity.[43] In a group of patients with a mean blood pressure of 160/104 mm Hg in whom medications had been discontinued for at least 3 weeks, Devereux and associates[11] found a close correlation between whole blood viscosity at high shear rates and left ventricular mass. This relationship was stronger than that between blood pressure and left ventricular mass. Finally, they noted that hypertensive patients with normal left ventricular mass had normal whole blood viscosity. They suggested several mechanisms by which increased viscosity could produce left ventricular hypertrophy, including increased arteriolar resistance independent of vasoconstriction, and blunting of the diurnal variation of blood pressure. Alternatively, a common as yet undefined mechanism may be responsible for both hemoconcentration and elevated peripheral vascular resistance.

SYSTOLIC FUNCTION OF THE HYPERTROPHIED LEFT VENTRICLE IN ESSENTIAL HYPERTENSION

The echocardiographic indices of left ventricular function have been well defined in essential hypertension. In adolescents and young adults with early hypertension, ejection fraction or fractional shortening is normal, despite the increase in afterload.[4,10,15,19,66,88] The ejection fraction may be depressed in severe established hypertension.[19] The functional reserve of the left ventricle, as assessed by the increase in ejection fraction with dynamic exercise, is normal.[24]

The velocity of circumferential fiber shortening, V_{cf}, is sensitive to the contractile state of the myocardium but is usually depressed by increasing afterload.[53] Thus, the finding by several investigators of supranormal V_{cf}[34] or normal V_{cf}[46,78,88] suggests that the left ventricle compensates adequately for the increased afterload. Ejection fraction, shortening fraction, and V_{cf} are inversely related to wall stress,[1,15,77,78] implying that if compensatory hypertrophy does not occur to decrease wall stress, ventricular performance tends to decrease.

Cardiac output or index, whether measured by indicator dilution, nuclear techniques, or echocardiography, is usually normal[17,18,23,78] in established hypertension or mildly elevated[48] in early borderline hypertension. Cardiac work or stroke work is increased in hypertension.[18,46] Peak dp/dt is increased, except in patients with ventricular dilatation or regional wall abnormalities.[78]

The wall stress-diameter relationship may be an index of contractility that incorporates afterload but is independent of preload.[64] Although similar in principle to the end-systolic pressure–volume relationship proposed by Sagawa,[62] the wall stress-diameter relationship has the further advantage of normalizing for ventricular size and wall thickness. Using this technique,

Takahashi and colleagues[79] demonstrated normal slope and intercept of the wall stress-diameter relationship in hypertensive patients with an end-diastolic wall thickness less than 1.3 cm. Only those patients with severe hypertrophy, an end-diastolic wall thickness greater than 1.3 cm, had depression of myocardial contractility with a decrease in the slope of the wall stress-diameter relationship.

Thus, patients with essential hypertension have normal left ventricular function at rest and with exercise. Only those patients with coronary artery disease or severe left ventricular hypertrophy with dilatation are expected to have ventricular dysfunction.

DIASTOLIC FUNCTION IN THE HYPERTROPHIED LEFT VENTRICLE IN ESSENTIAL HYPERTENSION

In contrast to systolic function, a number of abnormalities of diastolic ventricular function have been identified in patients with essential hypertension. Fouad and colleagues[23] found decreased diastolic filling velocity using gated blood pool studies. Smith and coworkers[74] showed that the rapid diastolic filling rate, as determined by a nonimaging nuclear probe, was 30 per cent less in patients with hypertension compared with normotensive controls and athletes with physiologic hypertrophy.[32] The rapid filling rate was inversely related to the left ventricular mass index. Similar findings were noted by Shapiro and McKenna[72] with moderate and severe hypertension (systolic blood pressure greater than 175 mm Hg). The echocardiographic left atrial emptying index, rapid atrial filling divided by total atrial emptying, is reduced in patients with hypertensive left ventricular hypertrophy.[62] The atrial emptying index did not correlate well with total peripheral resistance, which Dreslinski and associates[17] suggest indicates that left ventricular compliance is decreased secondary to the hypertrophy. Hartford and colleagues[36] measured isovolumic relaxation time (aortic closure to mitral valve opening) and found that it increased with the severity of the hypertension. They also noted prolonged relaxation times in several patients without left ventricular hypertrophy, suggesting that other factors in addition to wall thickness were affecting the relaxation time.

Although the preceding data imply that the left ventricular chamber compliance is abnormal in essential hypertension, they do not measure compliance directly and do not clarify the underlying mechanism for the impaired filling or abnormal compliance. Decreased chamber compliance may be due either to a shift upward along the diastolic pressure-volume curve or a change in the shape of the pressure-volume curve as a result of alterations in the intrinsic properties of the muscle. The former is most frequently the result of increased preload, and the latter is due to myocardial thickening, myocardial fibrosis, or incomplete relaxation. Although there is a paucity of data regarding the diastolic pressure-volume relationship of the hypertrophied heart in essential hypertension, data from patients with aortic stenosis suggest that chamber compliance is either normal or decreased. In contrast, the compliance of the myocardium itself, especially in the absence of fibrosis due to ischemia, is normal.[29,41]

The clinical importance of the diastolic filling abnormalities of the left ventricle and their pathogenesis remains to be elucidated. Perhaps they will serve as a marker for future morbidity or will be a sensitive guide to the efficacy of treatment in the normalization of the cardiovascular system.

LEFT VENTRICULAR HYPERTROPHY AND THE PREHYPERTENSIVE STATE

The possibility that left ventricular hypertrophy precedes the development of hypertension would have considerable impact on our concepts of the pathogenesis of left ventricular hypertrophy in essential hypertension and would provide a useful marker for those individuals who are likely to develop sustained hypertension. Sparrow and coworkers[76] prospectively followed 1090 normotensive men for 10 years and found that the eventual development of blood pressure greater than 159/94 mm Hg could be predicted from the amplitude of the left ventricular forces on the initial electrocardiogram and the body mass index. They concluded that the small increase in the R- and S-wave amplitudes could be an early manifestation of left ventricular hypertrophy and that there was a dissociation between blood pressure and hypertrophy. To further test this hypothesis, Nielsen and Oxhoj[52] studied 25 normotensive male offspring with at least one hypertensive parent. Echocardiographic left ventricular mass was increased and asymmetric septal hypertrophy was present in 17 per cent of those subjects, despite blood pressures that were comparable to those of the control group with a negative family history (Fig. 7). These early findings need to be followed by

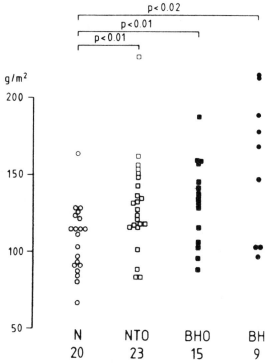

Figure 7. Left ventricular mass for normal subjects (N), normotensive offspring with a positive family history of essential hypertension (NTO), borderline hypertensive subjects with a positive family history of essential hypertension (BHO), and borderline hypertensive subjects on treatment (BH). *Shaded area* represents the 95 per cent confidence limits of the control group. (*From* Nielsen, J.R., and Oxhoj, H.: Echocardiographic variables in progeny of hypertensive and normotensive parents. Acta Med. Scand. (Suppl.), *693*:61–64, 1985; with permission.)

other studies, including ones that evaluate the left ventricular hypertrophy as a function of 24-hour ambulatory blood pressure and exercise blood pressure, in order to confirm the apparent dissociation between blood pressure and left ventricular hypertrophy.

SUMMARY AND CONCLUSIONS

The evidence is inescapable that even mild essential hypertension is associated with left ventricular hypertrophy, regardless of the age of the patient. Increased left ventricular afterload must play a major role in the pathogenesis of the hypertrophy; however, further proof of this awaits our improved understanding of the quantitation of afterload in the clinical setting.

Other factors, including the adrenergic nervous system and blood viscosity, may play an additional role, possibly mediated through alterations in afterload or by direct myocardial action.

Left ventricular hypertrophy exerts a positive benefit by normalizing wall stress in patients with hypertension. Especially in patients without coexistent coronary abnormalities, systolic function is normal and abnormalities of diastolic function are of uncertain clinical importance. Because echocardiography now provides a convenient and sensitive noninvasive means of following patients with left ventricular hypertrophy, long-term studies are now needed to document the incremental risk (or benefit) of left ventricular hypertrophy over blood pressure itself in the eventual morbidity of essential hypertension.

The recognition of left ventricular hypertrophy in a patient with borderline elevation of blood pressure poses a new clinical dilemma. Should treatment be instituted based on this additional finding? In view of the data correlating stress, exercise, and mean daily blood pressure with left ventricular hypertrophy and the reduction of left ventricular mass following lowering of blood pressure, it has been our practice to treat patients with left ventricular hypertrophy more readily than those without left ventricular hypertrophy. The rationale in this approach is not that left ventricular hypertrophy per se is harmful, but rather that it indicates a greater degree of afterload than may be evident from office blood pressure measurements.

REFERENCES

1. Abi-Sambra, F., Fouad, F.M., and Tarazi, R.C.: Determinants of left ventricular hypertrophy and function in hypertensive patients. Am. J. Med., 75:26–33, 1983.
2. Bouthier, J.D., De Luca, N., Safer, M.E., et al.: Cardiac hypertrophy and arterial distensibility in essential hypertension. Am. Heart J., 109:1345–1352, 1985.
3. Carter, W.A., and Estes, E.H.: Electrocardiographic manifestations of ventricular hypertrophy; a computerized study of ECG-anatomic correlations in 319 cases. Am. Heart J., 68:173–182, 1964.
4. Cohen, A., Hagan, A.D., Watkins, J., et al.: Clinical correlates in hypertensive patients with left ventricular hypertrophy diagnosed with echocardiography. Am. J. Cardiol., 47:335–341, 1981.
5. Corea, L., Bentivoglio, M., and Vedecchia, P.: Echocardiographic left ventricular hypertrophy as related to arterial pressure and plasma norepinephrine concentration in arterial hypertension. Hypertension, 5:837–843, 1983.
6. Covell, J.W., Pouleur, H., and Ross, J., Jr.: Left ventricular wall stress and aortic input impedance. Fed. Proc., 39:202–207, 1980.
7. Culpepper, W.S., Sodt, P.C., Messerli, F.H., et al.: Cardiac status in juvenile borderline hypertension. Ann. Intern. Med., 98:1–7, 1983.
8. Cutilletta, A.F., Benjamin, M., Culpepper, W.S., et al.: Myocardial hypertrophy and ventricular performance in the absence of hypertension in spontaneously hypertensive rats. J. Mol. Cell. Cardiol., 10:689–703, 1978.
9. Cutilletta, A.F., Erinoff, L., Heller, A., et al.: Development of left ventricular hypertrophy in young spontaneously hypertensive rats after peripheral sympathectomy. Circ. Res., 40:428–434, 1977.
10. Devereux, R.B.: Noninvasive evaluation of cardiac anatomy and function in patients with hypertension. Cardiovasc. Rev. Rep., 3:313–322, 1982.
11. Devereux, R.B., Drayer, J.I.M., Chien, S., et al.: Whole blood viscosity as a determinant of cardiac hypertrophy in systemic hypertension. Am. J. Cardiol., 54:592–595, 1984.
12. Devereux, R.B., Pickering, T.G., Harshfield, G.A., et al.: Left ventricular hypertrophy in patients with hypertension: Importance of blood pressure response to regularly recurring stress. Circulation, 68:470–476, 1983.
13. Devereux, R.B., and Reichek, N.: Echocardiographic determination of left ventricular mass in man. Circulation, 55:613–618, 1977.
14. Devereux, R.B., Savage, D.D., Drayer, J.I.M., et al.: Left ventricular hypertrophy and function in high, normal and low-renin forms of essential hypertension. Hypertension, 4:524–531, 1982.
15. Devereux, R.B., Savage, D.D., Sachs, I., et al.: Relation of hemodynamic load to left ventricular hypertrophy and performance in hypertension. Am. J. Cardiol., 51:171–176, 1983.
16. Dreslinski, G.R.: Identification of left ventricular hypertrophy: Chest roentgenography, echocardiography, and electrocardiography. Am. J. Med., 75:47–50, 1983.
17. Dreslinski, G.R., Frohlich, E.D., Dunn, F.G., et al.: Echocardiographic diastolic ventricular abnormality in hypertensive heart disease: Atrial emptying index. Am. J. Cardiol., 47:1087–1090, 1981.
18. Dreslinski, G.R., Messerli, F.H., Dunn, F.G., et al.: Early hypertension and cardiac work. Am. J. Cardiol., 50:149–151, 1982.
19. Dunn, F.G., Chandraratna, D., deCarvallo, J.G.R., et al.: Pathophysiologic assessment of hypertensive heart disease with echocardiography. Am. J. Cardiol., 39:789–795, 1977.
20. Dunn, R.A., Zenner, R.J., and Pipberger, H.V.: Serial electrocardiograms in hypertensive cardiovascular disease. Circulation, 56:416–423, 1977.
21. Fisher, J.E., Horst, J.D., and Kopin, I.J.: Norepinephrine metabolism in hypertrophied rat hearts. Nature, 207:951–953, 1965.
22. Fouad, F.M., Nakashima, Y., Tarazi, R.C., et al.: Reversal of left ventricular hypertrophy in hypertensive patients treated with methyldopa: Lack of association with blood pressure control. Am. J. Cardiol., 49:795–801, 1982.
23. Fouad, F.M., Tarazi, R.C., Gallagher, J.H., et al.: Abnormal left ventricular relaxation in hypertensive patients. Clin. Sci., 59:411s–414s, 1980.
24. Francis, C.K., Cleman, M., Berger, H.J., et al.: Left ventricular systolic performance during upright bi-

cycle exercise in patients with essential hypertension. Am. J. Med., 75:40–46, 1983.

25. Freis, E.D.: Electrocardiographic changes in the course of antihypertensive treatment. Am. J. Med., 75:111–115, 1983.

26. Frohlich, E.D.: Hemodynamics and other determinants in development of left ventricular hypertrophy. Fed. Proc., 42:2709–2715, 1983.

27. Frohlich, E.D., and Tarazi, R.C.: Is arterial pressure the sole factor responsible for hypertensive cardiac hypertrophy? Am. J. Cardiol., 44:959–963, 1979.

28. Gaasch, W.H.: Left ventricular radius to wall thickness ratio. Am. J. Cardiol., 43:1189–1194, 1979.

29. Gaasch, W.H., Bing, O.H.L., and Mirsky, I.: Chamber compliance and myocardial stiffness in left ventricular hypertrophy. Eur. Heart J., 3(Suppl. A):139–145, 1982.

30. Geva, B., Elkayam, U., Frishman, W., et al.: Determination of left ventricular wall thickening in patients with chronic systemic hypertension. Chest, 76:557–561, 1979.

31. Goldring, D., Hernandez, A., Choi, S., et al.: Blood pressure in a high school population. II. Clinical profile of the juvenile hypertensive. J. Pediatr., 95:298–304, 1979.

32. Granger, C.B., Karimeddini, M.K., Smith, V.E., et al.: Rapid ventricular filling in left ventricular hypertrophy. I. Physiologic hypertrophy. J. Am. Coll. Cardiol., 5:862–868, 1985.

33. Grossman, W., Jones, D., and McLaurin, L.P.: Wall stress in the normal and hypertrophied human left ventricle. J. Clin. Invest., 56:56–64, 1975.

34. Guazzi, M., Fiorentini, C., Olivari, M.T., et al.: Cardiac load and function in hypertension. Am. J. Cardiol., 44:1007–1012, 1979.

35. Hamer, J., Shinebourne, E., and Fleming, J.: Significance of electrocardiographic changes in hypertension. Br. Med. J., 1:79–82, 1969.

36. Hartford, M., Wikstrand, J., Wallentin, I., et al.: Diastolic function of the heart in untreated primary hypertension. Hypertension, 6:329–338, 1984.

37. Hartford, M., Wikstrand, J., Wallentin, I., et al.: The relation between cardiac hypertrophy and hypertension. Acta Med. Scand. (Suppl.),672:101–104, 1983.

38. Helak, J.W., and Reichek, N.: Quantitation of human left ventricular mass and volume by two-dimensional echocardiography: In vitro anatomic validation. Circulation, 63:1398–1407, 1981.

39. Henry, W.L., Ware, J., Gardin, J.M., et al.: Echocardiographic measurements in normal subjects: Growth-related changes that occur between infancy and early adulthood. Circulation, 57:278–285, 1978.

40. Kaliner, J.S., Williams, D., Gorwitt, J., et al.: Left ventricular performance in patients with left ventricular hypertrophy caused by systemic hypertension. Br. Heart J., 39:1239–1245, 1977.

41. Krayenbuehl, H.P., Hess, O., and Hirzel, H.: Pathophysiology of the hypertrophied heart in man. Eur. Heart J., 3(Suppl. A):125–131, 1982.

42. Laird, W.P., and Fixler, D.E.: Left ventricular hypertrophy in adolescents with elevated blood pressure: Assessment by chest roentgenography, electrocardiography, and echocardiography. Pediatrics, 67:255–259, 1981.

43. Letcher, R.L., Chien, S., Pickering, T.G., et al.: Direct relationship between blood pressure and blood viscosity in normal and hypertensive subjects. Role of fibrinogen and concentration. Am. J. Med., 70:1195–1202, 1981.

44. Mazzoleni, A., Wolff, R., Wolff, L., et al.: Correlation between component cardiac weights and electrocardiographic patterns in 185 cases. Circulation, 30:808–829, 1964.

45. Merillon, J.P., Fortenier, G.J., Lerallut, J.F., et al.: Aortic input impedance in normal man and arterial hypertension: Its modification during changes in aortic pressure. Cardiovasc. Res., 16:646–656, 1982.

46. Messerli, F.H., Sundgaard-Riise, K., Reisin, E.D., et al.: Dimorphic cardiac adaptation to obesity and arterial hypertension. Ann. Intern. Med., 99:757–761, 1983.

47. Messerli, F.H., Ventura, H., Aristimuno, G.G., et al.: Arterial compliance in systolic hypertension. Clin. Exp. Hypertension, 7:1037–1044, 1982.

48. Messerli, F.H., Ventura, H.O., Reisin, E., et al.: Borderline hypertension and obesity: Two prehypertensive states with elevated cardiac output. Circulation, 66:55–60, 1982.

49. Milnor, W.R.: Arterial impedance as ventricular afterload. Circ. Res., 36:565–570, 1975.

50. Nathwani, D., Reeves, R.A., Marquez-Julio, A., et al.: Left ventricular hypertrophy in mild hypertension: Correlation with exercise blood pressure. Am. Heart J., 109:386–387, 1985.

51. Nichols, W.W., and Pepine, C.J.: Left ventricular afterload and aortic input impedance: Implications of pulsatile blood flow. Prog. Cardiovasc. Dis., 24:293–306, 1982.

52. Nielsen, J.R., and Oxhoj, H.: Echocardiographic variables in progeny of hypertensive and normotensive parents. Acta Med. Scand (Suppl.), 693:61–64, 1985.

53. Quinones, M.A., Gaash, W.H., Cole, J.S., et al.: Echocardiographic determination of left ventricular stress-velocity relations in man. With reference to the effects of loading and contractility. Circulation, 51:1185–1190, 1975.

54. Randall, O.S.: Effect of arterial compliance on systolic blood pressure and cardiac function. Clin. Exp. Hypertension, 7:1045–1057, 1982.

55. Reichek, N., and Devereux, R.B.: Left ventricular hypertrophy: Relationship of anatomic, echocardiographic and electrocardiographic findings. Circulation, 63:1391–1398, 1981.

56. Reichek, N., Franklin, B.B., Chandler, T., et al.: Reversal of left ventricular hypertrophy by antihypertensive therapy. Eur. Heart J., 3(Suppl. A):165–169, 1982.

57. Ren, J., Hakki, A., Kotler, M.N., et al.: Exercise systolic blood pressure: A powerful determinant of increased left ventricular mass in patients with hypertension. J. Am. Coll. Cardiol., 5:1224–1231, 1985.

58. Romhilt, D.W., Bove, K.E., Norris, R.J., et al.: A critical appraisal of the electrocardiographic criteria for the diagnosis of left ventricular hypertrophy. Circulation, 40:185–195, 1969.

59. Ross, A.M., Pisarczyk, P., Calabresi, M., et al.: Echocardiographic and clinical correlations in systemic hypertension. J. Clin. Ultrasound, 6:95–99, 1978.

60. Rowlands, D.B., Ireland, M.A., Stallard, T.J., et al.: Assessment of left ventricular mass and its response to antihypertensive treatment. Lancet, 1:467–470, 1982.

61. Safer, M.E., Lehner, J.P., Vincent, M.I., et al.: Echocardiographic dimensions in borderline and sustained hypertension. Am. J. Cardiol., 44:930–935, 1979.

62. Sagawa, K.S.: The pressure-volume diagram revisited. Circ. Res., 43:677–687, 1977.

63. Sahn, D.J., DeMaria, A., Kisslo, J., et al.: Recommen-

dations regarding the quantitation in M-mode echocardiography: results of a survey of echocardiographic measurements. Circulation, *58*:1072–1083, 1978.

64. Sasayama, S., Franklin, D., Ross, J., Jr.: Hyperfunction with normal inotropic state of the hypertrophied left ventricle. Am. J. Physiol., *232*:H418–H425, 1977.

65. Sasayama, S., Ross, J., Jr., Franklin, D., et al.: Adaptations of the left ventricle to chronic pressure overload. Circ. Res., *38*:172–178, 1976.

66. Savage, D.D., Drayer, J.I.M., Henry, W.L., et al.: Echocardiographic assessment of cardiac anatomy and function in hypertensive subjects. Circulation, *59*:623–632, 1979.

67. Schieken, R.M., Clarke, W.R., and Lauer, R.M.: Left ventricular hypertrophy in children with blood pressures in the upper quintile of the distribution (The Muscatine Study). Hypertension, *3*:669–675, 1981.

68. Schlant, R.C., Feiner, J.M., Heymsfield, S.G., et al.: Echocardiographic studies of left ventricular anatomy and function in essential hypertension. Cardiovasc. Med., *2*:477–491, 1977.

69. Scott, R.C.: The correlation between the electrocardiographic patterns of ventricular hypertrophy and the anatomic findings. Circulation, *37*:509–517, 1968.

70. Sen, S., Tarazi, R.C., and Bumpus, F.M.: Cardiac hypertrophy and antihypertensive therapy. Cardiac Res., *11*:427–433, 1977.

71. Sen, S., Tarazi, R.C., Khairallah, P.A., et al.: Cardiac hypertrophy in spontaneously hypertensive rats. Circ. Res., *35*:775–781, 1974.

72. Shapiro, L.M., and McKenna, W.J.: Left ventricular hypertrophy. Relation of structure to diastolic function in hypertension. Br. Heart J., *51*:637–642, 1984.

73. Simpson, P.: Norepinephrine-stimulated hypertrophy of cultured rat myocardial cells is an alpha₁ adrenergic response. J. Clin. Invest., *72*:732–738, 1983.

74. Smith, V.E., Schulman, P., Karimeddini, M.K., et al.: Rapid ventricular filling in left ventricular hypertrophy. I. Pathologic hypertrophy. J. Am. Coll. Cardiol., *5*:869–874, 1985.

75. Sokolow, M., and Lyon, T.P.: The ventricular complex in left ventricular hypertrophy as obtained by unipolar precordial and limb leads. Am. Heart J., *37*:161–186, 1949.

76. Sparrow, D., Thomas, H.E., Jr., Rosner, B., et al.: The relationship of the baseline ECG to blood pressure change. J.A.M.A., *250*:1285–1288, 1983.

77. Strauer, B.E.: Functional dynamics of the left ventricle in hypertensive hypertrophy and failure. Hypertension, *6*:III-4–III-12, 1984.

78. Strauer, B.E.: Ventricular function and coronary hemodynamics in hypertensive heart disease. Am. J. Cardiol., *44*:999–1006, 1979.

79. Takahashi, M., Sasayama, S., Kawai, C., et al.: Contractile performance of the hypertrophied ventricle in patients with systemic hypertension. Circulation, *62*:116–126, 1980.

80. Tarazi, R.C., and Fouad, F.M.: Reversal of cardiac hypertrophy in humans. Hypertension, *6*:III-141–III-146, 1984.

81. Tarazi, R.C., and Levy, M.N.: Cardiac responses to increased afterload: State-of-the-art review. Hypertension, *4*:II-8–II-18, 1982.

82. Tarazi, R.C., Sen, S., Saragoca, M., et al.: The multifactorial role of catecholamines in hypertensive cardiac hypertrophy. Eur. Heart. J., *3*(Suppl. A):103–110, 1982.

83. Troy, B.L., Pombo, J., and Rackley, C.E.: Measurement of left ventricular wall thickness and mass by echocardiography. Circulation, *45*:602–611, 1971.

84. Weiss, L., and Lungren, Y.: Left ventricular hypertrophy and its reversibility in young spontaneously hypertensive rats. Cardiovasc. Res., *12*:635–638, 1978.

85. Wikman-Coffelt, J., Parmley, W.W., et al.: The cardiac hypertrophy process. Circ. Res., *45*:697–707, 1979.

86. Wikstrand, J.: Left ventricular function in early primary hypertension: Functional consequences of cardiovascular structural changes. Hypertension, *6*:III-108–III-116, 1984.

87. Yamori, Y., Mori, C., Nishio, T., et al.: Cardiac hypertrophy in early hypertension. Am. J. Cardiol., *44*:964–969, 1979.

88. Zahka, K.G., Neill, C.A., Kidd, L., et al.: Cardiac involvement in adolescent hypertension. Hypertension, *3*:664–668, 1981.

89. Zak, R., Kizu, A., and Bugaisky, L.: Cardiac hypertrophy: Its characteristics as a growth process. Am. J. Cardiol., *44*:941–946, 1979.

Division of Pediatric Cardiology
The Johns Hopkins Hospital
600 North Wolfe Street
Baltimore, Maryland 21205

Adverse Effects of
Risk Factor Reduction

Adverse Effects of the Treatment for Hyperlipidemia

M. Rene Malinow, M.D.*

This presentation deals with hyperlipidemias encountered in patients with plasma cholesterol* levels of 600 mg per dl or less or triglyceride levels of 1000 mg per dl or less. In patients with much higher lipid levels, such as those with chylomicron retention that might be associated with acute pancreatitis or those with homozygous familial hypercholesterolemia and premature atherosclerosis, management of life-threatening situations differs from that of the usual hyperlipidemia. In homozygous familial hypercholesterolemia, for instance, lipoprotein apheresis,[107] portacaval shunt,[105] and liver-heart transplantation[104] pose obvious hazards, but the risk posed by nontreatment may outweigh the risk posed by treatment.

There are no known adverse effects of reducing lipids toward more normal plasma levels. However, the agents or procedures utilized for the control of hyperlipidemia may have detrimental effects. As in other clinical circumstances, the risk-to-benefit ratio needs to be evaluated for each individual patient. Thus, although the benefits of reducing hypercholesterolemia have been demonstrated definitively,[61] possible harmful effects of lifelong interventions must be carefully taken into consideration in the therapeutic decision.

When hyperlipidemia is *not* reduced after a concerted intervention effort, certain patients are subject to adverse psychologic effects, in ad-

dition to long-term risk of atherosclerosis. Anxiety and depression can occur when expectations are not fulfilled, for example, when patients do not comply with prescribed interventions or when therapy is discontinued because of an inadequate response or intolerance. Patients in these circumstances should be given sympathetic understanding; it is sometimes useful to emphasize that current worldwide research is expected to produce more effective and better tolerated or accepted drugs.

RISKS OF PLASMA CHOLESTEROL LEVELS THAT ARE TOO LOW

Six prospective studies in men revealed an excessive number of deaths from colon cancer that were associated wtih lower-than-expected levels of blood cholesterol.[93] Although in short-term studies colon cancer occurred in the early years of the observation,[94] the negative correlation was still present when observations spanned 18 years;[119] therefore, it is unlikely that cancer was present but unsuspected during the early examination. In the Framingham experience, serum cholesterol level was inversely associated with the incidence of colon cancer and with cancer in other sites only in men; these associations were significant after adjustment for age, alcohol consumption, cigarette smoking, education, systolic blood pressure, and relative weight.[119] Pathogenetic mechanisms that might be involved in this negative correlation are unknown. However, because an increased inci-

---

*The term "cholesterolemia" will be used interchangeably with blood, plasma, or serum cholesterol levels.

*Professor, Division of Cardiology and Division of Metabolism and Clinical Nutrition, Oregon Health Sciences University, Portland; Senior Scientist, Division of Immune and Metabolic Diseases, Oregon Regional Primate Research Center, Beaverton, Oregon

dence of cancer was associated mainly with serum cholesterol levels lower than 190 mg per dl[119]—levels seldom attained after antihyperlipidemia regimens—it is likely that the high incidence of cancer observed during certain hyperlipidemia therapies (for example, clofibrate [Atromid-S]) was not related to the slightly reduced cholesterol levels but to effects of the drug itself.

ADVERSE EFFECTS OF DIETARY INTERVENTION

Food with reduced cholesterol, fat, and saturated fat content that has a polyunsaturated fat–to–saturated fat ratio around 1.0 is the mainstay of antihyperlipidemia regimens,[18] and it may contribute to the prevention of coronary heart disease (CHD).[50] A somewhat more stringent vegetarian diet with a polyunsaturated fat–to–saturated fat ratio of 2.0 or more arrested the progression of coronary atherosclerosis and even induced its regression in people with preexisting arterial plaques.[5] Although reductions in plasma cholesterol levels after dietary changes are usually less than 10 per cent,[61] more marked responses averaging 20 per cent reduction have been reported.[50]

Low-calorie diets aimed at controlling obesity are useful adjuncts to antihyperlipidemia regimens. Liquid protein diets are not recommended for rapid weight loss; sudden death in these circumstances has been associated with inflammatory changes in the heart.[102] Caloric intake in the range of 1000 to 1500 calories per day, with adequate intake of proteins, vitamins, and minerals, poses no harm and usually controls weight. It has been reported that during the early stages of weight reduction, a transitory rise in low-density lipoprotein (LDL) levels may occur, probably owing to reduced clearance of LDL,[31] but this phenomenon seems uncommon. In extreme caloric reduction, such as in anorexia nervosa, hypercholesterolemia may occur, and it could indicate retention of dietary cholesterol with decreased turnover of cholesterol and bile acids.[81] In these patients, hypercholesterolemia is reduced when body weight is increased.[79]

Pronounced weight loss in obese patients may be associated with supersaturated bile, and the risk of gallstones may be increased.[37] Diets rich in polyunsaturated fatty acids are also associated with an increased incidence of gallstones.[109] Grundy[37] has raised the question of whether administration of chenodeoxycholic acid, which opposes the occurrence of lithogenic bile, would

be a practical procedure in similar circumstances.

Increased polyunsaturated fat–to–saturated fat ratios brought about by dietary manipulation decreased high-density lipoprotein (HDL) cholesterol concentrations in several series of observations; however, the data, as well as increased LDL cholesterol-to-HDL cholesterol ratios, were not always consistent.[77] In addition, risks that might be associated with diets having increased polyunsaturated fatty acid content have received a great deal of attention, especially since epidemiologic intercountry data on food availability and mortality have shown that cancer of the breast and large bowel correlates positively with food fat.[20] However, putative associations with dietary polyunsaturated fatty acids need to be addressed independently from associations with total fat or saturated fat. Thus, the incidence of breast cancer does not correlate with intake of vegetable fat,[16] and the previous epidemiologic data therefore might indicate a positive correlation with the amount of dietary saturated fat. Findings that apparently contradict the previous observation were obtained in an 8-year study designed to test the hypothesis that dietary intervention alters the risk of CHD; the study included 424 men on an experimental diet and 422 men on a control diet. Diets high in polyunsaturated fatty acids, accounting for 11.4 per cent of the total calories, were associated with an increased incidence of cancer,[89] but these findings were not confirmed in four prospective studies involving 661 patients on a diet rich in polyunsaturated fatty acids and 765 patients on a usual diet who were followed from 1 to 7 years.[25] Similarly, food disappearance data from 20 industrialized countries showed a high degree of correlation between total fat, saturated fat, monounsaturated fat—but not polyunsaturated fat—or cholesterol and deaths from colon cancer.[62] Partial correlation coefficients were no longer significant when the dietary factors were adjusted for cholesterol. Furthermore, the estimated partial correlation coefficient between cholesterol and colon cancer was still significant ($p < 0.001$) when each of the other dietary factors was controlled. Thus, a diet low in fat, saturated fatty acids, and cholesterol, which is recommended for antihyperlipidemia regimens, should reduce the risk of colon cancer,[62] whereas small relative increases in polyunsaturated fatty acid content probably pose no cancer risk.[38]

The previous studies involved diets with predominantly ω-6 fatty acids from vegetable sources; because ω-3 and ω-6 polyunsaturated fatty acids may have different effects, the risk from diets rich in ω-3 fatty acids should be considered separately. Intake of predominantly ω-3 fatty acids of marine origin, advocated for patients with hypertriglyceridemia,[42] may prolong bleeding time and decrease the number of circulating platelets.[32] Serious side effects have not been reported with this therapy, but long-term observations are lacking. No undue incidence of gallstones or cancer was noted in a short series of postmortem examinations conducted in Eskimo populations naturally ingesting large amounts of marine lipids.[6,34]

ADVERSE EFFECTS OF EXERCISE

Long-term exercise programs are a useful adjunct to the treatment of patients with hyperlipidemia. In animals, muscular activity accelerates the incorporation of cholesterol into bile acids and its excretion into bile[69,73] and decreases the extent of coronary atherosclerosis.[59] Physical activity helps people lose weight, curbs appetite temporarily,[26] and is associated with decreases in plasma triglyceride levels, modest decreases in cholesterolemia, and increases in HDL cholesterol.[33,120] However, the effects of exercise on lipid levels, which are independent from body weight changes, are quite variable.[78] Moffat and Gilliam[78] reviewed 17 series totaling 721 patients who underwent physical training for periods of 3 weeks to 1 year. A reduction in plasma cholesterol was observed in nine series, whereas no changes occurred in eight series; LDL cholesterol decreased in two series and did not change in one series. An increase in HDL cholesterol was observed in two series, and no changes were found in one series. These discordant results may be due to differences in the initial lipid levels; the type of hyperlipidemia; the age and sex composition of the populations under study; the duration, intensity, and frequency of predominantly isometric or isotonic exercise; or other confounding factors such as diet composition and alcohol consumption.

Approximately 50 per cent of Americans report that they exercise;[103] hazards associated with exercise include heat injury, dehydration, sprains, fractures, and cardiovascular events.[74] Rhabdomyolysis also occurs; it generally involves muscle groups not usually stressed and happens in people with a prior sedentary background involved in exhausting exercise.[29] Deaths during strenuous prolonged exercise are not uncommon, especially in people with preexisting CHD,[117] but most deaths are related to the nature of the sport. Death rates range from 1.8 per 1000 participants in boxing to 29.6 per 1000 participants in air shows or air racing.[74] Other fatalities also occur by chance on a purely temporal basis owing to the high prevalence of CHD.[57] However, for apparently healthy adults engaged in recreational physical activity, the risk is low. The incidence of fatalities is one death per 396,000 man-hours of jogging, somewhat higher than the mortality rate of 0.29 per cent per year reported for more sedentary controls.[113] Similarly, a 10-year retrospective survey of sports offered by Young Men's Christian Associations (YMCAs) in the United States, including basketball, racquetball, handball, squash, swimming, jogging, weight lifting, and calisthenics, disclosed low rates of sudden death and cardiac arrests (approximately 1 per 3,000,000 and 1 per 2,000,000 person-hours, respectively).[68] Although deaths do occur during jogging,[114,118] even in marathons,[35] the benefits of increased physical activity seem to outweigh the risks.[58]

ADVERSE EFFECTS OF DRUG THERAPY

Antihyperlipidemia drug therapy reduced CHD in primary[61] and secondary[12] prevention clinical trials. However, the possibility of adverse effects necessitates careful consideration of benefit-to-risk ratios. Drug therapy should be instituted when the risk of hyperlipidemia is sufficiently high to justify exposing patients to medications for an indefinite period; only patients with primary hyperlipidemia who show elevated plasma lipid levels after an adequate dietary trial are candidates. Patients with secondary hyperlipidemia may be similarly considered after the primary disorder, for example, hypothyroidism, diabetes, or nephrosis, has been managed. In both instances, the specific therapeutic goals must be clear to patients and physicians alike.[60]

A number of drugs advocated for use against hypercholesterolemia can be considered harmless but useless, for example, lecithin;[28,36] others were initially considered useful but have since been shown to be harmful, for example, clofibrate (Atromid-S), estrogens,[112] and D-thyroxine.[112]

The adverse effects observed after short-term interventions with hypolipidemic drugs are commonly more annoying than serious. These side effects are generally dose-related and usually disappear once the drug is discontinued or the dose is reduced. Adverse effects associated with long-term medication are more difficult to detect and can be very serious. Not all hypolipidemic drugs have been studied adequately on a long-term basis, so that medications given for an indefinite period must be re-evaluated frequently. However, there are several agents that lower plasma lipid levels effectively and that have been used for more than two decades without serious side effects; it seems unlikely that unexpected adverse effects will be uncovered with their future use.

Finally, because drugs given to patients with hyperlipidemia may promote the fecal excretion of cholesterol and bile acids, the long-term effects of these substances on the colonic mucosa are of concern. It has been hypothesized that the gut microflora metabolize acid and neutral steroids to carcinogens active in the large bowel.[4,48] However, the fact that cholesterol has no colon tumor–promoting activity in germ-free or conventional rat models[91] suggests that neither cholesterol nor any cholesterol metabolite is a carcinogen or promoter of cancer in the colonic mucosa.[90] Although reportedly[62] there is a positive correlation between dietary cholesterol and colon cancer, other human data are contradictory: the excretion of neutral steroids in patients with colon cancer has been reported to be increased[49] or unchanged.[80] Similar contradictions are apparent with regard to fecal acid steroids: Even if lithocholic and chenodeoxycholic acids promote colon tumors in rats,[90] a long-term clinical trial with bile acid–binding resins has not shown increased cancer death rates.[61] Thus, diversion of cholesterol and bile acids to the gut by medication does not seem to increase the risk of cancer.

Clofibrate. The early reports[47,83] on consistent hypolipidemic responses to clofibrate (Atromid-S) led to large primary[84] and secondary[111] prevention clinical trials that established the occurrence of unacceptable adverse effects after prolonged intake. In the World Health Organization 5-year primary prevention trial,[84] Atromid-S intake effected about a 9 per cent mean reduction in the serum cholesterol level and reduced the incidence of nonfatal myocardial infarction by 25 per cent, but the number of deaths and crude death rates from all causes significantly exceeded those in the control groups. The greatest proportionate excess in the cancer death rate was related to the liver and the biliary and intestinal systems; the cholecystectomy rate for gallstones was also higher.[19] In the secondary prevention trial, which also lasted 5 years, effectiveness was not demonstrated, and although cancer deaths were not increased, the incidence of gallstones was higher than that in controls.[111] These results led to United States

Food and Drug Administration (FDA) restrictions on the use of Atromid-S in patients with hyperlipidemia, except those with primary disbetalipoproteinemia (type III hyperlipidemia).[82]

Gemfibrozil. Gemfibrozil (Lopid) is a phenoxy acid derivative with a structure somewhat similar to that of clofibrate; it is effective against hyperlipidemia. Clinical studies conducted for 5 years demonstrated good tolerance and acceptance.[101] Side effects were not very common; they mostly involved the gastrointestinal tract in 11.1 per cent of 496 patients.[17] These symptoms disappeared when the dose was reduced or when treatment was discontinued. Liver biopsies performed in nine patients receiving gemfibrozil for up to 27 months[21] and in 27 patients receiving the drug for up to 7 years[40] disclosed no microscopic abnormalities attributable to the drug. However, liver carcinoma and benign Leydig cell tumors have been induced in male rats through use of gemfibrozil in high doses.[17] Moreover, the similarities in chemical structure between gemfibrozil and clofibrate, as well as a possible cancer hazard associated with occupational exposure to phenoxy acid compounds,[41] indicate that caution should be exercised in long-term gemfibrozil use.

Nicotinic Acid. Nicotinic acid is an effective hypolipidemic agent that has been used since 1955[1] despite annoying side effects. The most common side effect is flushing, a reddening of the skin with the sensation of heat or itching, that mainly affects the upper body and face and occurs within 1 or 2 hours of ingestion. That these symptoms usually disappear after repeated administration of nicotinic acid suggests exhaustion of tissular mediator substances.[3] Flushing, which may reappear intermittently even in well-conditioned patients, may be decreased by (1) use of initial small doses and slow progression to higher doses over the course of several weeks;[44,45] (2) ingestion of nicotinic acid with meals; (3) use of retard compounds; and (4) prior administration of aspirin, which probably inhibits flushing by interfering with the release of prostaglandins.

Deterioration of oral glucose tolerance is commonly observed during therapy with nicotinic acid.[8] It is probably due to increased glycogen mobilization from the liver secondary to a reduction in the nonesterified fatty acid concentration.[2] Hyperuricemia also may be elicited by nicotinic acid, apparently through an increase in purine synthesis[10] and reduced renal uric acid clearance.[30] Liver dysfunction—elevation of serum transaminases, alkaline phosphatase, and bilirubin levels[22,85]—may lead the physician to discontinue therapy; the abnormalities then usually disappear.[88] Toxic amblyopia and acanthosis nigricans have also been reported under these circumstances.[44,45] Although intake of nicotinic acid was associated with a nonsignificant increase in the incidence of gallstones,[111] the drug did not raise the concentration of biliary cholesterol.[37]

Bile Acid Sequestrant Resins. Bile acid sequestrant resins (cholestyramine [Questran], colestipol [Colestid]) have been prescribed for hypercholesterolemia for more than 20 years[11,43] without serious side effects. Long-term compliance in a large series of patients resulted in decreased CHD morbidity and mortality without an increase in total mortality.[61] Because cholestyramine, used initially, and colestipol, used more recently,[108] have similar side effects, they will be discussed together. Both are equally disagreeable to patients. The most common complaint is a gritty, sandy sensation in the mouth and pharynx; it might be decreased if the drug were mixed with juice, a carbonated beverage, or applesauce. Other complaints involve the gastrointestinal tract, that is, constipation (counteracted with bulk laxatives), gastric fullness, and gastric pain; these may proscribe its use in patients with a gastroduodenal ulcer or obstructive disease.[13] Because bile acid sequestrant resins may aggravate anorectal disorders, they should be used with caution in patients with hemorrhoids.[13] In the presence of liver or bowel disease or when high doses are used, steatorrhea and impairment of absorption of fat-soluble vitamins may occur; large doses may produce hyperchloremia in small children.[13] These resins may also bind certain drugs (for example, thyroxine, digitalis glycosides, warfarin, thiazide diuretics, tetracycline, vancomycin, phenylbutazone, and phenobarbital) and interfere with their absorption; administration of drugs 1 hour before administration of the resin usually insures normal absorption.[45] There is no increase in cholelithiasis with the use of these agents,[61] probably because of a compensating increase in bile acid synthesis.[37] The raised triglyceridemia observed with the use of these compounds may indicate an increase in synthesis of very-low-density lipoprotein (VLDL), which, in most cases, returns to normal after a few weeks.[13]

The high cost of these agents must be considered by patients embarking on long-term treatment.

Probucol. Probucol (Lorelco) is a hypocholesterolemic drug that has been well tolerated in patients followed up to 9 years.[76] No deaths have been attributed to its use; diarrhea was observed

in 19.3 per cent of patients in the first year, and none was observed by the end of the seventh year.[76] A review of several controlled and open studies[46] involving more than 800 patients followed for 6 weeks to 5 years disclosed no serious adverse effects of probucol. The most frequently occurring side effects have been loose stools, mild diarrhea, nausea, and vomiting; about 3 per cent of patients have discontinued treatment during long-term (mean 3.6 years) administration.[110] In the aforementioned review, less common reactions, for which causative relationships were not always established, were mentioned. These included hyperhydrosis, pruritus, angioneurotic edema, dizziness, palpitations, and purpura. It is disturbing, though, that the levels of HDL cholesterol were decreased and that the LDL cholesterol–to–HDL cholesterol ratios were increased in patients receiving probucol.[53] Other investigators have not observed decreases in the HDL cholesterol concentration but have reported lowered levels of apolipoprotein-AI (Apo-AI) and apolipoprotein-AII (Apo-AII).[92]

Epinephrine-induced ventricular fibrillation observed in dogs given probucol seems to be species-specific.[75] The occurrence of a prolonged QT_c interval, ventricular arrhythmias, and death in monkeys receiving probucol and fed high-fat food (21 per cent of diet by weight) did not depend on the type of fatty acids; it was observed equally with hydrogenated coconut oil, medium-chain triglycerides, and corn oil.[24] Patients ingesting probucol showed prolonged QT_c intervals in proportion to serum concentrations of the drug; the average increase of 20 msec was not usually detected on ordinary electrocardiograms.[14]

Neomycin. Neomycin, first given as a hypocholesterolemic agent more than 25 years ago,[97] is useful for some patients.[98] The drug markedly reduces body cholesterol pools,[95,100] reduces cholesterol absorption, and increases fecal excretion of neutral steroids without changing the total excretion of bile acids.[56] At doses much lower than those necessary for antibiotic activity, it is well tolerated. However, enterocolitis due to resistant organisms can occur; otic, hepatic, renal, and bone marrow toxicity can appear, especially in patients with pre-existing bowel disease.

Mevinolin and Compactin. Two fungal metabolites, mevinolin (MK-803) and compactin (ML-263B), inhibit sterol synthesis and lower LDL concentrations very effectively.[39,115,116] Although no serious side effects have been reported,[55,115,116] their relatively recent use suggests caution because of the possibility of adverse effects with long-term administration.

Combined Drug Regimens. It is common to use combined-drug regimens in treating patients with hyperlipidemia when single drugs are ineffective. Such combinations include neomycin and clofibrate;[96] oxyphenol derivatives and nicotinic acid;[87] cholestyramine and neomycin;[27] colestipol and nicotinic acid;[54] colestipol and probucol;[23] cholestyramine and pectin;[99] colestipol, probucol, and nicotinic acid;[106] and neomycin and nicotinic acid.[52] Increased effectiveness may allow one to lower the dose of drugs used individually and thus theoretically decrease side effects. On the other hand, combined drugs may have the opposite effects on plasma lipids; for instance, cholestyramine plus neomycin decreases HDL levels unaffected or elevated by the bile acid sequestrant resin.[51]

Miscellaneous Interventions. Alfalfa meal,[72] as well as an extract of alfalfa meal operationally termed "alfalfa saponins,"[64] reduced hypercholesterolemia and induced regression of atherosclerosis in monkeys,[63] without any evidence of toxicity;[71] these compounds have not been approved for clinical use. Alfalfa seeds, ingested as food, were better accepted by people, and their short-term intake was associated with pronounced hypocholesterolemic effects,[65] but transitory pancytopenia developed in one man who ingested alfalfa seeds intermittently for 5 months.[66] The seeds induced a systemic lupus erythematosus–like syndrome in monkeys.[9] The substance responsible for the toxic effects was identified as L-canavanine, a nonprotein amino acid.[67] Destruction of L-canavanine in seeds by autoclaving preserves the hypocholesterolemic activity of the saponins while eliminating the toxic effects.[70,71] Clinical trials conducted with autoclaved alfalfa seeds are still in the early stage.[86]

An effective intervention in lowering cholesterolemia, partial ileal bypass,[15] is being evaluated with respect to its effects on the progression of atherosclerotic plaques.[7] Evaluation of the risk-to-benefit ratio must await analysis of the data.

CONCLUSIONS

A variety of treatments are available to lower elevated plasma lipid levels in patients with hyperlipidemia. Many of these procedures, for example, dietary modification, recreational physical exercise, and drug intervention, may be associated with adverse side effects that range from mere annoyances to uncommon, serious consequences.

The protracted therapeutic lowering of cholesterolemia in patients with hyperlipidemia may prevent the manifestations of CHD, arrest the progression of coronary atherosclerosis, and even induce its regression. However, as in other clinical circumstances, risk-to-benefit ratios must be taken into consideration before reaching a therapeutic decision. Therefore, the management of hyperlipidemia requires that the risk of nontreatment be weighed against the adverse effects that might arise from treatment.

ACKNOWLEDGMENT

This is publication #1439 of the Oregon Regional Primate Research Center, Supported in part by grants from the National Institutes of Health (RR–00163 and HL–116587).

REFERENCES

1. Altschul, R., Hoffer, A., and Stephen, J.D.: Influence of nicotinic acid on serum cholesterol in man. Arch. Biochem., 54:558–559, 1955.
2. Ammon, H.P.T., Estler, C.J., and Heim, F.: In Gay, K.F., and Carlson, L.A. (eds.): Metabolic Effects of Nicotinic Acid and Its Derivatives. Bern, Huber, 1971, p. 799.
3. Andersson, R.G., Aberg, G., Brattsand, R., et al.: Studies on the mechanism of flush induced by nicotinic acid. Acta Pharmacol. Toxicol., 41:1–10, 1977.
4. Aries, V., Crowther, J.S., Drasar, B.S., et al.: Bacteria and the etiology of cancer of the large bowel. Gut, 10:334–335, 1969.
5. Arntzenius, A.C., Kromhout, D., Barth, J., et al.: Diet, lipoproteins and the progression of coronary atherosclerosis. The Leiden Intervention Trial. N. Engl. J. Med., 312:805–811, 1985.
6. Arthaud, J.B.: Cause of death in 339 Alaskan natives as determined by autopsy. Arch. Pathol., 90:433–438, 1970.
7. Azen, S., Blankenhorn, D.H., and Nessim, S.: Status of controlled clinical trials in peripheral vessel atherosclerosis. In Malinow, M.R., and Blaton, V. (eds.): Regression of Atherosclerotic Lesions: Experimental Studies and Observations in Humans. New York, Plenum Press, 1984, pp. 277–288.
8. Balasse, E.O., and Neef, A.: Influence of nicotinic acid on the rates of turnover and oxidation of plasma glucose in man. Metabolism, 22:1193–1204, 1973.
9. Bardana, E.J., Malinow, M.R., Houghton, D.C., et al.: Diet-induced systemic lupus erythematosus (SLE) in primates. Am. J. Kidney Dis., 1:345–352, 1982.
10. Becker, M.A., Raivio, K.O., and Meyer, L.J.: The effects of nicotinic acid on human purine metabolism. Clin. Res., 21:616, 1973.
11. Berkowitz, D.: Selective blood lipid reductions by newer pharmacologic agents. Am. J. Cardiol., 2:834–840, 1964.
12. Brensike, J.R., Levy, R.I., Kelsey, S.F., et al.: Effects

of therapy with cholestyramine on progression of coronary arteriosclerosis: Results of the NHLBI Type II Coronary Intervention Study. Circulation, 69:313–324, 1984.

13. Brown, W.V., Goldberg, I.J., and Ginsberg, H.N.: Treatment of common lipoprotein disorders. Prog. Cardiovasc. Dis., 17:1–20, 1984.

14. Browne, K.F., Prystowsky, E.N., Heger, J.J., et al.: Prolongation of the QT interval induced by probucol: Demonstration of a method for determining QT interval change induced by a drug. Am. Heart J., 107:680–684, 1984.

15. Buchwald, H., Moore, R.B., and Varco, R.L.: Surgical treatment of hyperlipidemia. Circulation, 49(Suppl. 1):1-1–1-37, 1974.

16. Carroll, K.K.: Experimental evidence of dietary factors and hormone-dependent cancers. Cancer Res., 35:3374–3383, 1975.

17. Compendium of Pharmacological and Clinical Studies. Morris Plains, New Jersey, Warner-Lambert Company, 1982.

18. Connor, W.E., and Connor, S.L.: The dietary treatment of hyperlipidemia. Rationale, technique and efficacy. Med. Clin. North Am., 66:485–518, 1982.

19. Cooper, J., Geizerova, H., and Oliver, M.F.: Clofibrate and gallstones. Lancet, 1:1083, 1975.

20. Correa, P.: Epidemiological correlations between diet and cancer frequency. Cancer Res., 41:3685–3689, 1981.

21. De La Iglesia, F.A., Lewis, J.E., Buchanan, R.A., et al.: Light and electron microscopy of liver in hyperlipoproteinemic patients under long-term gemfibrozil treatment. Atherosclerosis, 43:19–37, 1982.

22. Dietman, K., and Stork, H.: Bilirubinamie nach Applikation von Nicotinsaure. Med. Klin, 71:1047–1050, 1976.

23. Dujovne, C.A., Krehbiel, P., Decoursey, S., et al.: Probucol with colestipol in the treatment of hypercholesterolemia. Ann. Intern. Med., 100:477–482, 1984.

24. Eder, H.A.: The effect of diet on the transport of probucol in monkeys. Artery, 10:105–107, 1982.

25. Ederer, F., Leren, P., Turpeinen, O., et al.: Cancer among men on cholesterol lowering diets. Lancet, 2:203–206, 1971.

26. Edholm, O.G., Fletcher, J.S., Widdowson, E.M., et al.: Energy expenditure and food intake of individual men. Br. J. Nutr., 9:286–300, 1955.

27. Faergeman, O.: Effects and side-effects of treatment of hypercholesterolemia with cholestyramine and neomycin. Acta Med. Scand., 194:165–167, 1973.

28. Fletcher, D.C.: Lecithin for hyperlipemia—harmless but useless. J.A.M.A., 238:64, 1977.

29. Geller, S.A.: Extreme exertion rhabdomyolysis. A histopathologic study of 31 cases. Human Pathol., 4:241–250, 1973.

30. Gershon, S.L., and Fox, I.H.: Pharmacologic effects of nicotinic acid on human purine metabolism. J. Lab. Clin. Med., 84:179–186, 1974.

31. Ginsberg, H., Le, N.-A., Gibson, J., et al.: Effect of weight reduction on very low density lipoprotein and low density lipoprotein apoprotein B metabolism. Clin. Res., 30:393A, 1982.

32. Goodnight, S.H.., Jr., Harris, W.S., Connor, W.E., et al.: Polyunsaturated fatty acids, hyperlipidemia, and thrombosis. Arteriosclerosis, 2:87–113, 1982.

33. Gordon, D.J., Witztum, J.L., Hunninghake, D., et al.: Habitual physical activity and high-density lipoprotein cholesterol in men with primary hypercholesterolemia. Circulation, 67:512–520, 1983.

34. Gottman, A.W.: A report of one hundred three autopsies on Alaskan natives. Arch. Pathol., 70:117–124, 1960.

35. Green, L.H., Cohen, S.I., and Kurland, G.: Fatal myocardial infarction in marathon racing. Ann. Intern. Med., 84:704–706, 1976.

36. Gretzen, H., Raetzer, H., Stiehl, A., et al.: The effect of polyunsaturated phosphatidylcholine on plasma lipids and fecal sterol excretion. Atherosclerosis, 36:81–88, 1980.

37. Grundy, S.M.: Biliary lipids, gallstones, and treatment of hyperlipidemia. Eur. J. Clin. Invest., 9:179–180, 1979.

38. Grundy, S.M.: Recommendations for the treatment of hyperlipidemia in adults. A joint statement of the Nutrition Committee and the Council on Arteriosclerosis of the American Heart Association. Arteriosclerosis, 4:445A–468A, 1984.

39. Haba, T., Mabuchi, H., Yoshimura, A., et al.: Effects of ML-236B (compactin) on sterol synthesis and low density lipoprotein receptor activities in fibroblasts of patients with homozygous familial hypercholesterolemia. J. Clin. Invest., 67:1532–1540, 1980.

40. Hanefeld, M., Kemmer, C.H., Leonhardt, W., et al.: Effects of p-chlorophenooxyisobutyric acid (CPIB) on the human liver. Atherosclerosis, 36:159, 1980.

41. Hardell, L., and Sandstrom, A.: Case-control study: Soft tissue sarcomas and exposure to phenoxyacetic acids or chlorophenols. Br. J. Cancer, 39:711–717, 1979.

42. Harris, W.S., Connor, W.E., and McMurry, M.P.: The comparative reduction of the plasma lipids and lipoproteins by dietary polyunsaturated fats: Salmon oil versus vegetable oils. Metabolism, 32:179–184, 1983.

43. Hashim, S.A., and Van Itallie, T.B.: Cholestyramine resin therapy for hypercholesterolemia: Clinical and metabolic studies. J.A.M.A., 192::289–293, 1965.

44. Havel, R.J.: Approach to the patient with hyperlipidemia. Med. Clin. North Am., 66:319–333, 1982.

45. Havel, R.J., and Kane, J.P.: Therapy of hyperlipidemic states. Annu. Rev. Med., 33:417–433, 1982.

46. Heel, R.C., Brogden, R.N., Speight, T.M., et al.: Probucol: A review of its pharmacological properties and therapeutic use in patients with hypercholesterolaemia. Drugs, 15:409–428, 1978.

47. Hellman, L., Zunoff, B., Kessler, G., et al.: Reduction of serum cholesterol and lipids by ethyl chlorophenoxyisobutyrate. Journal of Atheroscleroses Research, 3:454–466, 1963.

48. Hill, M.J., Drasar, B.S., Aires, V.C., et al.: Bacteria and etiology of cancer of the large bowel. Lancet, 1:95–100, 1971.

49. Hill, M.J., Drasar, B.S., Williams, R.E.O., et al.: Fecal bile acid and clostridia in patients with cancer of the large bowel. Lancet, 2:535–539, 1975.

50. Hjermann, I., Holme, I., Velve Byre, K., et al.: Effect of diet and smoking intervention on the incidence of coronary heart disease. Lancet, 2:1303–1310, 1981.

51. Hoeg, J.M., Maher, M.B., Bailey, K.R., et al.: Effects of combination cholestyramine-neomycin treatment on plasma lipoprotein concentrations in type II hyperlipoproteinemia. Am. J. Cardiol., 55:1282–1286, 1985.

52. Hoeg, J.M., Zech, L.A., Gregg, R.E., et al.: Combination of neomycin and niacin normalizes the

plasma lipoprotein concentrations in type II hyper-lipoproteinemia. Arteriosclerosis, 4:544a, 1984.

53. Hunninghake, D.B., Bell, C., and Olson, L.: Effect of probucol on plasma lipids and lipoproteins in type IIb hyperlipoproteinemia. Atherosclerosis, 37:469–474, 1980.

54. Illingworth, D.R., Phillipson, B.E., Rapp, J.H., et al.: Colestipol plus nicotinic acid in treatment of het-erozygous familial hypercholesterolemia. Lancet, 1:296–298, 1981.

55. Illingworth, D.R., and Sexton, G.J.: Hypocholester-olemic effects of mevinolin in patients with heter-ozygous familial hypercholesterolemia. J. Clin. In-vest., 74:1972–1978, 1984.

56. Kesaniemi, Y.A., and Grundy, S.M.: Turnover of low density lipoproteins during inhibition of cholesterol absorption by neomycin. Arteriosclerosis, 4:41–48, 1984.

57. Koplan, J.P.: Cardiovascular deaths while running. J.A.M.A., 242:2578–2579, 1979.

58. Koplan, J.P., Powell, K.E., Sikes, R.K., et al.: An epidemiologic study of the benefits and risks of run-ning. J.A.M.A., 248:3118–3121, 1982.

59. Kramsch, D.M., Aspen, A.J., Abramowitz, B.M., et al.: Reduction of coronary atherosclerosis by mod-erate conditioning exercise in monkeys on an ath-erogenic diet. N. Engl. J. Med., 305:1483–1489, 1981.

60. LaRosa, J.C.: The mechanism of action of lipid-low-ering drugs. Angiology, 33:562–576, 1982.

61. Lipid Research Clinic Program: The Lipid Research Clinics coronary primary prevention trial results. J.A.M.A., 252:351–364, 1984.

62. Liu, K., Moss, D., Persky, V., et al.: Dietary choles-terol, fat, and fibre, and colon cancer mortality. Lan-cet, 2:782–785, 1979.

63. Malinow, M.R., McLaughlin, P., Stafford, C., et al.: Effects of alfalfa saponins on regression of athero-sclerosis in monkeys. In Hauss, W.H., and Wissler, R.W. (eds.): Rheinisch-Westfalische Akademie der Wissenschaften, Abhandlung Band 70. Second Munster International Arteriosclerosis Symposium: Clinical Implications of Recent Research Results in Arteriosclerosis. Opladen, West Germany, West-deutscher Verlag 1983, pp. 241–254.

64. Malinow, M.R.: Triterpenoid saponins in mammals: Effects on cholesterol metabolism and atheroscle-rosis. In Nes, W.D., Fuller, G., and Tsai, L.S. (eds.): Biochemistry and Function of Isopentenoids in Plants. New York, Marcel Dekker, 1984, pp. 229–246.

65. Malinow, M.R.: Alfalfa seeds: Effect on cholesterol me-tabolism. Experientia, 36:562–563, 1980.

66. Malinow, M.R., Bardana, E.J., Jr., and Goodnight, S.H., Jr.: Pancytopenia during ingestion of alfalfa seeds. Lancet, 1:615, 1981.

67. Malinow, M.R., Bardana, E.J., Jr., Pirofsky, B., et al.: Systemic lupus erythematosus-like syndrome in monkeys fed alfalfa sprouts: Role of a nonprotein amino acid. Science, 216:415–417, 1982.

68. Malinow, M.R., McGarry, D.L., and Kuehl, K.S.: Is exercise testing indicated for asymptomatic active people? J. Cardiac Rehabil. 4:376–380, 1984.

69. Malinow, M.R., and McLaughlin, P.: Muscular activity and the degradation of cholesterol by the liver. Ath-erosclerosis, 15:153–162, 1972.

70. Malinow, M.R., McLaughlin, P., Bardana, E.J., Jr., et al.: Elimination of toxicity from diets containing

alfalfa seeds. Food Chem. Toxicol., 22:583–587, 1984.

71. Malinow, M.R., McLaughlin, P., McNulty, W.P., et al.: Lack of toxicity of alfalfa saponins in monkeys. J. Med. Primatol., 11:106–118, 1982.

72. Malinow, M.R., McLaughlin, P., Naito, H.K., et al.: Effect of alfalfa meal on shrinkage (regression) or atherosclerotic plaques during cholesterol feeding in monkeys. Atherosclerosis, 30:27–43, 1978.

73. Malinow, M.R., McLaughlin, P., Perley, A.M., et al.: The effect of muscular activity on bile acid excretion in rats. J. Appl. Physiol., 29:610–614, 1970.

74. Mann, G.V.: The Care and Feeding of Athletes. New York, Le Jacq Publishers, 1980, p. 92.

75. Marshall, F.N., and Lewis, J.E.: Sensitization to ep-inephrine-induced ventricular fibrillation produced by probucol in dogs. Toxicol. Appl. Pharmacol., 24:594–602, 1973.

76. McCaughan, D.: Nine years of treatment with prob-ucol. Artery, 10:56–70, 1982.

77. McGill, H.C., McMahan, C.A., and Wene, J.D.: Un-resolved problems in the diet-heart issue. Arterios-clerosis, 1:164–176, 1981.

78. Moffat, R.J., and Gilliam, T.B.: Serum lipids and lipo-proteins as affected by exercise: A review. Artery, 6:1–19, 1979.

79. Mordasini, R., Klose, G., and Greten, H.: Secondary type II hyperlipoproteinemia in patients with an-orexia nervosa. Metabolism, 27:71–79, 1978.

80. Moskovitz, M., White, C., and Floch, M.H.: Acid and neutral sterol excretion in carcinoma of the colon and control subjects. Clin. Res., 26:584A, 1978.

81. Nestel, P.J.: Cholesterol metabolism in anorexia ner-vosa and hypercholesterolemia. J. Clin. Endocrinol. Metab., 38:325–328, 1974.

82. New restrictions on clofibrate. Food and Drug Admin-istration Bulletin, 9:14–15, 1979.

83. Oliver, M.F.: Reduction of serum lipid and uric acid levels by an orally active androsterone. Lancet, 1:1321–1323, 1962.

84. Oliver,: M.R., Heady, J.A., Morris, J.N., et al.: A co-operative trial in the primary prevention of is-chaemic heart disease using clofibrate. Br. Heart J., 40:1069–1118, 1978.

85. Olsson, A.G., Oro, L., and Rossner, S.: Clinical and metabolic effects of pentaerythritol tetranicotinate (Perycit) and a comparison with plain nicotinic acid. Atherosclerosis, 19:61, 1974.

86. Olsson, A.G.: Personal communication.

87. Olsson, A.G., Erikson, U., Helmius, G., et al.: Regres-sion of femoral atherosclerosis in humans: Meth-odological and clinical problems associated with studies of femoral atherosclerosis development as assessed by angiograms. In Malinow, M.R., and Bla-ton, V. (eds.): Regression of Atherosclerotic Lesions: Experimental Studies and Observations in Humans. New York, Plenum Press, 1984, pp. 311–328.

88. Parsons, W.B., Jr.: The effect of nicotinic acid on serum lipids. Am. J. Clin. Nutr., 8:471, 1960.

89. Pearce, M.L., and Dayton, S.: Incidence of cancer in men on a diet high in polyunsaturated fat. Lancet, 1:464–467, 1971.

90. Reddy, B.S.: Dietary fat and its relationship to large bowel cancer. Cancer Res., 41:3700–3705, 1981.

91. Reddy, B.S., and Watanabe, K.: Effect of cholesterol metabolites and promoting effect of lithocholic acid in colon carcinogenesis in germ-free and conven-tional F344 rats. Cancer Res., 39:1521–1524, 1979.

92. Riesen, W.F., Keller, M., and Mordasini, R.: Probucol

in hypercholesterolemia. A double blind study. Atherosclerosis, *36*:201–207, 1980.

93. Rose, G., Blackburn, H., Keys, A., et al.: Colon cancer and blood cholesterol. Lancet, *1*:181–183, 1974.
94. Rose, G., and Shipley, M.J.: Plasma lipids and mortality: A source of error. Lancet, *1*:523–526, 1980.
95. Samuel, P., Holtzman, C.M., Meilman, E., et al.: Effect of neomycin on exchangeable pools of cholesterol in the steady state. J. Clin. Invest., *47*:1806–1818, 1968.
96. Samuel, P., Holtzman, C.M., Meilman, E., et al.: Reduction of serum cholesterol and triglyceride levels by the combined administration of neomycin and clofibrate. Circulation, *41*:109–114, 1970.
97. Samuel, P., and Steiner, A.: Effect of neomycin on serum cholesterol level of man. Proc. Soc. Exp. Biol. Med., *100*:193–195, 1959.
98. Samuel, P., and Waithe, W.I.: Reduction of serum cholesterol concentrations by neomycin, para-aminosalicylic acid, and other antibacterial drugs in man. Circulation, *24*:578, 1961.
99. Schwandt, P., Richter, W.O., Weisweiler, P., et al.: Cholestyramine plus pectin in treatment of patients with familial hypercholesterolemia. Atherosclerosis, *44*:379–383, 1982.
100. Sedaghat, A., Samuel, P., Crouse, J.R., et al.: Effects of neomycin on absorption, synthesis and/or flux of cholesterol in man. J. Clin. Invest., *55*:12–21, 1975.
101. Seed, M., Niththyananthan, R., and Wynn, V.: Long-term treatment of hyperlipidaemia with gemfibrozil. J. Inter. Biomed. Inf. Data, *3*:23–36, 1982.
102. Siegel, R.J., Cabeen, W.R., and Roberts, W.C.: Prolonged Q-T interval–ventricular tachycardia syndrome from massive rapid weight loss utilizing the liquid-protein-modified-fast diet: Sudden death in sinus node ganglionitis and neuritis. Am. Heart J., *102*:121, 1981.
103. Stamler, J.: Primary prevention of coronary heart disease: The last 20 years. Am. J. Cardiol., *47*:722–735, 1981.
104. Starzl, T.E., Bahnson, H.T., Hardesty, R.L., et al.: Heart-liver transplantation in a patient with familial hypercholesterolaemia. Lancet, *1*:1382–1383, 1984.
105. Starzl, T.E., Chase, H.P., Putnam, C.W., et al.: Portacaval shunt in hyperlipoproteinaemia. Lancet, *2*:940–944, 1973.
106. Stein, E.A., and Mellies, M.J.: Successful treatment of receptor defective homozygous familial hypercholesterolemia by combined drug therapy. Arteriosclerosis, *3*:485a, 1983.
107. Stoffel, W.: Specific extracorporeal LDL apheresis: Method and clinical application. *In* Carlson, L.A.,

and Olsson, A.G. (eds.): Treatment of Hyperlipoproteinemia. New York, Raven Press, 1984, pp. 137–140.

108. Stone, N.J.: Cholesterol, colestipol, and coronary heart disease. J. Chronic Dis., *31*:1–3, 1978.
109. Sturdevant, R.A.L., Pearce, M.L., and Dayton, S.: Increased prevalence of cholelithiasis in men ingesting a serum cholesterol lowering diet. N. Engl. J. Med., *288*:24–27, 1979.
110. Taylor, H.L., Nolan, R.B., Tedeschi, R.E., et al.: Combined results of the study of probucol at 1 gm/day in eight centers. Clin. Pharmcol. Ther., *23*:131, 1978.
111. The Coronary Drug Project Research Group: Clofibrate and niacin in coronary heart disease. J.A.M.A., *231*:360–381, 1975.
112. The Coronary Drug Project Research Group: The Coronary Drug Project: Initial findings leading to modifications of its research protocol. J.A.M.A., *214*:1303–1313, 1970.
113. Thompson, P.D., Funk, E.J., Carlton, R.A., et al.: Incidence of death during jogging in Rhode Island from 1975 through 1980. J.A.M.A., *247*:2535–2538, 1982.
114. Thompson, P.D., Stern, M.P., et al.: Death during jogging or running. J.A.M.A., *242*:1265–1267, 1979.
115. Tobert, J.A., Bell, D., Birtwell, J., et al.: Cholesterol-lowering effect of mevinolin, an inhibitor of 3-hydroxy-3-methylglutaryl-coenzyme A reductase, in healthy volunteers. J. Clin. Invest., *69*:913–919, 1982.
116. Tobert, J.A., Hitzenberger, G., Kukovetz, W.R., et al.: Rapid and substantial lowering of human serum cholesterol by mevinolin (MK-803), an inhibitor of hydroxymethylglutaryl-coenzyme A reductase. Atherosclerosis, *41*:61–65, 1981.
117. Vuvori, I., Makarainen, M., and Jaaskelainen, A.: Sudden death and physical activity. Cardiology, *63*:287–304, 1978.
118. Waller, B.F., and Roberts, W.C.: Sudden death while running in conditioned runners aged 40 years or over. Am. J. Cardiol., *45*:1292–1300, 1980.
119. Williams, R.R., Sorlie, P.D., et al.: Cancer incidence by levels of cholesterol. J.A.M.A., *245*:247–252, 1981.
120. Wood, P.D., Haskell, W.L., Stern, M.P., et al.: Plasma lipoprotein distributions in male and female runners. Ann. N.Y. Acad. Sci., *301*:748–763, 1977.

Oregon Regional Primate Research Center
505 N.W. 185th Avenue
Beaverton, Oregon 97006

Adverse Effects of Antihypertensive Treatment

Barry J. Materson, M.D. *

In the 1980s, antihypertensive drugs enjoy an exceptionally good benefit-to-risk ratio. Major advances in medicinal chemistry have completely changed the approach to treating patients with hypertension. Only 30 years ago, the benefit-to-risk ratio for available antihypertensive drugs was so poor that only the more severely ill hypertensive patients were identified and treated. Development of newer drugs, particularly the diuretics, permitted successful treatment of hypertensive patients far more safely. When the positive benefits of treatment were unequivocably demonstrated in 1967, massive screening of the population for hypertension and treatment of the patients thus identified became practical.[65]

The current therapeutic problem is not so much directed to the relatively easy task of lowering elevated blood pressure as it is to lowering blood pressure in a virtually asymptomatic population without causing symptomatic adverse effects. In addition, some drugs that are effective have metabolic consequences that, at least in theory, pose a cardiovascular risk by facilitating atherosclerosis or cardiac dysrhythmias. This has caused a major re-examination of the strategy for the treatment of uncomplicated hypertension.

Metabolic adverse effects are relatively easy to quantitate. Cardiac dysrhythmias can also be readily quantitated, although great attention must be given to methodologic detail. On the other hand, quantitation of those symptomatic adverse effects that conceivably could alter quality of life is extraordinarily difficult. There are major problems of objectivity. Psychometric testing instruments are not necessarily highly accurate, may be difficult to use, and are not universally accepted. In order to assess symptoms that have an impact on quality of life, it is mandatory that clinical trials be placebo-controlled, double-blinded, carefully randomized prospectively, and conducted by investigators who are aware of the numerous pitfalls of such trials. For example, we have seen mini-epidemics of specific adverse effects when patients participating in a given clinical trial were allowed to discuss their symptoms, both real and imagined, with each other in a common waiting room.

There is a clearly identified risk of labeling a patient with a diagnosis of hypertension.[6,29] Such patients may begin to perceive themselves as being ill, have a greater frequency of absenteeism from work, and have a greater background frequency of symptoms even without drug treatment. Such symptoms include headache, weakness, depression, and sexual dysfunction. Therefore, it is critical to consider the adverse effects that occur in patients taking blinded placebo in relation to those effects that occur in patients taking active drug.

An encyclopedic listing of adverse effects of each of the given antihypertensive drugs can be found in any standard textbook of pharmacology, the Physicians' Desk Reference, or the package insert for the specific drug. In this article, I shall select adverse effects that I believe to be clinically important with the perspective of attempting to prevent them, to deal with them if they do occur, or to avoid overreacting to them.

A common cause of adverse effects from antihypertensive drugs is overdose of the drug based

---

*Professor of Medicine, Department of Medicine, University of Miami School of Medicine; Acting Chief, Medical Service, Veterans Administration Medical Center, Miami, Florida

on inadequate or misleading information about the blood pressure. Some patients are notorious office hyperreactors, and it is necessary to base their treatment on the blood pressure that they have while under less terrifying conditions for them. If at all possible, a member of the family should be recruited to perform blood pressure measurements at home in order to provide the clinician with data that are likely to be more useful in the regulation of blood pressure. The clinician must ascertain that the surrogate practitioner is sufficiently skilled in making accurate determinations. That individual should also be cautioned against using home blood pressure readings to adjust medication dose without permission of the clinician and should be cautioned emphatically against using the device as a basis for sharing medications or prescribing for other relatives and neighbors.

Blood pressure readings may be elevated by pain, fear, a very cold room, emotional upset, and a full stomach, bowel, or bladder. To the extent possible, these conditions should be eliminated prior to determining the blood pressure in the office. Either the supine or seated blood pressure may be used, depending on which is most convenient. At least on the initial visit and once annually, blood pressure should be determined in both arms, and if a difference is detected, the higher reading should be used. Blood pressure must be determined at each visit with the patient standing. Significant orthostatic hypotension may be present for a wide variety of reasons, including the neuropathies of diabetes, uremia, alcohol abuse, and amyloidosis. Before drug treatment is initiated, it is crucial to determine the extent of blood pressure fall on standing. It is equally important to determine the effect of any given therapy on standing blood pressure in order to avoid administering drug doses that are likely to cause symptomatic orthostatic hypertension or even syncope.

Elderly patients, particularly those with isolated systolic hypertension, must be treated with special caution. Low doses of drugs should be used, upward titration should be made with care, and the temptation to overreact to the characteristic lability of blood pressure in this population[36] should be rejected. Pseudohypertension should be ruled out by means of Osler's maneuver.[48] The clinician must recognize that it may not be possible to achieve perfect control of a given elderly patient. Partial treatment is far better than no treatment, and the appropriate compromise must be reached.

DIURETICS

Volume Depletion. Extracellular fluid volume depletion is a goal of diuretic therapy. Indeed, one expects and desires a weight loss of approximately 1 to 3 pounds associated with diuretic treatment. Furthermore, reversal of that weight loss provides a clue to excessive intake of salt and water by the patient such that the prolonged natriuretic effect of the drug may be overwhelmed. Nevertheless, it is important to avoid excessive volume depletion to the extent of causing symptoms or decreasing renal function. The lowest effective dose of diuretic should be used, and it should be titrated upward only when it becomes evident that the initial dose is inadequate.[42] If goal blood pressure is being approached, it may be well worthwhile to continue to observe the patient for as long as 6 months until deciding to increase the dose further or add an additional drug.[57]

For patients with normal renal function at baseline, there should be either a trivial change or no change in serum creatinine after a diuretic drug is administered. Serum urea nitrogen concentration will be elevated routinely by a few mg per dl in almost all patients. This should be expected, and no countermeasures are required. Patients with moderate to severe degrees of renal failure may experience a greater increase in serum urea nitrogen, but this in itself should not be a cause for panic. Such changes should be viewed in the perspective of the patient's total well-being. Hypertension must be treated in these patients in order to delay progression of renal failure.[56] It may be necessary to accept a somewhat greater elevation of serum urea nitrogen, provided that it does not cause symptoms of uremia itself. Patients who are already volume-depleted because of vomiting, diarrhea, or other causes of extracellular fluid loss may be particularly sensitive to diuretic drugs. It may be necessary to discontinue the diuretic or to initiate treatment with a nondiuretic agent. It is also clear that diuretics potentiate the effect of other antihypertensive drugs and should be used with greater caution in those circumstances.

Hypokalemia. Any effective natriuretic drug will also be associated with increased potassium excretion. Potassium loss can be minimized by keeping the diuretic dose as low as possible and by moderate restriction of dietary sodium to 4 to 6 gm of salt per day (68 to 103 mEq of sodium). Potassium administration and blood tests add both risk and cost.[28,37] There is no uniformity of opinion about the lowest acceptable level of serum potassium concentration for hypertensive patients who are otherwise completely healthy. The majority of authorities would be unwilling to accept serum potassium levels of less than 3.0 mEq per L. Many authorities hold the opinion that even otherwise normal patients should not be permitted to experience serum potassium levels of less than 3.5 mEq per L. Our opinion is that a patient who is relatively young and free from all evidence of organic heart disease (including a completely normal electrocardiogram) can be permitted to have a serum potassium level as low as 3.0 mEq per L without problem. In contrast, patients taking digitalis, those who have edema, and those with any clinical evidence of organic heart disease (including nonspecific ST-T–wave changes on the electrocardiogram) should have their serum potassium level maintained in the normal range. The major reason for this is evidence that patients with organic heart disease are more susceptible to increased frequency and severity of ventricular ectopic activity when their serum potassium level is low.[8,45,60] Furthermore, diuretics (except those that spare potassium) also increase urinary magnesium loss. This may add an additional risk of cardiac dysrhythmias.[14,15]

When patients taking diuretic drugs experience weakness or muscle cramps, they sometimes benefit from bringing their serum potassium level back to normal. Our experience has been that this is not absolute; that is, some patients have weakness and muscle cramps even if they are not taking diuretic drugs and even with a perfectly normal serum potassium level. In others, these symptoms may not be corrected by the addition of potassium. However, there are many patients who will respond to administration of potassium, and it is worth the effort. Carbohydrate intolerance also may be related to decreased intracellular potassium levels. In patients who develop clinically important carbohydrate intolerance, an effort should be made to normalize the serum potassium level.[51]

Hyperuricemia. Serum uric acid levels will be increased from 1 to 1.5 mg per dl with the administration of diuretic drugs. This should be no reason for concern. It is uncommon for acute gout to be precipitated, but if that does occur, it should be treated in the usual fashion. The chances are excellent that the patient will never experience another attack. In contrast, the patient with known gout may experience problems when given diuretic drugs. It may be necessary to give allopurinol if that is not already being administered. Asymptomatic hyperuricemia associated with diuretic drugs does not automatically require treatment. Uric acid levels of more than 10 mg per dl can be readily tolerated without fear of precipitating renal disease or stones.[22]

Hyponatremia. Hyponatremia is a very uncommon but potentially lethal complication of diuretic therapy and deserves close scrutiny. The population at risk generally is composed of elderly women who tend to drink large quantities of water. Because diuretics interfere with the excretion of sodium-free water (free water clearance), these excess water drinkers may cause rather rapid dilution of their serum sodium. Symptoms of headache, nausea, vomiting, and changes in mental status should trigger immediate measurement of serum sodium. If the serum sodium is low, the diuretic should be stopped immediately and treatment given as indicated. As a general rule, this problem can be avoided by telling all patients who are started on a new drug to call immediately if any unusual reaction occurs. Some patients who had their initial symptoms misinterpreted as those of a viral syndrome later died of severe hyponatremia.[4,23]

Photosensitivity. Dermatologists occasionally see erythematous eruptions in patients taking hydrochlorothiazide.[27] We have changed such patients to metolazone in the mistaken belief that metolazone did not have an ultraviolet absorption band within the sunlight spectrum. Despite our error in logic, the patients fully recovered. The exact mechanism remains unknown, but for practical purposes, an attempted continuation of diuretic treatment might be made with an alternative drug.

Sulfa Sensitivity. All of the diuretic drugs, with the exception of ethacrynic acid and the potassium-sparing diuretics, are sulfonamide derivatives. An allergy to one agent generally conveys an allergic response to all, with the exception of those without a sulfamoyl group. Such sensitivity may be manifested by such peculiar complaints as generalized weakness, muscle aches, or even abdominal pain. We have successfully changed such patients to ethacrynic acid.

Ototoxicity. This very rare complication generally can be avoided by not using large pulsed doses of loop diuretics in patients with renal failure who are also receiving aminoglycosides.

Nephrotoxicity. Diuretics used alone are rarely associated with interstitial nephritis. They may, however, potentiate the ability of other drugs to cause interstitial nephritis. In particular, the combination of triamterene with nonsteroidal anti-inflammatory drugs should be avoided.[21]

Hyperkalemia. The potassium-sparing diuretics are associated occasionally with hyperkalemia. This can be readily avoided by being certain that patients do not take previous prescriptions for potassium replacement medications or consume large quantities of potassium-containing fruit juices or excessive quantities of potassium-containing salt substitutes. They should also be used with additional caution in those patients who are concomitantly taking beta-adrenergic blocking agents or converting enzyme inhibitors. The risk in patients with renal failure is obvious. Patients with hyporeninemic hypoaldosteronism, who frequently have mild to moderate renal failure and diabetes mellitus and are elderly, are particularly susceptible to hyperkalemia. Serum potassium concentrations greater than 5.0 mEq per L can be associated with a risk of increased frequency of ventricular tachycardia and/or fibrillation after a myocardial infarction approximately equal to that induced by serum potassium levels less than 3.5 mEq per L.[58]

Renal Calculi. There are a number of reports that suggest that triamterene either may be the nidus for renal calculus formation or may, because of its relative insolubility, constitute a calculus in and of itself.[19] It is difficult to ascertain the true incidence of this phenomenon. One study suggests that the frequency of stone formation in patients taking triamterene is not higher than that in patients taking other diuretic drugs.[20]

Hyperlipidemia. The use of diuretics is associated with an increase in total cholesterol and triglycerides and a decrease in HDL cholesterol.[46,52,71] Although an association with increased incidence of atherosclerosis has not been proved, many have suggested this as one of the reasons for failure of diuretic drug treatment to reduce the incidence of coronary heart disease more substantially in patients who have been treated for hypertension. The data are not clear because the alterations in plasma lipids are not necessarily long-lived and there may be a substantial element of dose response.[24,46] In addition, the effect of diuretics on specific HDL subtypes needs to be elucidated. Dietary reduction of fat and cholesterol intake may blunt or eliminate diuretic-associated increases in serum lipids.

In summary, the diuretic drugs that were responsible for the revolutionary advances in antihypertensive therapy are associated with a small but real risk. Most of these risks can be anticipated and either counteracted or eliminated. Nevertheless, this extra degree of surveillance has prompted the recommendation that the stepped-care algorithm requiring diuretics first be modified. The most recent recommendation places diuretics and beta-adrenergic blocking agents as coequal for consideration for initial treatment of hypertension.[35] However, many other drugs may also be suitable for initial therapy. It is probable that recommendations and practice habits will be changed as new information becomes available.

CENTRALLY ACTING AGENTS

Each of this class of drugs that works either partially or completely by agonism of central alpha$_2$ receptors is capable of causing sedation and dry mouth. Both symptoms may be minimized by beginning with low drug doses and gradually titrating upward as needed. If the initial or larger dose is given before bedtime, much of the sedative effect may have dissipated by the time of awakening. These drugs may increase serum prolactin levels and are capable of causing galactorrhea. The allegation that reserpine was associated with an increased risk of breast cancer in women has not been substantiated. If abnormal secretions from the breast do occur, they should not be explained away as due to the drug. If microscopic examination of the secreted fluid reveals red blood cells, careful work-up for occult mammary carcinoma should be made. One of our patients who developed galactorrhea while taking reserpine had red blood cells identified in her breast secretions and subsequently was found to have a small curable ductal carcinoma. Methyldopa is unique in this group in that it can cause a peculiar hypersensitivity-type hepatitis that may be associated with fever. The hepatitis generally reverses upon withdrawal of the drug. Methyldopa is also associated with a positive Coombs' reaction in approximately 20 per cent of the patients taking it. Rarely, however, is this reaction associated with hemolytic anemia.

ALPHA$_1$-ANTAGONISTS

Prazosin is the only currently available drug in this class, but a number of similar drugs may become available soon. Prazosin has the advantage of being free from most of the adverse effects that characterize the diuretics and beta-adrenergic blocking drugs. Syncope following the first dose of the drug occurs uncommonly if that first dose is not greater than 1 mg and the patient's extracellular fluid volume is not depleted. Some authorities recommend giving the first dose at bedtime in order to avoid syncope. If this is done, the patient must be advised not to drink fluids before bedtime and to empty his or her bladder before going to bed. The patient who awakes at night with a full bladder, having taken an initial dose of prazosin, might be subject not only to the first-pass syncope but also to "micturition syncope." One of the more important adverse effects of prazosin is dizziness that is not necessarily orthostatic and that persists throughout treatment.[66] Prazosin was originally thought to be free from problems of sexual dysfunction, but this has turned out not to be the case. Prazosin has been associated with incompetence of the urinary sphincters resulting in urinary incontinence.[62] Urologists have taken advantage of this adverse effect by treating patients with urinary sphincter spasm with prazosin.[30]

BETA-ADRENERGIC ANTAGONISTS

The beta-adrenergic blocking agents only recently have achieved coequal status in the United States with diuretics for the initial treatment of hypertension, although they have been the first-line agent in Europe for many years. There is little question about their overall efficacy and safety, but like the diuretics, even their relatively small percentage of symptomatic and biochemical adverse effects is becoming less acceptable for the treatment of the large population of asymptomatic, mildly hypertensive patients.

All of the beta-adrenergic blocking agents reduce cardiac output, and they all have a negative chronotropic effect. Drugs that possess intrinsic sympathomimetic activity tend to reduce the heart rate less and may be of value in those few patients who develop symptomatic bradycardia from one of the other drugs. Those patients who depend on maximum sympathetic drive for compensation of congestive cardiac failure may experience pulmonary edema upon the addition of the beta-blocker. Additive negative effects also may occur when a beta-blocker is combined with a calcium-entry blocker.

All of the beta-antagonists, with the possible exception of those having intrinsic sympathomimetic activity, increase total peripheral resistance because of unopposed alpha-mediated vasoconstriction. This likely accounts for such associated symptoms such as Raynaud's phenomenon, cold extremities, and aggravation of intermittent claudication. Patients who are salt-and water-replete and who likely have low plasma renin activity at baseline, such as the elderly and blacks, actually may experience a substantial increase in both systolic and diastolic pressure. This is much more likely to occur in black patients than in white patients.[67]

Bronchoconstriction in susceptible individuals is a major risk with the beta-adrenergic blocking agents. Even though this risk may be reduced by the use of beta$_1$-specific agents, that specificity is incomplete, tends to disappear with increased doses, and carries the potential for serious or even lethal reactions. It is my personal policy not to use any beta-adrenergic blocking agents in patients with a history of bronchospastic disease.

Carbohydrate homeostasis is beta-receptor–dependent at the levels of the pancreas, liver, and skeletal muscles. Both hyperglycemia and hypoglycemia have been reported, and there may well be a tendency for more prolonged disturbance of carbohydrate homeostasis after cessation of beta-blockers when compared with diuretics.[70] Beta-antagonists may also block the premonitory symptoms of hypoglycemia. I generally select a beta$_1$-specific blocking agent for diabetic patients who require this type of treatment.

All of the beta-antagonists are capable of penetrating the blood-brain barrier and causing central adverse effects such as excessive tiredness, weakness, sleep disorders, nightmares, and even depression. The more lipid-soluble drugs appear to be associated with these central effects much more than the water-soluble drugs. Even so, the water-soluble drugs are capable of causing these effects.[54,55,61]

Much has been written about the renal effects of beta-adrenergic blocking drugs. There is no question that propranolol is capable of decreasing the glomerular filtration rate, but it is not clear that this is of clinical significance. This problem has been reviewed in detail elsewhere.[5,18]

COMBINED ALPHA-BETA–ANTAGONISTS

Labetalol is the first of what is likely to be a series of drugs that counter the problem of increased alpha-mediated peripheral resistance associated with beta-adrenergic blocker therapy by adding peripheral alpha$_1$-antagonist effect to the molecule. This molecular manipulation has produced drugs of therapeutic efficacy, but as might be predicted, orthostatic hypotension is a problem.

Other adverse effects are those associated with both alpha- and beta-adrenergic blockade. In addition, peculiar paresthesias, including tingling of the scalp, have been reported. Sexual dysfunction, characterized by failure of ejaculation, can occur. Labetalol has some beta$_2$-agonist effect, and this may be responsible for an increase in the incidence of tremor when it is administered together with tricyclic antidepressants.[1]

DIRECT VASODILATORS

Hydralazine and minoxidil are the two direct vasodilators available for treatment of ambulatory patients.

Hydralazine. Hydralazine enjoyed a resurgence as an effective drug for a number of reasons since its introduction in 1951. Its therapeutic efficacy was markedly enhanced and its general dose was reduced by the availability of concomitant diuretic use. A rational approach to the tachycardia associated with hydralazine use was made possible by the addition of beta-adrenergic blocking drugs. Combined diuretic, hydralazine, and beta-blocker achieved the status of standard triple therapy.[77] Additional impetus for the use of the drug was given when cardiologists found it to be useful for afterload reduction in patients with severe congestive heart failure. Finally, although much less well appreciated, hydralazine plus a diuretic appears to be a very useful combination for the treatment of elderly hypertensive patients. Patients over the age of 50 years are not likely to experience the tachycardia from hydralazine associated with use of the drug in younger patients.[66] Keeping the dose less than 200 mg per day minimizes the risk of drug-associated lupus.

Minoxidil. Minoxidil traditionally has been reserved for treatment of patients with very severe hypertension, and its use has been limited by adverse effects. Marked fluid retention demands the use of concomitant diuretic drugs, even to the extent, on occasion, of the necessity of combining diuretics such as furosemide and metolazone.[17] Even then, pleural and pericardial effusions may occur. Tachycardia associated with minoxidil is striking and occurs even in older patients. It is difficult to use the drug without concomitant beta-adrenergic blockade. Hair growth occurs in most patients who take the drug.[74] Because of the availability of alternative drugs, we almost never use minoxidil in women.

We and others have had considerable success in reducing the required dose of minoxidil by using it with a diuretic plus captopril.[63] Early reports of specific atrial lesions associated with minoxidil have not been substantiated.

PERIPHERAL ANTIADRENERGIC AGENTS

Of the available antihypertensive oral drugs, guanethidine probably has the lowest benefit-to-risk ratio, and it is used much less frequently because of the introduction of safer, more effective agents. Its most important adverse effects are orthostatic hypotension, diarrhea, and sexual dysfunction. Guanadrel is a similar but shorter-acting drug that has a different profile for arteriolar and venodilatation. Although its adverse effects are similar to those of guanethidine, they occur much less frequently, so that the benefit-to-risk ratio is better.[13]

Trimethaphan used to be one of the major drugs for the treatment of hypertensive emergencies. Because its major adverse effects include paralytic ileus, urinary retention, and blurred vision, it has largely given way to sodium nitroprusside and other drugs.

CONVERTING ENZYME INHIBITORS

The angiotensin-converting enzyme inhibitors may have the best benefit-to-risk ratio of all the antihypertensive drugs when they are used properly.[68,69] It appears that all of these drugs, when used in equivalent doses and equivalent patient populations, will have very similar qualitative and quantitative adverse effect profiles.[43,44] Hypotension generally can be avoided by not giving too large an initial dose and by not administering these agents to volume-depleted patients or those receiving high doses of diuretics or other antihypertensive drugs. Placing the patient on a diuretic holiday for a day or two may be a very effective measure. A more rapidly acting drug such as captopril can be tested in the office by giving 6.25 mg orally and checking the blood pressure every half hour or so for the next hour and a half. If hypotension does not occur in this situation, it is unlikely to do so. On the other hand, almost all patients being treated with converting enzyme inhibitors for severe congestive heart failure are at risk for hypotension. Special attention must be given to the balance between the use of diuretics and the converting enzyme inhibitors in this situation.

Hyperkalemia can occur if the drug is given to patients with severe renal failure, those taking potassium-sparing diuretics and/or potassium supplements, or those who have hyporeninemic hypoaldosteronism. On the other hand, converting enzyme inhibitors ameliorate the hypokalemia and hyperuricemia associated with thiazide diuretic drugs.[72] Neutropenia has been exceptionally well studied with captopril.[9] The risk of neutropenia in an otherwise healthy population with normal renal function is approximately 0.01 per cent. Other than a baseline white blood cell count, no additional surveillance measures are required. In patients with decreased renal function, the incidence of neutropenia is 0.17 per cent. Patients who have scleroderma or systemic lupus erythematosus and renal failure have a risk of neutropenia of about 3.7 per cent, which requires intensive monitoring.[34] However, this should not be an absolute contraindication to the use of converting enzyme inhibitors, because the risk of drug adverse effect may be far less than the risk of the untreated disease.

Renal failure can occur in two basic situations. The most common setting for this uncommon adverse effect is the patient who becomes markedly dehydrated because of prolonged vomiting, diarrhea, or fluid deprivation. Because the angiotensin-converting enzyme inhibitors interfere with the normal homeostatic countermeasures for maintaining glomerular filtration rate, acute renal failure may ensue. The treatment simply consists of stopping the drug and replenishing volume. The renal failure is reversible. Reversible acute renal failure may also occur in a very small percentage (about 6 per cent) of patients with bilateral renal artery stenosis.[33] These patients uniformly have increased serum creatinine levels at baseline and therefore appear to constitute the population at risk. My personal opinion is that acute renal failure in such a patient should serve as a marker for the possible presence of bilateral renal artery stenosis and should trigger arteriographic investigation with an aim toward corrective balloon dilatation or surgery. This entity may also occur in patients who have a single functioning kidney supplied by a single stenotic renal artery. This situation occurs occasionally in patients who have had renal transplants.

Membranous glomerulopathy that was originally attributed to captopril now appears to have been diagnosed improperly.[7,39] Proteinuria occurs so frequently in the hypertensive population that it is exceedingly difficult to determine what apparently new proteinuria is or is not drug-related. I have seen full-blown nephrotic syndrome occur in patients who were receiving blinded placebo. Therefore, this level of "background noise" makes it extraordinarily difficult to determine true drug effect.

Skin rash is one of the most common problems associated with angiotensin-converting enzyme inhibitors, although it can be minimized by keeping the drug dose low. Most of these rashes are so evanescent that they are reported to the clinician after they have come and gone. For those patients who experience uncomfortable pruritus, an antihistamine usually is adequate to control that symptom until the rash disappears spontaneously. Urticaria is far less common, but because of its potentially more serious consequences, it should be followed very closely and the drug stopped if there is even a hint of possible angioedema.

Taste disturbances appear to be more related to decreased renal function than to drug dose. They are a very infrequent cause of drug discontinuation. Occasionally, dysgeusia is associated with weight loss. Oral ulcers have also been reported with or without associated dysgeusia. It is important to note, however, that such ulcers may occur in patients with collagen vascular diseases and/or renal failure.

A dry, hacking cough may be associated with angiotensin-converting enzyme inhibitors. Although it is a rare cause of drug discontinuation, clinicians should be aware that it is likely due to bradykinin increases in pulmonary tissue.

In summary, despite the relatively long list of potential problems with the angiotensin-converting enzyme inhibitors, in reality they are among the safest of the antihypertensive drugs.

CALCIUM ENTRY–BLOCKING AGENTS

Calcium entry–blocking agents are a group of very dissimilar drugs that have the same ultimate mechanism of action. There are substantial differences in the effects of each of the drugs as well as in their adverse effects. Of the currently available drugs, verapamil has the most potent negative inotropic, chronotropic, and dromotropic effects. These specific advantages for treatment of supraventricular dysrhythmias become a liability in terms of contraindication to concomitant use with beta-adrenergic blocking drugs. Verapamil also is associated with a fairly high incidence of constipation.[47]

Nifedipine represents the opposite end of the spectrum in that it has mostly vasodilating effects with relatively little effect on the conduction system. It can be used concomitantly with beta-blockers. On the other hand, it has adverse effects that are similar to those associated with the direct vasodilating agents, including reflex tachycardia, headache, and flushing. Patients may also experience a peculiar tingling paresthesia. Edema of the lower extremities may occur and may be annoying. The edema generally is not responsive to diuretic treatment. The preparation available in the United States at this time is best suited for treatment of angina pectoris in that it acts very rapidly. The sustained-release tablet that is available in Europe is more suitable for treatment of hypertension.[31]

Diltiazem is also a potent coronary and peripheral vasodilator; it has a somewhat greater effect on the conduction system than nifedipine but less of an effect than verapamil. It can be used concomitantly with beta-adrenergic blocking drugs and angiotensin-converting enzyme inhibitors. It is associated with little in the way of reflex tachycardia, flushing, or headache and, indeed, seems to have the lowest incidence of adverse effects of the three drugs.[26,76]

OTHER COMPLICATIONS OF THERAPY

Neurologic Disturbances. The vast majority of hypertensive patients can have their blood pressure lowered safely without fear of neurologic sequelae. However, rapid reduction from markedly elevated levels may be associated with temporary or permanent neurologic damage.[59]

Effect on Exercise. Many young, otherwise healthy hypertensive patients are actively engaged in vigorous physical exercise and wish to continue that activity while receiving treatment. In general, the beta-adrenergic blocking drugs impair performance to some degree and may cause the individual to have an overall feeling of lassitude or weakness.[41] The remainder of the antihypertensive drugs seem to have little or no effect on exercise performance or tolerance. Angiotensin-converting enzyme inhibitors have been used with considerable success in professional athletes.[12,25]

Hypertension and Anesthesia. Whenever possible, hypertension existing prior to an operative procedure should be controlled by drug therapy. Antihypertensive therapy should be continued up to and, if possible, through the operative procedure itself and should be reinitiated as soon as possible after surgery. Numerous adverse effects and drug interactions may occur during anesthesia, and the anesthesiologist must be fully aware of the antihypertensive

medications in order to cope with these successfully.[11]

Sexual Dysfunction. All of the antihypertensive drugs are capable of causing sexual dysfunction. Drugs such as guanethidine, guanadrel, and labetalol are more likely to cause retrograde ejaculation than complete impotence. Drugs that have an effect within the central nervous system are more likely to decrease libido and cause generalized erectile failure. The angiotensin-converting enzyme inhibitors appear to be the least likely to interfere with libido or sexual function.[50,64] Diabetic patients, who already have an extraordinary incidence of sexual dysfunction, are at even higher risk for additional problems associated with the antihypertensive drugs.[19]

Abrupt Discontinuation of Therapy. Patients with very mild hypertension tend to return very slowly to their baseline blood pressure after discontinuation of therapy. In contrast, patients with very severe blood pressure who require high doses of medication for control tend to rebound to their baseline level quickly, often within a few hours. Some patients, particularly those treated with clonidine and clonidine-like drugs, may experience a rebound phenomenon characterized by excess sympathetic nervous system discharge. The most appropriate treatment for this syndrome is usually reinstitution of the drug that was abruptly discontinued, unless there is some specific contraindication to doing so. Discontinuation of beta-adrenergic blocking agents that have been used for treatment of angina pectoris with concomitant hypertension incurs the risk of precipitating severe angina or even myocardial infarction. Discontinuation in these patients should be gradual, and the patients should be instructed to resume their treatment level of exercise and physical activity very slowly and cautiously.[32,73]

Psychiatric Considerations. As mentioned earlier, most of the antihypertensive medications have the capability of causing some alterations in mental status and feeling of well-being. There has been considerable question about the intellectual performance of patients taking antihypertensive medications.[49,75] The Veterans Administration Cooperative Study Group on Antihypertensive Agents has just completed a major study of treatment of patients 65 years of age and older with a variety of drugs. The preliminary indication is that all of the drugs used successfully lowered blood pressure in this population and did not have an adverse effect on intellectual function, affect, mechanical skills, or activities of daily living.

Psychiatric patients who have concomitant hypertension are at special risk for drug interactions and adverse effects.[3] Such drug combinations as diuretics and lithium should be avoided. Many of the major psychiatric tranquilizers and tricyclic antidepressant drugs themselves have an effect on the blood pressure. This effect must be determined for each individual patient. Our experience has been that the angiotensin-converting enzyme inhibitors and the calcium entry–blocking agents are the safest to use in this circumstance.[16,61]

SUMMARY AND CONCLUSIONS

Elevated blood pressure can be lowered safely in the vast majority of patients by selecting the single drug most likely to be efficacious in that patient. Skillful management with full knowledge of drug pharmacology should provide the patient with the maximum opportunity to benefit from normalization of blood pressure while at the same time having little or no impact on quality of life.

REFERENCES

1. Abramowicz, M. (ed.): Labetalol for hypertension. The Medical Letter, *26*:83–85, 1984.
2. Ahearn, D.J., and Grim, C.E.: Treatment of malignant hypertension with sodium nitroprusside. Arch. Intern. Med., *133*:187–191, 1974.
3. Alexander, H.E., Jr., McCarty, K., and Giffen, M.B.: Hypotension and cardiopulmonary arrest associated with concurrent haloperidol and propranolol therapy. J.A.M.A., *252*:87–88, 1984.
4. Ashraf, N., Locksley, R., and Arieff, A.I.: Thiazide-induced hyponatremia associated with death or neurologic damage in outpatients. Am. J. Med., *70*:1163–1168, 1981.
5. Bauer, J.H.: Adrenergic blocking agents and the kidney. J. Clin. Hypertension, *1*:199–221, 1985.
6. Bulpitt, C.J., Dollery, C.T., and Carne, S.: Change in symptoms of hypertensive patients after referral to hospital clinic. Br. Heart J., *38*:121–128, 1976.
7. Captopril Collaborative Study Group: Does captopril cause renal damage in hypertensive patients? Lancet, *1*:988–990, 1982.
8. Caralis, P.V., Materson, B.J., and Perez-Stable, E.C.: Potassium and diuretic-induced ventricular arrhythmias in ambulatory hypertensive patients. Miner. Electrolyte Metab., *10*:148–154, 1984.
9. Cooper, R.A.: Captopril-associated neutropenia. Who is at risk? Arch. Intern. Med., *143*:659–660, 1983.
10. Cottrell, J.E., Casthely, P., Brodie, J.D., et al.: Prevention of nitroprusside-induced cyanide toxicity with hydroxocobalamin. N. Engl. J. Med., *298*:809–811, 1978.
11. Craig, D.B., and Bose, D.: Drug interactions in anaesthesia: Chronic antihypertensive therapy. Can. Anaesth. Soc. J., *31*:580–588, 1984.
12. Crow, R.S., Sopko, G., Jacobs, D.R., Jr., et al.: Effective antihypertensive medications on physical work capacity. J. Cardiac Rehabil., *4*:55–61, 1984.
13. Dunn, M.I., and Dunlap, J.L.: Guanadrel: A new antihypertensive drug. J.A.M.A., *245*:1639–1642, 1981.
14. Dyckner, T., and Wester, P.O.: Ventricular extrasystoles and intracellular electrolytes before and after potassium and magnesium infusions in patients on diuretic treatment. Am. Heart J., *97*:12–18, 1979.
15. Dyckner, T., and Wester, P.O.: Intracellular magnesium loss after diuretic administration. Drugs, *28*(Suppl. 1):161–166, 1984.
16. Editorial: Intellectual performance in hypertensive patients. Lancet, *1*:87, 1984.
17. Epstein, M., Lepp, B.A., Hoffman, D.S., et al.: Potentiation of furosemide by metolazone in refractory edema. Curr. Ther. Res., *21*:656–667, 1977.
18. Epstein, M., and Oster, J.R.: Beta blockers and renal function: A reappraisal. J. Clin. Hypertension, *1*:85–99, 1985.
19. Ettinger, B., Weil, E., Mandel, N.S., et al.: Triamterene-induced nephrolithiasis. Ann. Intern. Med., *91*:745–746, 1979.
20. Ettinger, B.: Excretion of triamterene and its metabolite in triamterene stone patients. J. Clin. Pharmacol., *25*:365–368, 1985.
21. Faure, L., Glasson, P., and Vallotton, M.B.: Reversible acute renal failure from combined triamterene and indomethacin: A study in healthy subjects. Ann. Intern. Med., *96*:317–320, 1982.
22. Fessel, W.J.: Renal outcomes of gout and hyperuricemia. Am. J. Med., *67*:74–82, 1979.
23. Fichman, M.P., Vorherr, H., Kleeman, C.R., et al.: Diuretic-induced hyponatremia. Ann. Intern. Med., *75*:853–863, 1971.
24. Flamenbaum, W.: Metabolic consequences of antihypertensive therapy. Ann. Intern. Med., *98*(Part 2):875–880, 1983.
25. Graham, D.I.: Ischaemic brain damage following emergency blood pressure lowering in hypertensive patients. Acta Med. Scand. [Suppl.], *678*:61–69, 1982.
26. Guazzi, M.D., Decesare, N., Galli, C., et al.: Calcium-channel blockade with nifedipine and angiotensin converting-enzyme inhibition with captopril in the therapy of patients with severe primary hypertension. Circulation, *70*:279–284, 1984.
27. Harber, L.C., Lashinsky, A.M., and Baer, R.L.: Photosensitivity due to chlorothiazide and hydrochlorothiazide. N. Engl. J. Med., *261*:1378–1381, 1959.
28. Harrington, J.T., Isner, J.M., and Kassirer, J.P.: Our national obsession with potassium. Am. J. Med., *73*:155–159, 1982.
29. Haynes, R.B., Sackett, D.L., Taylor, D.W., et al.: Increased absenteeism from work after detection and labeling of hypertensive patients. N. Engl. J. Med., *299*:741–744, 1978.
30. Hedlund, H., Andersson, K.-E., and Ek, A.: Effects of prazosin in patients with benign prostatic obstruction. J. Urol., *130*:275–278, 1983.
31. Hornung, R.S., Gould, B.A., Jones, R.I., et al.: Nifedipine tablets for systemic hypertension: A study using continuous ambulatory intraarterial recording. Am. J. Cardiol., *51*:1323–1327, 1983.
32. Houston, M.C.: Abrupt discontinuation of antihypertensive therapy. South. Med. J., *74*:1112–1123, 1981.
33. Hricik, D.E., Browning, P.J., Kopelman, R., et al.: Captopril-induced functional renal insufficiency in patients with bilateral renal-artery stenoses or renal-

artery stenosis in a solitary kidney. N. Engl. J. Med., *308*:373–376, 1983.

34. Jenkins, A.C., Dreslinski, G.R., Tadros, S.S., et al.: Captopril in hypertension: Seven years later. J. Cardiovasc. Pharmacol., 7:S96–S101, 1985.

35. Joint National Committee on Detection, Evaluation, and Treatment of High Blood Pressure: The 1984 report of the Joint National Committee on Detection, Evaluation, and Treatment of High Blood Pressure. Arch. Intern. Med., *144*:1045–1057, 1984.

36. Kannel, W.B., Sorlie, P., and Gordon, T.: Labile hypertension: A faulty concept? Circulation, *61*:1183–1187, 1980.

37. Kaplan, N.M., Carnegie, A., Raskin, P., et al.: Potassium supplementation in hypertensive patients with diuretic-induced hypokalemia. N. Engl. J. Med., *312*:746–749, 1985.

38. Koch-Weser, J.: Diazoxide. N. Engl. J. Med., *294*:1271–1274, 1976.

39. Lewis, E.L., and Captopril Collaborative Study Group: Proteinuria and abnormalities of the renal glomerulus in patients with hypertension. Clin. Exp. Pharmacol. Physiol., 7(Suppl.):105–115, 1982.

40. Lipson, L.G.: Treatment of hypertension in diabetic men: Problems with sexual dysfunction. Am. J. Cardiol., *53*:46A–50A, 1984.

41. Lowenthal, T.J., Saris, S., Falkner, B., et al.: The clinical pharmacology of cardiovascular drugs during exercise. J. Cardiac Rehabil., *3*:829–837, 1983.

42. Materson, B.J., Oster, J.R., Michael, U.F., et al.: Dose response to chlorthalidone in patients with mild hypertension. Efficacy of a lower dose. Clin. Pharmacol. Ther., *24*:192–198, 1978.

43. Materson, B.J.: Angiotensin converting enzyme inhibitors in the treatment of hypertension. Compr. Ther., *9*:14–20, 1983.

44. Materson, B.J.: Monotherapy of hypertension with angiotensin converting enzyme inhibitors. Am. J. Med., *77*:128–134, 1984.

45. Materson, B.J., and Caralis, P.V.: Risk of cardiac arrhythmias in relation to potassium imbalance. J. Cardiovasc. Pharmacol., *6*(Suppl. 3):S493–S497, 1984.

46. Materson, B.J., Freis, E.D., Reda, D., et al.: Dose-dependent metabolic perturbations by HCTZ and propranolol. *In* Puschett, J.B., and Greenberg, A. (eds.): Diuretics: Chemistry, Pharmacology, and Clinical Applications. New York, Elsevier Science Publishing Company, Inc., 1984.

47. McCall, D., Walsh, R.A., Frohlich, E.D., et al.:Calcium entry blocking drugs: Mechanisms of action, experimental studies and clinical uses. Curr. Probl. Cardiol., *10*:6–80, 1985.

48. Messerli, F.H., Ventura, H.O., and Amodeo, C.: Osler's maneuver and pseudohypertension. N. Engl. J. Med., *312*:1548–1551, 1985.

49. Miller, R.E., Shapiro, A.P., King, H.E., et al.: Effect of antihypertensive treatment on the behavioral consequences of elevated blood pressure. Hypertension, *6*:202–208, 1984.

50. Papadopoulos, C.: Cardiovascular drugs and sexuality. Arch. Intern. Med., *140*:1341–1345, 1980.

51. Perez-Stable, E.C., and Caralis, P.V.: Thiazide-induced disturbances in carbohydrate, lipid, and potassium metabolism. Am. Heart J., *106*:245–251, 1983.

52. Perez-Stable, E.C., Caralis, P.V., and Materson, B.J.: Secondary drug related risk factors. Relevance of biochemical homeostasis. *In* Bergener, M., and Grobecker, H. (eds.): Hypertonie im Alter: Normvariante

oder Krankheit? Stuttgart, Schattauer, 1984, pp. 207–222.

53. Ram, C.V.S., and Kaplan, N.M.: Individual titration of diazoxide dosage in the treatment of severe hypertension. Am. J. Cardiol., *43*:627–630, 1979.

54. Russell, J.W., and Schuckit, M.A.: Anxiety and depression in patient on nadolol. Lancet, *2*:1286–1287, 1982.

55. Salem, S.A., and McDevitt, D.G.: Central effects of beta-adrenoceptor antagonists. Clin. Pharmacol. Ther., *33*:52–57, 1982.

56. Shimamatsu, K., Onoyama, K., Harada, A., et al.: Effect of blood pressure on the progression rate of renal impairment in chronic glomerulonephritis. J. Clin. Hypertension, *1*:239–244, 1985.

57. Soghikian, K., and Bartenbach, D.E.: Influence of dosage and duration of therapy on the rate of response to methyclothiazide in essential hypertension. South. Med. J., *70*:1397–1404, 1977.

58. Solomon, R.J., and Cole, A.G.: Importance of potassium in patients with acute myocardial infarction. Acta Med. Scand. [Suppl.], *647*:87–93, 1980.

59. Strandgaard, S., Andersen, G.S., Ahlgreen, P., et al.: Visual disturbances and occipital brain infarct following acute, transient hypotension in hypertensive patients. Acta Med. Scand., *216*:417–422, 1984.

60. Struthers, A.D., Whitesmith, R., and Reid, J.L.: Prior thiazide diuretic treatment increases adrenaline-induced hypokalemia. Lancet, *1*:1358–1361, 1983.

61. Swift, R.M., and Black, H.R.: Essential hypertension: Psychiatric aspects and use of psychotropics. Psychosomatics, *25*:737–745, 1984.

62. Thien, T.H., Dalaere, K.P.J., Debruyne, F.M.J., et al.: Urinary incontinence caused by prazosin. Br. Med. J., *1*:622–623, 1978.

63. Traub, Y.M., and Levey, B.A.: Combined treatment with minoxidil and captopril in refractory hypertension. Arch. Intern. Med., *143*:1142–1144, 1983.

64. Van Arsdalen, K.N., and Wein, A.J.: Drug-induced sexual dysfunction in older men. Geriatrics, *39*:63–70, 1984.

65. Veterans Administration Cooperative Study Group on Antihypertensive Agents: I. Results in patients with diastolic blood pressure averaging 115 through 129 mm Hg. J.A.M.A., *202*:116–122, 1967.

66. Veterans Administration Cooperative Study Group on Antihypertensive Agents: Comparison of prazosin with hydralazine in patients receiving hydrochlorothiazide. A randomized double-blind clinical trial. Circulation, *64*:772–779, 1981.

67. Veterans Administration Cooperative Study Group on Antihypertensive Agents: Comparison of propranolol and hydrochlorothiazide for the initial treatment of hypertension. I. Results of short-term titration with emphasis on racial differences in response. J.A.M.A., *248*:1996–2003, 1982.

68. Veterans Administration Cooperative Study Group on Antihypertensive Agents: Low-dose captopril for the treatment of mild to moderate hypertension. II. Long-term results. Hypertension, 5(Suppl. III):III-139–III-144, 1983.

69. Veterans Administration Cooperative Study Group on Antihypertensive Agents: Low-dose captopril for the treatment of mild to moderate hypertension. I. Results of a 14-week trial. Arch. Intern. Med., *144*:1947–1953, 1984.

70. Veterans Administration Cooperative Study Group on Antihypertensive Agents: Comparison of propranolol and hydrochlorothiazide for the initial treatment of

hypertension. IV. Effect on plasma glucose and tolerance. Hypertension, 7:1008–1016, 1985.

71. Weidmann, P., Uehlinger, D.E., and Gerber, A.: Antihypertensive treatment and serum lipoproteins. J. Hypertension, 3:297–306, 1985.

72. Weinberger, M.H.: Comparison of captopril and hydrochlorothiazide alone and in combination in mild to moderate essential hypertension. Br. J. Clin. Pharmacol., *14*:127S–131S, 1982.

73. Whitsett, T.L.: Abrupt cessation of treatment with centrally acting antihypertensive agents: A review. Chest, *83*(Suppl. 2):400–402, 1983.

74. Wilburn, R.L., Blaufuss, A., and Bennett, C.M.: Long-term treatment of severe hypertension with minoxidil, propranolol and furosemide. Circulation, 52:706–713, 1975.

75. Wilkie, F., and Eisdorfer, C.: Intelligence and blood pressure in the aged. Science, *172*:959–962, 1971.

76. Yamakado, T., Oonishi, N., Kondo, S., et al.: Effects of diltiazem on cardiovascular responses during exercise in systemic hypertension and comparison with propranolol. Am. J. Cardiol., 52:1023–1027, 1983.

77. Zacest, R., Gilmore, E., and Koch–Weser, J.: Treatment of essential hypertension with combined vasodilation and beta-adrenergic blockade. N. Engl. J. Med., *286*:617–622, 1972.

Veterans Administration Medical Center (III)
1201 N.W. 16th Street
Miami, Florida 33125

Adverse Effects of Antihypertensive Drug Therapy on Glucose Intolerance

*Mark C. Houston, M.D., F.A.C.P.**

Glucose intolerance and diabetes mellitus are well-recognized risk factors for the accelerated development of coronary heart disease (CHD).[62,98–101] The risk for CHD and other cardiovascular complications increases even within the normal range of glucose levels, but dramatic increases occur at higher levels exceeding 140 mg per dl (Fig. 1).[62,98–101] In the Whitehall Study,[62] patients with a normal fasting glucose level but an abnormal glucose tolerance test had a twofold greater incidence of CHD. Even mild glucose elevations have biologic significance,[29,63] with elevations in glycohemoglobin[29,78,106] and other biochemical and clinical abnormalities, as well as a secondary hyperlipoproteinemia[171] (increase in total cholesterol, triglycerides, very-low-density lipoprotein [VLDL], and low-density lipoprotein [LDL] and decrease in high-density lipoprotein [HDL]), which further increases CHD risk.[4,22,98–101,168,171] Glucose intolerance, hyperlipoproteinemia, and hypertension are independent risk factors for CHD and other cardiovascular diseases, but their combination is not only additive but also synergistic to this risk[98–101] (Fig. 2). It is crucial to the management of the hypertensive patient that antihypertensive drug selection does not exacerbate glucose intolerance or other CHD risk factors that could potentially negate the beneficial effects of a reduced blood pressure. *Optimal* risk reduction for CHD should be a major goal of antihypertensive therapy.

This article will discuss the effects of the antihypertensive drugs on glucose intolerance in both nondiabetic and diabetic patients with primary essential hypertension and how these may affect CHD and other cardiovascular risks and complications.

CORONARY HEART DISEASE RISKS: HYPERTENSION, HYPERGLYCEMIA, HYPERLIPOPROTEINEMIA

The probability of CHD developing during a 6-year period if cholesterol levels and systolic blood pressure are elevated and glucose intolerance is present is shown in Table 1. If a particular antihypertensive drug induces glucose intolerance and hypercholesterolemia (7 per cent increase over baseline) despite a reduction in systolic blood pressure of 12 per cent, the risk of CHD actually increases statistically from 7.6 per cent to 8.8 per cent.[3] The morbidity and mortality from CHD, myocardial infarction, congestive heart failure, cerebrovascular accidents, peripheral vascular disease, and renal disease are more common in the patient with glucose intolerance and diabetes mellitus plus hypertension than in the patient with glucose intolerance and diabetes mellitus or hypertension *alone*.[39,140] Table 2 shows the relative incidence of these complications in the diabetic patient without hypertension.[42,76,144] The incidence would be even greater in the hypertensive diabetic patient. Ischemic heart disease or CHD is the leading cause of death,[140] and 75 per cent of all deaths in diabetes mellitus are due to vascular disease.[39,140] The average life expectancy of the diabetic is two thirds that of a nondiabetic.[39,140]

---

*Assistant Professor of Medicine; Co-Director, Medical Intensive Care Unit; and Medical Director, Cooperative Care Center, Vanderbilt University Medical Center, Nashville, Tennessee

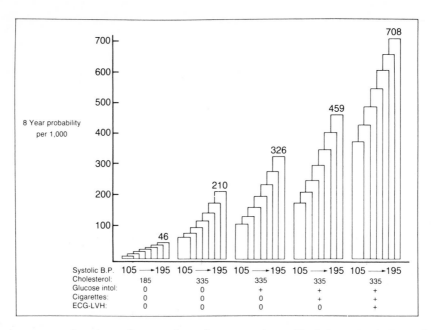

Figure 1. Average annual incidence of coronary heart disease according to blood glucose level. Framingham Study, 16-year follow-up of men and women 45 to 74 years of age. (Source: monograph section no. 26, Table 1–6-B, National Institutes of Health.) (1) Risk increases even within the normal range of glucose levels but increases dramatically at high levels (diabetes mellitus). (2) Women show more correlation than men. (3) Even mild elevations of glucose level have biologic significance resulting in an elevated glycohemoglobin and have positive correlation with elevated serum lipids (cholesterol, triglycerides) in an adverse manner. (*From* Castelli, W.P.: Epidemiology of CHD: The Framingham Study. Am. J. Med., 76(2A):4–12, 1984; with permission.)

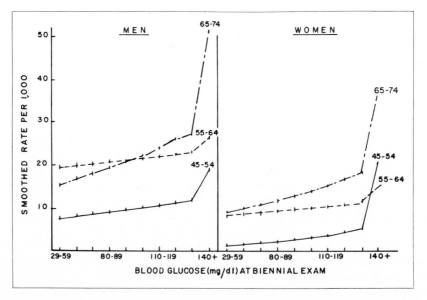

Figure 2. Risk of cardiovascular disease according to systolic blood pressure at specified levels of other risk factors. Framingham Study, 18-year follow-up, men aged 40 years. Additional risk factors *compound* total risk. (*From* Castelli, W.P.: Epidemiology of CHD: The Framingham Study. Am. J. Med., 76(2A):4–12, 1984; with permission.)

Table 1. *Probability of Coronary Heart Disease Developing in 6 Years During Treatment with an Antihypertensive Agent That Induces Glucose Intolerance and Hypercholesterolemia*

	BEFORE THERAPY	DURING THERAPY
Cholesterol	217 mg per dl	235 mg per dl
Systolic blood pressure	151 mm Hg	133 mm Hg
Glucose intolerance	No	Yes
Probability of CHD	7.6%	8.8%

From Ames, R.P.: Negative effects of diuretic drugs on metabolic risk factors for coronary heart disease: Possible alternative drug therapies. Am. J. Cardiol., *51*:632–638, 1983; with permission.

PREVALENCE AND INCIDENCE OF DIABETES MELLITUS AND HYPERTENSION

Hypertension and diabetes mellitus occur frequently together, and the coincidence is higher than expected from individual prevalence rates.[16,39,66,76,94,120,121,140,157] The incidence of hypertension in the diabetic is two to three times that in the nondiabetic[120] and varies from 41 per cent to 80 per cent,[39,76,157] with the incidence being greater in women than in men.[39,76,157] There are 35 to 60 million hypertensive individuals, 6 to 9 million diabetics, and 3 to 4 million diabetics with hypertension in the United States.[66,121] Hypertension is seen primarily in type II non–insulin-dependent diabetes mellitus and correlates with age,[16,39,76] weight,[76] duration of diabetes,[16,39,76] presence of proteinuria,[39] and declining renal function.[76] Hypertension is also common in type I insulin-dependent diabetes mellitus.[76]

DIFFERENTIAL DIAGNOSIS OF HYPERGLYCEMIA

Hyperglycemia or glucose intolerance may be due to diabetes mellitus, various endocrine dis-

Table 2. *Frequency of Complications in Individuals with Diabetes Mellitus Compared with the Normal Population*

	FREQUENCY IN DIABETES MELLITUS ($\times$ that in NP)
Acute myocardial infarction	$2\times$
Coronary heart disease	$2\times$–$4\times$
Congestive heart failure	$2\times$
Cerebrovascular accident	$2\times$
Peripheral vascular disease	$5\times$
Renal insufficiency	$17\times$

NP = normal population

eases, pancreatic insufficiency, obesity, electrolyte disorders, chronic renal insufficiency, or one of numerous drugs[48,149,167] (Table 3). The antihypertensive agents most commonly associated with glucose intolerance are thiazide and thiazide-like diuretics,[2–5, 13, 25, 45, 50, 57, 60, 65, 68, 69, 72, 77, 86, 87, 90, 102, 107, 117, 128, 152, 159, 165, 179, 185, 188, 189, 191, 192] chlorthalidone,[4,13,18,44,45,130,178] loop diuretics (furosemide),[4,13,25,30,73,122,126,154,175,177] diazoxide,[35,65,192] and the beta-blockers.[23, 64, 65, 72, 80, 133, 180, 181, 194] The relative effects of these and other antihypertensive agents on glucose intolerance will be discussed in detail later.

METABOLIC CONSEQUENCES AND CLINICAL EFFECTS OF HYPERGLYCEMIA

In addition to the increased CHD and cardiovascular risk induced by glucose intolerance, there are many other adverse metabolic, biochemical, and clinical effects of hyperglycemia (Table 4). Hypertension is positively correlated with blood glucose levels due to hypervolemia and with an expanded intravascular volume due to movement of interstitial fluid, sodium, and

Table 3. *Differential Diagnosis of Hyperglycemia*

1. Diabetes mellitus
2. Endocrine diseases
   Cushing's syndrome
   Acromegaly
   Hyperthyroidism and thyrotoxicosis
   Primary hyperaldosteronism
   Pheochromocytoma
   Glucagonoma or somatostatinoma
3. Pancreatic insufficiency
4. Obesity
5. Electrolyte disorders
   Hypokalemia
   Hypomagnesemia
   Hypophosphatemia
6. Chronic renal insufficiency
7. Drug-induced
   Corticosteroids
   Diphenylhydantoin
   Thiazide and thiazide-like diuretics (common)
   Chlorthalidone (common)
   Loop diuretics (uncommon)
   Beta-blockers (common)
   Estrogens and oral contraceptives
   Indomethacin
   Nicotine
   Niacin—nicotinic acid
   Phenothiazines and tricyclic antidepressants
   Streptozotocin
   Sympathomimetic agents
   Thyroid hormone
   Ethyl alcohol
   Caffeine
   L-Dopa

Table 4.   *Metabolic, Biochemical, and Clinical Effects of Hyperglycemia*

Hypertension[16,76,92]
Hypervolemia[37,83,119]
Hypovolemia
Hyperlipoproteinemia[4,83,197]
Postprandial atherogenesis[197]
Glycosylation of tissue proteins and glycohemoglobin[3,25,29,78,106,138]
Accumulation of sorbitol in nervous tissue (neuropathy)[63,100,140] and lens of the eye (cataracts)[63]
Platelet dysfunction with enhanced platelet aggregation and adhesion[105,160]
Decreased fibrinolysis and increased incidence of thromboembolic disease[105,160]
Microangiopathy accelerated[22,168]
Predisposition to infections due to reduced chemotaxis, phagocytosis, and other changes[149]
Fluid, electrolyte, and acid-base abnormalities[149]

water into the hyperosmolar intravascular space.[37,83,92,119] A secondary hyperlipoproteinemia is common with increased total cholesterol, triglyceride, VLDL, and LDL levels and reduced HDL cholesterol levels.[4,16,83,119,197] Marked postprandial glucose elevations accelerate atherosclerosis in diabetes mellitus[197] and possibly in latent diabetics or nondiabetics who develop hyperglycemia because of one of the causes listed in Table 3. Glycosylation of tissue proteins[29] may lead to metabolic dysfunction,[3,25,29,78,106,138] as may the elevated glycohemoglobin. Accumulation of sorbitol in nervous tissue may cause neuropathy,[62,100,140] and in the lens, it leads to cataracts[140] or, with microvascular changes, to retinopathy.[98–100,140] Abnormal platelet function with increased platelet aggregation and adhesion may exacerbate CHD or other cardiovascular disorders (for example, cerebrovascular accident or myocardial infarction).[105,160] A reduction in fibrinolytic activity may lead to an increased tendency of thromboembolic complications.[105,160] A predisposition to infections may be due to impaired chemotaxis, phagocytosis, and other causes.[149] Lastly, fluid, electrolyte, and acid-base derangements may occur with chronic hyperglycemia, hyperosmolar states, diabetic ketoacidosis, and dehydration.[149]

ALPHA- AND BETA-ADRENERGIC CONTROL OF INSULIN SECRETION AND GLUCOSE

There is excellent evidence that the alpha- and beta-adrenergic receptors in the pancreas, liver, and peripheral tissues play a major role in the control of insulin secretion and serum glu-

cose levels.[26,34,97,137,162,166] Beta$_2$-adrenergic stimulation with drugs such as isoproterenol, metaproterenol, and albuterol will increase insulin secretion and may reduce serum glucose in the long term.[97] On the other hand, beta-blockade with nonselective and cardioselective beta-blockers in high doses will inhibit insulin secretion, elevate serum glucose and growth hormone, and reduce fat mobilization.[26,34,97,137,162,166] Alpha-blockade with phentolamine increases secretion of insulin by 31 ± 23 per cent and reduces serum glucose.[34,166]

ANTIHYPERTENSIVE DRUG THERAPY: EFFECT ON GLUCOSE INTOLERANCE

There have been several recent reviews on the effects of antihypertensive drugs on carbohydrate metabolism and their use in the diabetic and nondiabetic patient with hypertension.[38,40,59,119] In the following sections, the effects of each class of antihypertensive drugs (Table 5) on glucose intolerance will be discussed in detail. The mechanism of glucose intolerance, a review of clinical studies, and suggestions on how to avoid, reduce, or treat the hyperglycemia and its associated problems will be reviewed for each antihypertensive drug. It should be noted that the various methods to determine glucose intolerance, such as fasting glucose, postprandial glucose, oral and intravenous glucose tolerance test, 24-hour urine glucose, and hemoglobin A$_1$C determinations, have not been used consistently in all the studies and that normal values in one parameter (for example, fasting glucose) do *not* necessarily imply that the other monitoring techniques are normal as well.[25] This was demonstrated by Bloomgarden and associates[25] in patients with insulin-dependent diabetes mellitus and hypertension treated with thiazide and loop diuretics in whom a significant elevation in hemoglobin A$_1$C occurred but was associated with a normal fasting glucose when compared with untreated patients. This implies that some antihypertensive-induced hyperglycemia is associated with a greater postprandial glycemic excursion but has less effect on the postabsorptive glycemic levels.[25] The glucose intolerance tests suggest the same response.

Diuretics

Thiazide Diuretics

Since the first description that chlorothiazide diuretics impair glucose tolerance,[190] numerous

Table 5. *Antihypertensive Drugs*

I. Diuretics
  A. Thiazides (benzothiadiazine derivatives)
    1. Hydrochlorothiazide (Oretic, Esidrix, HydroDiuril, Zide)
    2. Chlorothiazide (Diuril)
    3. Cyclothiazide (Anhydron)
    4. Benzthiazide (Exna, Aquatag)
    5. Polythiazide (Renese)
    6. Hydroflumethiazide (Saluron, Diucardin)
    7. Bendroflumethiazide (Naturetin)
    8. Trichlormethiazide (Naqua, Metahydrin)
    9. Methyclothiazide (Enduron, Aquatensen)
  B. Chlorthalidone (phthalimidine derivatives)
    1. Hygroton
    2. Thalitone
  C. Loop diuretics
    1. Furosemide (Lasix)
    2. Ethacrynic Acid (Edecrin)
    3. Bumetanide (Bumex)
  D. Potassium-sparing diuretics
    1. Triamterene (Dyrenium)
    2. Amiloride (Midamor)
    3. Spironolactone (Aldactone)
  E. Combination diuretics
    1. Dyazide
    2. Moduretic
    3. Aldactazide
    4. Maxzide
  F. Quinazoline diuretic derivatives
    1. Quinethazone (Hydromox)
    2. Metolazone (Zaroxolyn, Diulo)
  G. Indoline diuretic derivatives
    1. Indapamide (Lozol)
II. Central Nervous System Alpha-Agonists
  A. Clonidine (Catapres)
  B. Methyldopa (Aldomet)
  C. Guanabenz (Wytensin)
III. Postganglionic Neuron Inhibitors
  A. Reserpine and rauwolfia alkaloids (Serpasil) and others
  B. Guanethidine (Ismelin)
  C. Guanadrel (Hylorel)

IV. Alpha-Adrenergic Blockers
  A. Phentolamine (Rogitine)
  B. Phenoxybenzamine (Dibenzyline)
  C. Prazosin (Minipress) (see Indirect Vasodilators)
  D. Labetalol (Trandate, Normodyne) (see Beta-Adrenergic Blockers)
V. Beta-Adrenergic Blockers
  A. Propranolol (Inderal)
  B. Metoprolol (Lopressor)
  C. Nadolol (Corgard)
  D. Atenolol (Tenormin)
  E. Timolol (Blocadren)
  F. Pindolol (Visken)
  G. Labetalol (Trandate, Normodyne—alpha- and beta-blocker
  H. Acebutolol (Sectral)
VI. Vasodilators
  A. Direct vasodilators
    1. Hydralazine (Apresoline)
    2. Minoxidil (Loniten)
    3. Diazoxide (Hyperstat)
    4. Sodium nitroprusside (Nipride)
  B. Indirect vasodilators (alpha$_1$-blockers)
    1. Prazosin (Minipress)
VII. Ganglionic Blockers
  A. Trimethaphan (Arfonad)
  B. Pentolinium (Anolysen)
  C. Mecamylamine (Inversine)
VIII. Angiotensin-Converting Enzyme Inhibitors
  A. Saralasin (Sarenin)
  B. Captopril (Capoten)
  C. Enalapril (Vasotec)
IX. Calcium-Channel Blockers
  A. Diltiazem (Cardizem)
  B. Nifedipine (Procardia)
  C. Verapamil (Calan, Isoptin)

---

other studies have documented that carbohydrate intolerance is impaired by benzothiadiazine diuretics in nondiabetic subjects[57, 60, 65, 77, 87, 107, 117, 165, 188, 189, 191, 196] and in diabetic patients.[25, 32, 60, 65, 68, 102, 152, 159, 185, 189, 192] The effects have included elevated fasting and postprandial serum glucose levels,[2-5, 13, 44, 69, 72, 86, 90, 117, 179] decreased tolerance to oral and intravenous glucose tolerance tests,[3,5,69,86,90,117,128] overt diabetes mellitus,[44,69,86,90,128] nonketotic hyperosmolar coma,[45,50,189] and elevated hemoglobin A$_1$C.[3,5,25]

Mechanism of Thiazide-Induced Glucose Intolerance. Numerous mechanisms have been proposed to explain thiazide-induced glucose intolerance[15,19,56,61,70,71,74,79,82,104,152,163,165,188] (Table 6). Diuretic-induced hypokalemia leads to a higher secretion ratio of proinsulin to insulin; proinsulin has less biologic activity compared with insulin.[71] This in effect leads to decreased insulin secretion secondary to hypokalemia.[2,60,79,152,158] Potassium enhances beta-adrenergic secretory activity,[81] and there is an excellent correlation between reduction in total body potassium and the defect in insulin secretion.[158] Replacement of potassium (for example, with dietary measures, potassium salts, or potassium-sparing diuretics) minimizes the incidence and severity of thiazide diuretic–induced hyperglycemia.[60,79,74,152] When potassium losses were prevented in seven normal men taking 100 mg per day of hydrochlorothiazide by administration of 80 mEq of potassium chloride (KCl) per day for 10 days, there was no significant alteration in glucose tolerance, beta cell sensitivity to glucose, or beta cell sensitivity or tissue sensitivity to insulin.[79] Correction of potassium balance may obviate the need for hypoglycemic drugs or insulin in some of these patients.[60,74]

Table 6.   *Proposed Mechanisms of Thiazide-Induced Glucose Intolerance*

1. Diuretic-induced hypokalemia and indirect reduction in insulin secretion
2. Direct diuretic inhibition of insulin secretion
3. Decreased tissue sensitivity to insulin (insulin resistance)
4. Effects on enteropancreatic axis
5. Impaired glucose utilization due to blockade of the metabolic phosphorylation process
6. Alteration in hepatic glucose metabolism
7. Increased chronic insulin secretion, accelerating the development of insulin depletion in the prediabetic state (high insulin levels with insulin resistance)

A direct thiazide inhibition of pancreatic insulin secretion is also quite likely.[56,60,61,65,82,163] Other proposed mechanisms include actual insulin resistance due to decreased tissue sensitivity to insulin,[3,15,19,188] effects on the enteropancreatic axis,[70] impaired glucose utilization due to a blockade of the metabolic phosphorylation process,[65] alteration in hepatic glucose metabolism,[70] and chronic insulin secretion and elevated insulin levels accelerating the development of insulin depletion in the prediabetic state.[3,23,165]

Clinical Studies of Thiazide-Induced Glucose Intolerance. Many short- and long-term studies in normal, healthy individuals, nondiabetic and diabetic normotensive individuals, and nondiabetic and diabetic hypertensive individuals have demonstrated conclusively the frequency, onset, duration, and extent of glucose intolerance.[2–5,13,25,44,72,86,117,128,179] In the Medical Research Council Trial on Hypertension,[72] 7 to 9 per cent of both men and women treated with bendrofluazide, 5 mg q.d. to b.i.d., had significantly impaired glucose tolerance. In another study,[117] prolonged use of thiazides was not associated with elevated fasting glucose at 1 year but caused a 13 per cent average increase in fasting glucose in nondiabetic hypertensive patients at 6 years, and 22 per cent had an abnormal glucose tolerance test. Ames[3] found a significant increase in fasting glucose level, abnormal glucose tolerance tests, and glycohemoglobin levels despite an increased insulin response in the fasting state and during the glucose tolerance test. The elevated glucose level was positively correlated with increased serum lipid levels. Others have demonstrated a 30 per cent incidence of glucose intolerance in hypertensive patients treated with thiazide diuretics.[2] Abnormal glucose tolerance tests developed in 22 to 33 per cent[128] after 6 years of therapy with thiazides. About 9 per cent of these patients developed overt diabetes mellitus if there was

a recognized predisposition, such as a positive family history, obesity, or a pretreatment abnormal glucose tolerance test.[128] This familial relationship to the development of diabetes mellitus with thiazides was shown by Marks and colleagues.[128] In their study of 40 patients treated for more than 10 years with thiazides, 4 patients with an elevated glucose level and an abnormal glucose tolerance test had a positive family history of diabetes mellitus.

The European Working Party on Hypertension in the Elderly showed a 9.6 per cent increase in glucose at 2 years on thiazides compared with a 3.1 mg per dl decrease with placebo.[2] In the Veterans Administration Cooperative Study[179] of hypertensive patients, at 2 years, 30 per cent of thiazide-treated patients had a fasting glucose level of more than 110 mg per dl, compared with 17 per cent of placebo-treated patients.

Bloomgarden and coworkers[25] studied 89 patients with insulin-dependent diabetes mellitus and hypertension taking hydrochlorothiazide, furosemide, or no diuretic and found that hydrochlorothiazide, but not furosemide or placebo, caused a significant increase in hemoglobin A_1C and LDL levels but not the fasting glucose level. This suggests that hydrochlorothiazide is associated with a greater postprandial glycemic excursion than its effect on the postabsorptive glucose level.

Ames and Hill[5] withdrew thiazide diuretics in 35 hypertensive nondiabetic patients for 7 weeks and found improved fasting glucose levels (decreased 9.5 per cent) and glucose tolerance tests (reduced glucose levels 14 per cent), reduced glycohemoglobin levels (9 per cent), a decrease in serum lipids (total cholesterol decreased 18 mg per dl; LDL decreased 9 mg per dl; triglyceride decreased 27 mg per dl; VLDL decreased 8 mg per dl), and the total cholesterol–to–HDL ratio fell from 5.1 to 4.5.

Hollifield[86] suggests that the greater the initial glucose level, the greater the change with thiazide diuretics. If the fasting glucose is less than 100 mg per dl, there is minimal nonsignificant hyperglycemia, but if the fasting glucose is greater than 150 mg per dl, a 48 to 270 mg per dl increase occurs.[86] The hyperglycemic effect is dose-dependent,[86,151] age-dependent,[2,117] and duration-dependent.[2,117,128] In elderly patients, it takes less time (1 to 2 years or less) to develop glucose intolerance[2] compared with younger patients, in whom it may take more than 5 years.[117] In nondiabetic hypertensive patients, the fasting glucose may be normal at 1 year but become abnormal at 6 years and be associated with an abnormal glucose tolerance test.[117]

Chlorthalidone

Chlorthalidone is a long-acting thiazide-like diuretic that has been shown to induce glucose intolerance,[4,13,18,33,44,130,178] nonketotic hyperosmolar coma,[45] and adverse lipid changes[4,13,18] in both nondiabetic and diabetic patients with or without hypertension. The hyperglycemic effect is dose-related,[33,130,178] but the antihypertensive effect is not[33,130,178] and plateaus at a dose of 25 mg per day. The mechanism of hyperglycemia is thought to be similar to that of the thiazide diuretics.[3,15,19,23,56,60,61,65,70,82,163,165,188]

In a group of 37 nondiabetic patients with mild to moderate hypertension given progressively increased doses of chlorthalidone (25 to 200 mg per day) over 8 weeks, the antihypertensive effects were similar at high and low doses, but the adverse changes in serum glucose, potassium, chloride, and uric acid levels were dose-related.[178] The changes in fasting glucose from placebo were 5.2 ± 10 mg per dl at 25 mg per day, 10.1 ± 12 mg per dl at 50 mg per day, 11.8 ± 25 mg per dl at 100 mg per day, and 14.4 ± 20.4 mg per dl at 200 mg per day.[178] Other studies demonstrated the same antihypertensive potency of chlorthalidone at 25 mg and 100 mg per day but a dose-related increase in adverse effects on glucose, potassium, uric acid, and bicarbonate levels.[33,130] In the Hypertension Detection and Follow-up Program, about 2 per cent of those patients taking chlorthalidone developed elevated fasting glucose levels or overt diabetes mellitus.[44] Hyperosmolar, hyperglycemic, nonketotic coma or precoma may occur in predisposed patients such as those with overt or latent diabetes, those with a positive family history of diabetes mellitus, and those who are obese, elderly, or severely hypokalemic.[45] Several studies have shown a direct correlation between elevations in serum glucose level and adverse serum lipid changes.[4,18] In the Veterans Administration Study, 329 men with a diastolic blood pressure of 90 to 114 mm Hg treated with 25 to 50 mg of chlorthalidone per day for 12 weeks had a significant elevation in serum glucose, total cholesterol, and triglyceride levels. Ames and Hill[4] demonstrated elevations in glucose (p < 0.001), total cholesterol (222 mg per dl to 237 mg per dl, p < 0.001), and triglyceride (110 mg per dl to 146 mg per dl, p < 0.001) in a group of mildly hypertensive patients.

Loop Diuretics

Furosemide. Furosemide has been reported to induce mild glucose intolerance,[4,13,73,126,154] abnormal glucose tolerance tests,[154] glycosuria,[122,177] nonketotic hyperosmolar coma,[30] precoma,[175] mild elevations in hemoglobin A_1C,[25] and adverse lipid changes (total cholesterol, triglyceride, HDL)[4] occasionally in some patients. The mechanism is thought to be direct inhibition of glucose transport,[95] with no change in insulin levels, glucagon, or growth hormone.[154] The actual incidence of furosemide-induced glucose intolerance is unknown[154] but probably is uncommon.[73] Only 2 of 2367 patients followed on furosemide developed glucose intolerance.[73] Furosemide causes less hyperglycemia and alterations in hemoglobin A_1C and LDL in patients with insulin-dependent diabetes mellitus and hypertension than hydrochlorothiazide and is similar to placebo.[25] In fact, in other studies, there was no significant change in fasting glucose in patients without diabetes mellitus,[154] with insulin-dependent diabetes mellitus,[25] or with non–insulin-dependent diabetes mellitus[154] treated with 40 to 80 mg of furosemide per day and no significant change in glucose tolerance test in diabetics[96] treated for 6 weeks or longer.

The antihypertensive effect of furosemide is less than that of an equivalent dose of a thiazide (40 mg of furosemide versus 50 mg of hydrochlorothiazide per day),[12,28] but the adverse effects on the parameters to assess glucose intolerance are less with furosemide.[25,73,96,126]

Ethacrynic Acid. Ethacrynic acid is unlikely to affect the fasting glucose level,[32,90] glucose tolerance test,[96,126] or 2-hour postprandial glucose level in nondiabetics[90] or diabetics,[90] has a much lower frequency of these measures of glucose intolerance compared with thiazide diuretics[90] at equivalent doses of 50 to 100 mg per day over a 1-week[96,126] to 8-week treatment period,[90] and has an effect similar to that of placebo.[90] A study of 42 patients[90] with or without diabetes mellitus but with essential hypertension who were given ethacrynic acid, 50 mg b.i.d., hydrochlorothiazide, 50 mg b.i.d., or placebo demonstrated that in diabetics, ethacrynic acid had the same effect on glucose level as placebo (mean fasting glucose level of 137 mg per dl in both groups) but less than that which occurred with hydrochlorothiazide (mean fasting glucose level of 137 mg per dl for ethacrynic acid and 163 mg per dl for hydrochlorothiazide). In the 24 nondiabetic hypertensive patients[90] receiving ethacrynic acid, only 3 had a fasting glucose level over 100 mg per dl (107, 110, and 135 mg per dl), which was the same incidence as in the placebo-treated group. Ethacrynic acid, however, may be associated with more ototoxicity, which could limit its usefulness, particularly in higher doses.[28]

Bumetanide. Bumetanide has been shown to cause minimal to no change in fasting glucose level or glucose tolerance test in normal patients treated with 2 mg per day over 8 days[154] or in patients with non–insulin-dependent diabetes mellitus treated for 6 weeks.[126] No changes in insulin, glucagon, or growth hormone levels have been reported.[126,154] It should also be noted that 80 per cent of bumetanide is absorbed orally compared with only 50 per cent of furosemide.[28] This could alter the necessary antihypertensive or diuretic dose when changing from an intravenous to oral form with either drug, but more so with furosemide.

Conclusions. All loop diuretics have similar efficacy in treating hypertension[28] but in equipotent doses are less effective compared with thiazide or thiazide-like diuretics.[12,28] Glucose intolerance occurs less frequently with all loop diuretics compared with thiazide diuretics, and ethacrynic acid apparently has the least effect of the three loop diuretics.[25,28] In hypertensive patients, the loop diuretics should be reserved for those who have significant glucose intolerance or adverse lipid changes on thiazides, who have renal insufficiency with a creatinine clearance of less than 30 to 35 ml per minute (a point at which thiazide diuretics are ineffective), or have demonstrated lack of efficacy or adverse effects.[28]

Potassium-Sparing Diuretics

Triamterene. No known adverse effects on glucose tolerance have been demonstrated with triamterene,[43,65] but elevations in serum potassium may occur in normal individuals and especially in patients with diabetes mellitus and renal insufficiency.[43] It is a weak antihypertensive agent.

Amiloride. Amiloride does not induce glucose intolerance[65,112,135] but will elevate serum potassium in normal individuals, diabetics, and patients with renal insufficiency;[112,135] it will also increase uric acid and blood urea nitrogen (BUN).[112,135] It is a weak antihypertensive agent.

Spironolactone. Spironolactone has no adverse effects on serum glucose[6,41,65,89] or serum lipid levels.[4,6,65] In a study by Ames and Peacock,[6] 11 of 23 men with hypertension treated with hydrochlorothiazide or chlorthalidone, 50 to 100 mg per day, and diet were switched to spironolactone, 50 to 100 mg a day, for 2 to 4

months. In the spironolactone-treated patients, there was a significant reduction of total cholesterol of 24 mg per dl (compared with a reduction of 3 mg per dl with thiazides), a reduction of triglyceride of 58 mg per dl (compared with a reduction of 10 mg per dl with thiazides), a nonsignificant decrease in glucose of 4 mg per dl, and a nonsignificant increase in potassium of 0.9 mEq per liter. Spironolactone may cause hyperkalemia in normal patients or those with diabetes mellitus or renal insufficiency.[89] Hyperuricemia is rare.[6,41,89] The antihypertensive effects are similar to those of equal doses of thiazide diuretics and chlorthalidone.[6]

Indapamide

Although indapamide is reported to not induce adverse changes in glucose,[14,126,145,176] lipoprotein,[126,145,176] potassium,[126,145,176] or uric acid levels,[14,126,145,176] there is some controversy, depending on the dose and patient population selected.[1] There may be less hyperglycemia, hypokalemia, and hyperlipidemia with indapamide compared with thiazides,[176] but this must be balanced against other conflicting data[1,14] and the high cost of indapamide compared with thiazides. In a study of 30 black hypertensive patients with insulin-dependent diabetes mellitus[14] receiving 2.5 mg of indapamide per day for 2 to 3 months, there was a significant fall in systolic blood pressure (159 to 142 mm Hg), diastolic blood pressure (102 to 87 mm Hg), and serum potassium but no significant change in fasting glucose, BUN, or chloride levels. In a group of 29 patients with hypertension and renal insufficiency, some on hemodialysis,[1] there was a significant increase in fasting glucose (87 to 129 mg per dl), total cholesterol (172 to 179 mg per dl), triglyceride (100 to 131 mg per dl), and uric acid (8.2 to 8.6 mg per dl) and a decrease in serum potassium (5.5 to 4.5 mEq per liter).

Conclusions and Recommendations for Use of Diuretics

Thiazide and thiazide-like diuretics (chlorthalidone, metolazone) and indapamide have equal antihypertensive potency if given in equal doses but are superior to loop diuretics for the treatment of hypertension.[12,28] Lower doses of thiazide and thiazide-like diuretics have equal antihypertensive efficacy compared with higher doses, which plateaus at an equivalent dose of 25 mg of hydrochlorothiazide per day.[11,20,33,124,130,178] Doses exceeding this level increase adverse effects such as hyperglycemia and glucose intolerance, hypokalemia, hypomagnesemia, hyperuricemia, hyperlipidemia, hypercalcemia, elevated BUN, and other electrolyte disorders[33,68,130,151] without enhancing efficacy. Hyperglycemia and glucose intolerance and possibly hyperlipidemia are more common with thiazide diuretics, chlorthalidone, metolazone, and probably indapamide compared with the loop diuretics and potassium-sparing diuretics. However, triamterene and amiloride are weak antihypertensive agents compared with spironolactone and other diuretics.

The onset of glucose intolerance with thiazide diuretics, chlorthalidone, metolazone, and indapamide is immediate (days to 1 week) or years,[62,63,98–101] depending on age,[2,117] family history of diabetes mellitus,[128,132] duration of treatment,[2,117,130,132] dose,[86,124,132,151] premorbid fasting glucose level,[86,128,132] presence of diabetes mellitus,[128,132] glucose tolerance test abnormalities,[128,132] weight,[128] and the presence of congestive heart failure.[128] In normal patients, glucose intolerance may occur within 2 to 5 years, whereas in prediabetics, it may start in 8 weeks, and in overt diabetes mellitus, within 1 to 2 weeks.[130,132] Sulfonamide-based diuretics have the most adverse effects on glucose tolerance, and their effects may last for 2 weeks to 6 months after the diuretic is stopped.[6]

If glucose intolerance does occur with any diuretic agent that increases CHD or other cardiovascular risk and induces other complications in the hypertensive patient, it would be advisable to reduce the dose, switch to another class of diuretics with equal efficacy but no adverse effects, or discontinue the diuretic completely and use one of the nondiuretic antihypertensive agents that does not alter glucose tolerance, such as clonidine, guanabenz, prazosin, captopril, or a calcium-channel blocker[132] (see later discussion). It would be less advisable to give an oral hypoglycemic agent or insulin. With regard to low-dose diuretic therapy, it has been demonstrated that 80 per cent of the antihypertensive effect of thiazide diuretics is achieved at a dose of 12.5 mg per day or its equivalent and that 100 per cent of the antihypertensive effect is achieved at 25 mg per day.[11,20,33,124,130] Further increases to 50 mg, 100 mg, or 200 mg do not lower the blood pressure in most patients but will increase side effects. Doses as low as 6.25 mg of hydrochlorothiazide may be effective in some patients in combination with other nondiuretic antihypertensive agents.[11] Chlorthalidone demonstrates a similar antihypertensive dose response curve at 25 mg per day.[33,130,178]

It would seem prudent to monitor glucose levels in all patients treated with diuretics, particularly those listed in Table 7, and to make the appropriate changes in the therapeutic regimen as noted previously.

Central Alpha-Agonists

The three central alpha-agonists available in the United States for the treatment of hypertension are clonidine, guanabenz, and methyldopa. None of the agents has a significant effect on glucose tolerance, but they do differ in their effects on other biochemical parameters and their clinical use.[4, 17, 21, 24, 65, 75, 88, 93, 103, 108, 111, 134, 142, 150, 169, 173, 186, 187, 195] Each of these antihypertensive drugs will be discussed in detail.

Clonidine

Despite reports and studies of transient clonidine-induced hyperglycemia in some laboratory animals,[27,85,91,127,153,164] the effects have not occurred in other animals[27,131] or in in vitro pancreatic islet cell preparations.[113] In most studies, the doses given orally, intravenously, intra-arterially, or intracisternally were excessive and well beyond those used clinically in humans.[27] In one study,[27] 10 μg per kg of clonidine administered into the vertebral artery of cats produced hyperglycemia, but the blood pressure fell 40 to 50 per cent. Intravenous injections and lower infusion doses had no effect on blood glucose.[27] Therefore, the doses used in experimental animal studies that suggest a hyperglycemic response to clonidine were excessively high, greater than those required to reduce blood pressure, and the effect on glucose tolerance is not clinically important.[27] In addition, clonidine-

Table 7.   *Subgroups of Patients in Whom Glucose Monitoring is Advisable During Diuretic Therapy*[2,117,128,132]

1. Patients receiving chronic treatment
2. Patients receiving thiazide and thiazide-like diuretics, chlorthalidone, indapamide, and metolazone particularly (more so than with loop diuretics and spironolactone)
3. Patients with latent or overt diabetes mellitus
4. Patients with an abnormal glucose tolerance test before treatment
5. Patients with an elevated pretreatment fasting glucose level
6. Patients with a positive family history of diabetes mellitus
7. Obese patients
8. Patients with congestive heart failure
9. Elderly patients
10. Patients receiving high-dose diuretics

induced glucose intolerance is rare in humans. Human studies have shown that chronic administration of clonidine does not cause significant hyperglycemia[24,88,111,134,142,150,169,173,186,195] and that it is useful in the treatment of the hypertensive patient with diabetes mellitus.[24,75,88]

The proposed mechanism of the transient hyperglycemia response noted in some studies includes a central effect on alpha-receptors in the hypothalamus and pituitary,[27,84] alpha-receptor suppression of pancreatic insulin release (dose-dependent),[84] increased growth hormone levels[84,161] with no effect on prolactin-releasing, luteinizing, follicle-stimulating, or thyroid-stimulating hormones,[161] and a dual dopaminergic and noradrenergic mechanism increase of growth hormone and glucose.[161]

Numerous human studies after oral and intravenous administration of clonidine have demonstrated no significant acute or chronic glucose intolerance in normal individuals,[161] hypertensive normal individuals (nondiabetics),[24, 75, 88, 108, 111, 134, 142, 150, 169, 173, 195] or hypertensive diabetics[75,88,150] as measured by fasting glucose, glucose tolerance test, 24-hour urine glucose, postprandial glucose, and glycosylated hemoglobin.[161] Intravenous administration of clonidine to normal patients results in an average 12 mg per dl increase (not significant [NS]) in serum glucose at 15 minutes, which returned to baseline at 90 minutes.[161] In another group of nine nondiabetic mildly to moderately hypertensive patients given 0.4 mg of clonidine per day (0.1 mg q.i.d.) for 6 weeks, the fasting glucose level increased from 92 to 99 mg per dl (NS),[173] and there was no difference in the glucose tolerance test compared with that in patients given placebo.[173] However, if chlorthalidone, 60 mg per day, was added to the clonidine, the fasting glucose increased from 92 ± 5 mg per dl to 103 ± 5 mg per dl. In another study of 25 nondiabetic hypertensive patients treated for 3 to 8 months, there was no change in carbohydrate metabolism[111]; a similar group of 188 patients receiving 0.2 to 0.8 mg of clonidine per day had no change in glucose level or glucose tolerance test over 6 months.[108,134] In patients treated with clonidine, there is also a favorable lipid profile, with a reduction in total cholesterol, triglyceride, and LDL and an increase in HDL.[93,108,186] Guthrie[75] studied 10 patients with mild hypertension (a diastolic blood pressure of 90 to 104 mm Hg) and non–insulin-dependent diabetes mellitus receiving clonidine, 0.1 mg b.i.d., for 10 weeks and found no significant changes in fasting glucose, 24-hour urine glucose, or glycosylated hemoglobin levels.

Methyldopa

Clinical studies with methyldopa in patients with hypertension have shown no significant adverse effects on glucose tolerance,[4,21,65] but there was a definite increase in one study that did not achieve statistical significance.[21] Benfield and Hunter[21] compared 10 patients with hypertension and insulin-dependent diabetes mellitus in a 12-week randomized, double-blind, cross-over study with monotherapy with oxprenolol or methyldopa up to 1500 mg per day. The fasting glucose level increased from 176.4 mg per dl (mean) to 219.6 mg per dl (mean), but as mentioned, this did not reach statistical significance. However, triglyceride levels increased from 105 mg per dl to 133.5 mg per dl (p < 0.01) and free fatty acid levels fell from 1.03 mEq per liter to 0.45 mEq per liter (p < 0.05). Changes in HDL and total cholesterol were not significantly different from pretreatment values. The study by Ames and Hill[4] showed a significant reduction in HDL (p < 0.05) and the total cholesterol–to–HDL ratio (p < 0.02).

Guanabenz

Guanabenz has been reported to cause no significant change in fasting glucose in some studies[75] or a significant increase in fasting glucose in other human studies.[17] A group of 188 hypertensive patients given 8 to 64 mg per day of guanabenz over 6 months had no significant change in glucose level and a significant 20 per cent reduction in total cholesterol.[186] However, another study[17] of 40 hypertensive men receiving 8 to 12 mg per day of guanabenz showed a significant increase in fasting glucose at 3 to 6 weeks (98 to 105 mg per dl) and at 6 months (98 to 111 mg per dl) (p < 0.025). The total cholesterol and LDL are significantly reduced on guanabenz,[103,186,187] without change in VLDL, triglycerides, or HDL.[103]

Postganglionic Neuron Inhibitors

There has been no reported adverse effects on glucose tolerance with reserpine,[65,143] guanethidine,[65,193] or guanadrel.[54] In the Veterans Administration Study[18] of 329 men with a diastolic blood pressure of 90 to 114 mm Hg treated for 12 weeks with chlorthalidone, 25 to 50 mg per day, there was a slight but insignificant reduction in fasting glucose and triglyceride levels and a significant reduction in total cholesterol when reserpine, 0.05 to 0.25 mg per day, was added. However, other significant clinical side effects, such as severe orthostatic hypotension and impotence with guanethidine[65,193] and guanadrel[54] and a high incidence of depression with reserpine,[65] make these agents less desirable for modern-day treatment of hypertension.

Direct and Indirect Vasodilators

The indirect vasodilator prazosin (a peripheral alpha-blocker)[18,65,108,114,139] and the direct vasodilators hydralazine[65,110] and minoxidil[31,65,118] have no adverse effects on glucose tolerance. However, diazoxide may induce marked hyperglycemia or hyperosmolar nonketotic hyperglycemic coma.[35,65,192] Neither hydralazine nor minoxidil can be used as monotherapy for hypertension because of reflux tachycardia, exacerbation of ischemic heart disease, and tachyphylaxis due to reflex volume retention.[65] Prazosin, on the other hand, may be effective as monotherapy in hypertensive patients without diabetes mellitus[18,65,108,114,139] and with diabetes mellitus[114,139] without adverse effects on glucose tolerance, although its antihypertensive effects are enhanced by low-dose diuretic administration. In doses up to 20 mg per day for 8 weeks, prazosin caused no significant change in fasting serum glucose but a reduction in total cholesterol.[108] Other studies have also confirmed the favorable effects on serum lipids, including a reduction in total cholesterol, triglycerides, VLDL, LDL and an increase in HDL.[3,114,139] Bauer and associates[18] demonstrated a short-term (3 to 6 weeks) significant reduction in fasting glucose levels (81 to 72 mg per dl) in 14 male hypertensive patients receiving 1 to 10 mg per day of prazosin. However, with chronic therapy (5 to 6 months), fasting glucose levels returned to pretreatment levels (about 86 mg per dl).

Beta-Blockers

All the beta-blockers approved for clinical use in the United States have been shown to induce glucose intolerance in hypertensive or normal patients,[7,13,17,23,64,72,80,133,180,181,192,194] to induce nonketotic hyperosmolar hyperglycemic coma,[65,148] and to induce overt diabetes mellitus[23] or to exacerbate hyperglycemia in patients with diabetes mellitus,[194] as well as to have adverse effects on serum lipids.[13,51,64,65,72,93,115,120,194] Nonselective beta-blockers (that is, propranolol, nadolol, and timolol)[155,182,194] and high-

dose cardioselective beta-blockers (that is, atenolol and metoprolol)[141,194] are most likely to have an adverse effect on glucose tolerance, whereas beta-blockers with intrinsic sympathomimetic activity (that is, pindolol and acebutolol) have a minimal effect.[13,46,47,116,146] The effects of propranolol on insulin secretion and glucose intolerance have been the best studied and will be reviewed in detail to serve as a prototype for the other beta-blockers.

Mechanism of Glucose Intolerance with Beta-Blockers. Numerous mechanisms have been proposed to explain the glucose intolerance that occurs with beta-blockers (Table 8). Beta-blockade inhibits pancreatic insulin secretion (by 38 ± 15 per cent), possibly because of reduced granulation or membrane-stabilizing effects,[26,97,133,166,180,194] and glucose levels increase. Other mechanisms include increased hepatic glycogenolysis,[194] inhibition of peripheral glucose utilization,[23] increased growth hormone,[125] and reduced tissue sensitivity to insulin.[23]

Propranolol. The hyperglycemia induced by propranolol is equal to that caused by diuretics,[180,181] particularly hydrochlorothiazide.[180] In the Veterans Administration Cooperative Study on Hypertension,[180] 683 men receiving either propranolol (up to 640 mg per day) or hydrochlorothiazide (up to 200 mg per day) titrated to a diastolic blood pressure of less than 90 mm Hg had equivalent increases in fasting glucose levels from 103 to 110 mg per dl. About 3 per cent of hypertensive patients in the Medical Research Council Trial on Hypertension[72] developed impaired glucose tolerance. The Cleveland Clinic Study[133] of 40 nondiabetic hypertensive patients receiving 160 to 320 mg per day of propranolol for 6 months found a 57.5 per cent incidence of overt or latent diabetes mellitus on a 4-hour glucose tolerance test associated with blunted insulin secretion. After propranolol was discontinued in the patients with overt diabetes mellitus, 7 patients had reduced insulin requirement or stopped insulin completely. In 9 of 16 patients with latent diabetes mellitus, the 4-hour glucose tolerance test returned to normal within 3 to 6

Table 8. *Proposed Mechanisms of Glucose Intolerance with Beta-Blockers*

1. Beta-blockade inhibition of insulin secretion
2. Increased hepatic glycogenolysis secondary to reduced insulin secretion and relative preponderance of alpha-receptor–mediated glycogenolysis during beta-blockade
3. Inhibition of peripheral glucose utilization
4. Decreased peripheral sensitivity to insulin
5. Elevation of growth hormone levels

months after propranolol was discontinued.[133] Other studies have documented significant increases in fasting glucose,[64] 88.8 to 102 mg per dl on 80 mg b.i.d. for 8 weeks (12.8 per cent increase), overt diabetes mellitus,[23] or nonketotic hyperglycemic hyperosmolar coma.[65,148] In the Oslo Study,[80] the combination of a thiazide (hydrochlorothiazide, 50 mg per day) and propranolol (40 to 160 mg b.i.d.) caused a more significant increase in serum glucose (p < 0.001) and triglyceride (p < 0.001), more than any other antihypertensive drug combination. In a study of 20 hypertensive diabetic patients, the fasting glucose and postprandial glucose levels increased by 18 to 27 mg per dl[194] and triglyceride increased unrelated to the glucose change while they were taking propranolol, 80 mg b.i.d., for 12 weeks. There were no changes in insulin concentrations, and the glucose intolerance did not correlate with the plasma propranolol level. Propranolol-induced glucose intolerance was greater than that induced by metoprolol.[194] Numerous other studies have reported glucose intolerance in normal hypertensive and diabetic patients receiving propranolol[13,17,65,72,192] that is dose- and duration-related and in which the glucose intolerance may take 3 to 6 months to return to normal after beta-blockade is stopped.

Nadolol. Nadolol has effects on glucose intolerance that are virtually identical to those of propranolol.[182] In the Veterans Administration Cooperative Study of 489 men, with administration of nadolol alone, the fasting glucose level increased from 97 to 103 ± 2 mg per dl in 12 weeks and the triglyceride level increased 23 per cent.[182]

Timolol. Timolol elevated blood glucose by 75 mg per dl (p < 0.05) in 173 hypertensive patients over a 54-week study period.[182]

Metoprolol. In a group of hypertensive patients given 150 to 450 mg of metoprolol per day, there was no significant change in fasting glucose level, glucose tolerance test, or insulin level.[55] However, in 20 patients with diabetes mellitus and hypertension given metoprolol, 100 mg b.i.d., for 12 weeks, the fasting glucose and postprandial glucose levels increased significantly by 18 to 27 mg per dl,[194] as did triglyceride levels. There was no significant change in insulin concentration.

Atenolol. Atenolol had a minimal effect on serum glucose in one long-term study,[141] but in higher doses, the beta-adrenergic cardioselectivity is lost, and glucose intolerance may be similar to that of nonselective beta-blockers.

Pindolol. Pindolol does not usually alter carbohydrate metabolism or increase glucose in normal, prediabetic, or diabetic patients,[146] although it still may induce mild hyperglycemia in some patients.[13]

Acebutolol. Acebutolol has minimal to no effect on glucose intolerance.[46,47,116] When compared with hydrochlorothiazide, acebutolol produced fewer biochemical changes in glucose, lipids, potassium, and uric acid.[116]

Labetalol. Although labetalol is reported to cause minimal to no alteration in glucose levels,[123] other studies[7] in nondiabetic hypertensive men treated for 4 weeks with 300 to 1200 mg per day of labetalol showed a significant increase in fasting glucose of 95 to 106 mg per dl (p < 0.01) but no significant change in the oral glucose tolerance test.

Angiotensin-Converting Enzyme Inhibitors

Captopril causes no significant elevation in glucose or serum lipid levels in hypertensive normal or diabetic patients[58,109,183] and may actually improve glucose tolerance in both patients with insulin-dependent diabetes mellitus and those with non–insulin-dependent diabetes mellitus.[58] In 24 male patients with a diastolic blood pressure of 95 to 115 mm Hg for 8 weeks, there was no significant change in serum glucose or lipid levels on doses of captopril of 100 mg b.i.d.[109] In a similar study, 495 men with a diastolic blood pressure of 92 to 109 mm Hg who were treated with captopril, 50 mg t.i.d., for 14 weeks had no change in glucose or lipid levels.[183] In a group of four hypertensive patients[58] with diabetes mellitus (three with insulin-dependent diabetes mellitus and one with non–insulin-dependent diabetes mellitus), the three patients with insulin-dependent diabetes mellitus had hypoglycemia while receiving captopril and the patient with non–insulin-dependent diabetes mellitus had to stop taking oral hypoglycemics while receiving captopril. A follow-up study of nine patients (three with non–insulin-dependent diabetes mellitus, one with insulin-dependent diabetes mellitus, and five nondiabetics) given 50 mg b.i.d. of captopril demonstrated that the average blood glucose level was similar before and after treatment, but the glucose disposal rate was higher on captopril as measured by a euglycemic glucose-clamp method.[58] It is suggested that there may be enhanced insulin sensitivity induced by captopril, possibly secondary to decreased serum catecholamine levels or a direct yet unproven effect on the insulin or postinsulin receptor.[58]

Calcium-Channel Blockers

Studies of isolated pancreatic islet cells show reduced insulin secretion (regulated by calcium influx) when exposed to calcium antagonists.[129,170] High intravenous doses of verapamil in dogs inhibit insulin secretion.[52] In humans, similar increases in glucose and reduction in insulin secretion may occur with diltiazem,[174] nifedipine,[36,67] and verapamil.[10,49,156] Other studies, however, have demonstrated that basal insulin secretion in normal healthy patients is not influenced by diltiazem,[174] nifedipine,[36,53] or verapamil.[8–10,156] The effect on insulin secretion and glucose level can be demonstrated in normal patients only with high intravenous doses when stimulated by sulfonylureas.[36,49,67,156,174] In the usual therapeutic doses, there are no effects on insulin secretion in humans with a normal pancreas.[8,67,156] In fact, the glucose tolerance may actually improve in patients with non–insulin-dependent diabetes mellitus and normal patients[67] with nifedipine[53] and verapamil.[9] If an elevation in the blood glucose level occurs, it is usually transient[53] and probably secondary to extrahepatic causes,[10,67,156] such as elevated sympathetic nervous system activity.[10] There are no reports of adverse serum lipid changes with calcium-channel blockers.[129,172]

In 15 hypertensive patients, poorly controlled on atenolol and bendrofluazide, the addition of 10 to 30 mg t.i.d. of nifedipine resulted in an insignificant change in fasting glucose (104 to 109 mg per dl) but a significant fall in potassium (3.9 to 3.6 mEq per liter) (p < 0.05).[136] Eight patients with angina treated with diltiazem, 360 mg per day, for 12 to 16 months had no significant alteration in serum glucose or lipid levels.[147] In 15 patients given verapamil, 80 to 160 mg t.i.d., for 3 months, there was no change in glucose or lipid levels (total cholesterol, triglycerides, and HDL).[172,184]

SUMMARY, CONCLUSIONS, AND RECOMMENDATIONS

Antihypertensive drug therapy ultimately should reduce short- and long-term cardiovascular morbidity and mortality in patients with primary essential hypertension. *Optimal* reduction of *all* CHD risk factors, including blood pressure, should be a primary goal of the clinician, as CHD remains the major cause of death in the United States. Adverse changes in certain risk factors for CHD, such as serum glucose, lipids, electrolytes, and exercise capacity by some antihypertensive agents (particularly beta-blockers and diuretics) may partially or completely negate the beneficial effects of blood pressure reduction as it relates to CHD risk and its subsequent complications. In addition, antihypertensive drug therapy should reverse the primary hemodynamic abnormality in essential hypertension, an elevated systemic vascular resistance, without causing an adverse reduction in cardiac output. Further derangements of these hemodynamic abnormalities occur with such antihypertensive agents as beta-blockers without intrinsic sympathomimetic activity, reserpine, guanethidine, and guanadrel. Finally, the selected antihypertensive agent should not have an unfavorable influence on concomitant medical problems or diseases in the hypertensive patient.

Glucose intolerance is a well-documented risk factor for CHD. Significant elevations in the fasting glucose level or abnormalities in the glucose tolerance test are correlated positively with increased CHD risk. Antihypertensive medications that induce significant glucose intolerance may partially negate some of the beneficial effects on CHD risk, despite a reduction in blood pressure. The antihypertensive agents most frequently associated with this glucose intolerance include the thiazide and thiazide-like diuretics, chlorthalidone, and metolazone, with less adverse effects with the loop diuretics and indapamide. The potassium-sparing diuretics do not induce glucose intolerance. All the beta-blockers may induce glucose intolerance to some degree, which depends in part on characteristics such as cardioselectivity and intrinsic sympathomimetic activity. Nonselective and high-dose cardioselective beta-blockers induce the most glucose intolerance, whereas low-dose cardioselective beta-blockers, those with intrinsic sympathomimetic activity, and labetalol, comparatively speaking, have less of an adverse effect.

The central alpha-agonists, direct and indirect vasodilators (peripheral alpha-blockers), angiotensin-converting enzyme inhibitors, and calcium-channel blockers cause no significant increase in glucose intolerance in most clinical studies and are also appropriate in patients with diabetes mellitus.

All patients placed on antihypertensive drug therapy should have several biochemical parameters followed to assure that CHD risk factors such as glucose, lipids, and electrolytes are not affected adversely. Certain subsets of patients most likely to develop glucose intolerance include those receiving chronic high-dose thiazide treatment with or without hypokalemia and beta-blocker therapy, patients with latent or overt diabetes mellitus (elevated fasting glucose, abnormal glucose tolerance test, positive family history of diabetes mellitus), obese patients, the elderly, and those with congestive heart failure. Should significant glucose intolerance occur, it may be advisable to switch to another antihypertensive agent or to lower the dose of the offending agent if replacement of potassium does not correct the hyperglycemia.

It is no longer acceptable to monitor only blood pressure and attempt to reduce it without following the changes in biochemical parameters in the patient in order to achieve maximal reduction of the incidence of CHD.

REFERENCES

1. Acchiardo, S.R., and Skoutakis, V.A.: Clinical efficacy, safety, and pharmacokinetics of indapamide in renal impairment. Am. Heart. J., *106*:237–244, 1983.
2. Amery, A., Berthaux, P., Bulpitt, C., et al.: Glucose intolerance during diuretic therapy. Results of trial by the European Working Party on Hypertension in the Elderly. Lancet, *1*:681–683, 1978.
3. Ames, R.P.: Negative effects of diuretic drugs on metabolic risk factors for coronary heart disease: Possible alternative drug therapies. Am. J. Cardiol., *51*:632–638, 1983.
4. Ames, R.P., and Hill, P.: Antihypertensive therapy and the risk of coronary heart disease. J. Cardiovasc. Pharmacol.,*4*(Suppl. 2):S206–S212, 1982.
5. Ames, R.P., and Hill, P.: Improvement of glucose tolerance and lowering of glycohemoglobin and serum lipid concentrations after discontinuation of antihypertensive drug therapy. Circulation, *65*:899–904, 1982.
6. Ames, R.P., and Peacock, P.B.: Serum cholesterol during treatment of hypertension with diuretic drugs. Arch. Intern. Med., *144*:710–714, 1984.
7. Andersson, D., Berglund, G., and Hansson, L.: Antihypertensive action, time of onset and effects of carbohydrate metabolism of labetalol. Br. J. Clin. Pharmacol., *3*(Suppl. 3):757–761, 1976.
8. Andersson, D.E.H., and Röjdmark, S.: Effect of verapamil on blood glucose and serum insulin in patients with hyper- and hypothyroidism. Acta Med. Scand., *208*:375–379, 1980.
9. Andersson, D.E.H., and Röjdmark, S.: Improvement of glucose tolerance by verapamil in patients with non–insulin dependent diabetes mellitus. Acta Med. Scand., *210*:27–33, 1981.
10. Andersson, D.E.H., Röjdmark, S., Hed, R., et al.: Effect of verapamil on glucose response to glucagon during intravenous infusion of somatostatin. Horm. Metab. Res., *12*:554–555, 1980.
11. Andren, L., Weiner, L., and Svensson, A.: Enalapril with either "very low" or "low" dose hydrochlorothiazide is equally effective in essential hypertension. A double-blind trial in 100 hypertensive patients. J. Hypertension, *1*:384–386, 1983.
12. Araoye, M.A., Chang, M.Y., Khatri, I.M., et al.: Furosemide compared with hydrochlorothiazide: Long term treatment of hypertension. J.A.M.A., *240*:1863–1866, 1978.
13. Arnesen, E., Thelle, D.S., Førde, O.H., et al.: Serum lipids and glucose concentrations in subjects using antihypertensive drugs: Finnmark 1977. J. Epidemiol. Community Health, *37*:141–144, 1983.
14. Bam, W.J., and Bouwer, C.: Hypertension in diabetic patients—an evaluation of indapamide treatment. S. Afr. Med. J., *63*:802–803, 1983.
15. Barnett, C.A., and Whitney, J.E.: The effect of diazoxide and chlorothiazide on glucose uptake in vitro. Metabolism, *15*:88–93, 1966.
16. Barrett-Connor, E., Criqui, M.H., Klauber, M.R., et al.: Diabetes and hypertension in a community of older adults. Am. J. Epidemiol., *113*:276–284, 1981.
17. Bauer, J.H., and Burch, R.N.: Comparative studies: Guanabenz versus propranolol as first step therapy for the treatment of primary hypertension. Cardiovasc. Rev. Rep., *4*:329–339, 1983.
18. Bauer, J.H., Jones, L.B., and Gaddy, P.: Effects of prazosin therapy on BP, renal function and body fluid composition. Arch. Intern. Med., *144*:1196–1200, 1984.
19. Beardwood, D.M., Alden, J.S., Graham, C.A., et al.: Evidence for a peripheral action of chlorothiazide in normal man. Metabolism, *14*:561–567, 1965.
20. Beerman, B., and Groschinsky-Grind, M.: Antihypertensive effect of various doses of hydrochlorothiazide and its relation to the plasma level of the drug. Eur. J. Clin. Pharmacol., *13*:195–201, 1978.
21. Benfield, G.F., and Hunter, K.R.: Oxprenolol, methyldopa and lipids in diabetes mellitus. Br. J. Clin. Pharmacol., *13*:219–222, 1982.
22. Bergenstal, R.M., and Rubenstein, A.H.: Metabolic control and complications in diabetic patients. J.A.M.A., *245*:735–736, 1981.
23. Berglund, G., and Andersson, O.: Beta-blockers or diuretics in hypertension? A six year follow-up of blood pressure and metabolic side effects. Lancet, *1*:744–747, 1981.
24. Bhandarkar, S.D., and Vernekar, K.S.: Clonidine as an antihypertensive drug in diabetics. J. Postgrad. Med., *24*:182–185, 1978.
25. Bloomgarden, Z.T., Ginsberg-Fellner, Rayfield, E.J., et al.: Elevated hemoglobin A_1C and low density lipoprotein cholesterol levels in thiazide treated diabetic patients. Am. J. Med., *77*:823–827, 1984.
26. Blum, I., Doron, M., Laron, Z., et al.: Prevention of hypoglycemic attacks by propranolol in a patient suffering from insulinoma. Diabetes, *24*:535–537, 1975.
27. Bock, J.U., and VanZwieten, P.A.: The central hyperglycemic effect of clonidine. Eur. J. Pharmacol., *16*:303–310, 1971.
28. Brater, D.C.: Clinical use of loop diuretics. Hospital Formulary, *18*:962–975, 1983.
29. Brownlee, M., Vlassara, H., and Cerami, A.: Nonenzymatic glycosylation and the pathogenesis of diabetic complications. Ann. Intern. Med., *101*:527–537, 1984.
30. Burke, G.J.: Nonketotic, hyponatremic, normosmolar, diabetic coma and moderate furosemide therapy. S. Afr. Med. J., *50*:2118, 1976.
31. Canaday, B.: Minoxidil. South. Med. J., *73*:59–64, 1980.
32. Cannon, P.J.: Diuretics: Their mechanism of action and use in hypertension. Cardiovasc. Rev. Rep., *4*:649–666, 1983.
33. Carney, S., Gillies, A.I., and Morgan, T.: Optimal dose of a thiazide diuretic. Med. J. Aust., *2*:692–693, 1976.
34. Cerasi, E., Luft, R., and Efendic, S.: Effect of adre-

nergic blocking agents on insulin response to glucose infusion in man. Acta Endocrinol., 69:335–346, 1972.

35. Charles, M.A., and Danforth, E.: Monketoacidotic hyperglycemia and coma during intravenous diazoxide therapy in uremia. Diabetes, 20:501–503, 1971.

36. Charles, S., Ketelslegers, J.M., Buysschaert, M., et al.: Hyperglycaemic effect of nifedipine. Br. Med. J., 283:19–20, 1981.

37. Christlieb, A.R.: The hypertensions of diabetes. Diabetes Care, 5:50–58, 1982.

38. Christlieb, A.R.: Diabetes and hypertension. Cardiovasc. Rev. Rep., 1:609–616, 1980.

39. Christlieb, A.R.: Diabetes and hypertensive vascular disease: Mechanisms and treatment. Am. J. Cardiol., 32:592–606, 1973.

40. Christlieb, A.R.: Management of hypertension in the patient with diabetes mellitus. Pract. Cardiol., 8:94–103, 1982.

41. Crane, M.G., and Harris, J.J.: Effect of spironolactone in hypersensitive patients. Am. J. Med. Sci., 260:311–330, 1970.

42. Crofford, O.: Report of the National Commission on Diabetes. DHEW Publication No. (NIH) 76-1018. Washington, D.C., Government Printing Office, 1975.

43. Crosley, A.P., Jr., Ronquillo, L.M., Strickland, W.H., et al.: Triamterene, a new natriuretic agent. Preliminary observations in man. Ann. Intern. Med., 56:241–251, 1962.

44. Curb, J.D., Borhani, N.O., Blaszkowski, T.P., et al.: Long-term surveillance for adverse effects of antihypertensive drugs. J.A.M.A., 253:3263–3268, 1985.

45. Curtis, J., and Horrigan, F.: Chlorthialidone-induced hyperosmolar hyperglycemic nonketotic coma. J.A.M.A., 220:1592–1593, 1972.

46. Davidov, M.: Acebutolol in essential hypertension: Result of two multicenter studies against placebo and propranolol. Am. Heart J., 109(Suppl. 2):1158–1167, 1985.

47. DeBono, G., Kaye, C.M., Roland, E., et al.: Acebutolol: Ten years of experience. Am Heart J., 109(Suppl. 2):1211–1224, 1985.

48. DeFronzo, R.A., and Lang, R.: Hypophosphatemia and glucose intolerance: Evidence for tissue insensitivity to insulin. N. Engl. J. Med., 303:1259–1262, 1980.

49. DeMarinus, L., and Barbarino, A.: Calcium antagonists and hormone release. I. Effects of verapamil on insulin release in normal subjects and patients with islet-cell tumor. Metabolism, 29:599–604, 1980.

50. Diamond, M.T.: Hyperglycemic hyperosmolar coma associated with hydrochlorothiazide and pancreatitis. N.Y. State J. Med., 72:1741–1742, 1972.

51. Diehm, C., and Morl, H.: Lipid metabolism and antihypertensive treatment. In Weber, M.A., Drayer, J.I.M., and Kolloch, R. (eds.): Low Dose Oral and Transdermal Therapy of Hypertension. New York, Springer-Verlag, 1985, pp. 31–38.

52. Dominic, J.A., Miller, R.E., and McAllister, R.C.: Impairment of glucose tolerance by verapamil in the conscious dog. Diabetes, 28(Suppl.):438, 1979.

53. Donnely, T., and Harrower, A.D.B.: Effect of nifedipine on glucose tolerance and insulin secretion in diabetic and nondiabetic patients. Curr. Med. Res. Opin., 6:690–693, 1980.

54. Dunn, M.I., and Dunlap, J.L.: Guanadrel. A new antihypertensive drug. J.A.M.A., 245:1639–1642, 1981.

55. Ekberg, G., and Hansson, B.G.: Glucose tolerance and insulin release in hypertensive patients treated with the cardioselective beta-receptor blocking agent metoprolol. Acta Med. Scand., 202:393–397, 1977.

56. Fajans, S.S., Floyd, J.C., Knopf, R.F., et al.: Benzothiadiazine suppression of insulin release from normal and abnormal islet cell tissue in man. J. Clin. Invest., 45:481–493, 1966.

57. Ferguson, M.J.: Saluretic drugs and diabetes mellitus. Am. J. Cardiol., 7:568–569, 1961.

58. Ferriere, M., Lachkar, H., Richard, J.L., et al.: Captopril and insulin sensitivity. Ann. Intern. Med., 102:134–135, 1985.

59. Flamenbaum, M.: Metabolic consequences of antihypertensive therapy. Ann. Intern. Med., 98:875–880, 1983.

60. Freis, E.D.: Treatment of mild hypertension. Resident and Staff Physician, 21:55–69, 1975.

61. Frerichs, H., and Creutzfeldt, W.: Insulin release from pancreas of the rat, the rabbit, and miniature pig in vitro. Diabetologia, 1:80A, 1965.

62. Fuller, J.H., Shipley, M.J., Rose, G., et al.: Coronary-heart-disease risk and impaired glucose tolerance. Lancet, 1:1373–1376, 1980.

63. Gabbay, K.N.: The sorbitol pathway and the complications of diabetes. N. Engl. J. Med., 288:831–836, 1973.

64. Gemma, G., Montanari, G., Suppa, G., et al.: Plasma lipid and lipoprotein changes in hypertensive patients treated with propranolol and prazosin. J. Cardiovasc. Pharmacol., 4(Suppl. 2):S233–S237, 1982.

65. Gerber, J.G., and Nies, A.S.: Pharmacology of antihypertensive drugs. In Genest, J., Kuchel, O., Hamet, P., et al. (eds.): Hypertension. Edition 2. New York, McGraw-Hill, 1983, pp. 1093–1127.

66. Gerber, L.M., Wolf, A.M., Braham, R.L., et al.: Effects of sample selection on the coincidence of hypertension and diabetes. J.A.M.A., 247:43–46, 1982.

67. Giugliano, D., Torella, R., Cacciapioti, F., et al.: Impairment of insulin secretion in man by nifedipine. Eur. J. Clin. Pharmacol., 18:395–398, 1980.

68. Goldner, M.G., Zarowitz, H., and Akgun, S.: Hyperglycemia and glucosuria due to thiazide derivatives administered in diabetes mellitus. N. Engl. J. Med., 262:403–405, 1960.

69. Goodfellow, R., and Wesberg, B.: The treatment of high blood pressure in the elderly: A multi-centre evaluation of a fixed combination of methoprolol and hydrochlorothiazide ('Co-Betaloc') in general practice. Curr. Med. Res. Opin., 57:536–542, 1981.

70. Gordon, P.: Glucose intolerance with hypokalemia. Diabetes, 22:544–551, 1973.

71. Gorden, P., Sherman, B.M., and Simonpoulos, A.P.: Glucose intolerance with hypokalemia: An increased proportion of circulating preinsulin-like component. J. Clin. Endocrinol. Metab., 34:235–240, 1972.

72. Greenberg, G., Brennan, P.J., and Miall, W.E.: Effects of diuretic and beta blocker therapy in the Medical Research Council Trial. Am. J. Med., 76:45–51, 1984.

73. Greenblatt, D.J., Duhme, D.W., Allen, M.D., et al.: Clinical toxicity of furosemide in hospitalized patients. A report from the Boston Collaborative Drug Surveillance Program. Am. Heart J., 94:6–13, 1977.

74. Grunfeld, C., and Chappell, D.A.: Hypokalemia and diabetes mellitus. Am. J. Med., 75:553–554, 1983.

75. Guthrie, G.P.: Diabetes and hypertension: Clonidine monotherapy. In Weber, M.A., Drayer, J.I.M., and

132   Mark C. Houston

Kolloch, R. (eds.): Low Dose Oral and Transdermal Therapy of Hypertension. New York, Springer-Verlag, 1985, pp. 39–43.

76. Hamet, P.: Metabolic aspects of hypertension. In Genest, J., Kuchel, O., Hamet, P., et al. (eds.): Hypertension. Edition 2. New York, McGraw-Hill, 1983.

77. Hauman, R.L., and Weller, J.M.: Hyperglycemic effect of chlorothiazide. Clin. Res., 9:180A, 1961.

78. Health and Public Policy Committee: Glycosylated hemoglobin assay in the management and diagnosis of diabetes mellitus. Ann. Intern. Med., 101:710–713, 1984.

79. Helderman, J.H., Elahi, D., Anderson, D.K., et al.: Prevention of glucose intolerance of thiazide diuretics by maintenance of body potassium. Diabetes, 32:106–111, 1983.

80. Helgeland, A., Leren, P., Foss, O.P., et al.: Serum glucose levels during long-term observation of treated and untreated men with mild hypertension: The Oslo Study. Am. J. Med., 76:802–805, 1984.

81. Hiatt, N., Davidson, M.B., Chapman, L.W., et al.: Epinephrine enhancement of potassium-stimulated immunoreactive insulin secretion. Diabetes, 27:550–553, 1978.

82. Hiers, B.H., Ward, J.D., Jarrett, R.J., et al.: A controlled study of clopamine, clorexolone and hydrochlorothiazide in diabetes. Metabolism, 22:101–109, 1973.

83. Hodges, R.E., and Rebello, T.: Carbohydrates and blood pressure. Ann. Intern. Med., 98:838–841, 1983.

84. Hofkle, W.: Clonidine. In Scriabine, A. (ed.): Pharmacology of antihypertensive agents. New York, Raven Press, 1980, pp. 55–78.

85. Hofkle, W., and Kobinger, W.: Pharmakologische wirkunjen des 2-(2,6-dichlorphenylamino)-2-imidazolinhydrochloride einer neuen antihypertensiven substanz. Arzneimittelforsch, 16:1038–1050, 1966.

86. Hollifield, J.: Biochemical consequences of diuretic therapy in hypertension. J. Tenn. Med. Assoc., 71:757–758, 1978.

87. Hollis, W.C.: Aggravation of diabetes mellitus during treatment with chlorothiazide. J.A.M.A., 176:947–949, 1961.

88. Houston, M.C.: Clonidine hydrochloride. South. Med. J., 75:713–721, 1982.

89. Hunyor, S.N., Zweifler, A.J., Hansson, L., et al.: Effect of high dose spironolactone and chlorthalidone in essential hypertension. Relation to plasma renin activity and plasma volume. Aust. N.Z. J. Med., 5:17–24, 1975.

90. Hutchinson, J.C.: The hypotensive action of ethacrynic acid. Vasc. Dis., 5:104–117, 1968.

91. Iwata, Y.: Hyperglycemic action of 2-(2,6-dichlorphenylamino)-2-imidazoline hydrochloride in relation to its hypertensive effect. Jpn. J. Pharmacol., 19:249–259, 1969.

92. Jarrett, R.J., Kent, H., McCartney, M., et al.: Glucose tolerance and blood pressure in two population samples: Their relation to diabetes mellitus and hypertension. Int. J. Epidemiol., 7:15–24, 1978.

93. Johnson, B.E.: The emerging problem of plasma lipid changes during antihypertensive therapy. J. Cardiovasc. Pharmacol., 4(Suppl. 2):S213–S221, 1982.

94. Johnson, M.D., and Lipson, L.G.: Prevalence of hypertension and sexual dysfunction in diabetic women. Clin. Res., 32:49, 1984.

95. Jung, C.Y., and Mookerjee, B.K.: Inhibitory effect of furosemide on glucose transport. J. Lab. Clin. Med., 87:960–966, 1976.

96. Káldor, A., Gachályi, B., and Sebestyén, K.: Diabetogenic affect of oral diuretics in asymptomatic diabetics. Int. J. Clin. Pharmacol. Biopharm., 11:232–234, 1975.

97. Kaneto, A., Miki, E., and Kosaka, K.: Effect of beta and beta$_2$ adrenoreceptor stimulants infused intrapancreatically on glucagon and insulin secretion. Endocrinology, 97:1166–1173, 1975.

98. Kannel, W.B., Castelli, W.P., and McNamara, P.M.: The coronary profile: 12 year follow-up in the Framingham Study. J. Occup. Med., 9:611–619, 1967.

99. Kannel, W.B., Gordon, I., and Schwartz, M.J.: Systolic versus diastolic blood pressure and risk of coronary heart disease. Am. J. Cardiol., 27:335–346, 1971.

100. Kannel, W.B., Hjortland, M., and Castelli, W.P.: Role of diabetes in congestive heart failure: The Framingham Study. Am. J. Cardiol., 34:29–34, 1974.

101. Kannel, W.B., Wolf, P.A., and Verter, J.: Epidemiological assessment of the role of blood pressure in stroke. The Framingham Study. J.A.M.A., 214:301–310, 1970.

102. Kansal, P.C., Buse, J., Buse, M.G.: Thiazide diuretics and control of diabetes mellitus. South. Med. J., 62:1374–1379, 1969.

103. Kaplan, N.M.: Effects of guanabenz on plasma lipid levels in hypertensive patients. J. Cardiovasc. Pharmacol., 6:S841–S846, 1984.

104. Kaplan, N.M.: Systemic hypertension therapy. In Braunwald, E. (ed.): Heart Disease: A Textbook of Cardiovascular Medicine. Edition 1. Philadelphia, W.B. Saunders Company, 1980, pp. 2922–2951.

105. Katayama, S., and Lee, J.B.: Hypertension in experimental diabetes mellitus. Renin-prostaglandin interaction. Hypertension, 7:554–561, 1985.

106. Kennedy, A.L., and Merimee, T.J.: Glycosylated serum protein and hemoglobin A$_1$ levels to measure control of glycemia. Ann. Intern. Med., 95:56–58, 1981.

107. Khan, F., and Spergel, G.: Diabetogenic drugs. Lancet, 1: 808, 1976.

108. Kirkendall, W.M., Hammond, J.J., Thomas, J.C., et al.: Prazosin and clonidine for moderately severe hypertension. J.A.M.A., 240:2553–2556, 1978.

109. Kochar, M.S., Kaur, M., Zeller, J.R., et al.: Treatment of essential hypertension with a twice-daily dose of captopril. Curr. Ther. Res., 35:905–912, 1984.

110. Koch-Weser, J.: Hydralazine. N. Engl. J. Med., 295:320–323, 1976.

111. Kramer, D., Krause, W., and Renner, H.: Report on a long term trial of 2-(2,6-dichlorphenylamino)-2-imidazoline hydrochloride with special consideration of the effect on blood pressure and on carbohydrate metabolism. Arzneimittelforsch, 20:519–521, 1970.

112. Laragh, J.H.: Amiloride, a potassium-conserving agent new to the USA: Mechanisms and clinical relevance. Curr. Ther. Res., 32:173–178, 1982.

113. Leclercq-Meyer, V., Herchuelz, A., Valverde, I, et al.: Mode of action of clonidine upon islet function. Dissociated effects upon the time course and magnitude of insulin release. Diabetes, 29:193–200, 1980.

114. Leichter, S.B., and Baumgardner, B.: Effects of chronic prazosin therapy on intermediary metabolism in diabetic patients. J. Cardiovasc. Med., 6(Suppl.):38–42, 1981.

115. Leren, P., Foss, P.O., Helgeland, A., et al.: Effect of

propranolol and prazosin on blood lipids. The Oslo Study. Lancet, 2:4–6, 1980.

116. Lewis, J.E.: Comparison of acebutolol and hydrochlorothiazide in essential hypertension. Am. Heart J., *109*:(Suppl. 2):1168–1174, 1985.

117. Lewis, P.J., Kohner, E.M., Petrie, A., et al.: Deterioration of glucose tolerance in hypertensive patients on prolonged diuretic treatment. Lancet., *1*:564–566, 1976.

118. Linas, S.L., and Nies, A.S.: Minoxidil. Ann. Intern. Med., *94*:61–65, 1981.

119. Lipson, L.G.: Special problems in treatment of hypertension in the patient with diabetes mellitus. Arch. Intern. Med., *144*:1829–1831, 1984.

120. Lipson, L.G.: Treatment of hypertension in diabetic men: Problems with sexual dysfunction. Am. J. Cardiol., *53*:46A–50A, 1984.

121. Lipson, L.G., Moore, D., and Pope, A.M.: Sexual dysfunction in diabetic men. J. Cardiovasc. Med., *6*(Suppl.):30–37, 1981.

122. Lowe, J., Gray, Henry, D., et al.: Adverse reactions to furosemide in hospital inpatients. Br. Med. J., *2*:360–362, 1979.

123. Lunell, N.O., Hjemdahl, P., Fredholm, B.B., et al.: Circulatory and metabolic effects of a combined alpha- and beta-adrenoceptor blocker (labetalol) in hypertension of pregnancy. Br. J. Clin. Pharmacol., *12*:345–348, 1981.

124. MacGregor, G.A., Banks, R.A., Markandu, N.D., et al.: Lack of effect of beta-blocker on flat dose response to thiazide in hypertension: Efficacy of low dose thiazide combined with beta-blocker. Br. Med. J., *286*:1535–1538, 1983.

125. Maclaren, N.K., Taylor, G.E., and Raiti, S.: Propranolol-augmented, exercise-induced human growth hormone release. Pediatrics, *56*:804–807, 1975.

126. Maclean, D., and Tudhope, G.: Modern diuretic treatment. Br. Med. J., *286*:1419–1422, 1983.

127. Maling, H.M., Cho, A.K., Horakova, Z., et al.: The pharmacological effects of ST-155 (Catapres) and related imidazolines in the rat. Pharmacology, *2*:337–351, 1969.

128. Marks, P., Nimalasuriya, A., and Anderson, J.: The glucose tolerance test in hypertensive patients treated long term with thiazide diuretics. Practitioner, *225*:392–393, 1981.

129. Massie, B.M., Hirsch, A.T., Inouye, I.K., et al.: Calcium channel blockers as antihypertensive agents. Am. J. Med., *77*:135–142, 1984.

130. Materson, B.J., Oster, J.R., Michael, U.F., et al.: Dose response to chlorthalidone in patients with mild hypertension. Efficacy of a lower dose. Clin. Pharmacol. Ther., *24*:192–198, 1978.

131. Maxwell, G.M.: The effects of 2-(2,6-dichlorphenylamine)-2-imidazoline hydrochloride (Catapres) upon the systemic and coronary haemodynamics and metabolism of intact dogs. Arch. Int. Pharmacodyn. Ther., *181*:7–14, 1969.

132. McMahon, F.G.: Management of Essential Hypertension: The New Low-Dose Era. Edition 2. New York, Futura Publishing Company, 1984.

133. Mohler, H., Bravo, E.L., and Tarazi, R.C.: Long-term use of beta blockers may precipitate diabetes. Am. Fam. Physician, *20*:128, 1979.

134. Mroczek, W.J., Davidov, M., and Finnerty, F.A., Jr.: Prolonged treatment with clonidine. Comparative antihypertensive effects alone and with a diuretic agent. Am. J. Cardiol., *30*:536–541, 1972.

135. Multicenter Study Group: Multiclinic comparison of amiloride, hydrochlorothiazide and hydrochlorothiazide plus amiloride in essential hypertension. Arch. Intern. Med., *141*:482–486, 1981.

136. Murphy, M.B., Anthony, J.I., Scriven, M.B., et al.: Efficacy of nifedipine as a step 3 antihypertensive drug. Hypertension, 5(Suppl. II):II-118–II-121, 1983.

137. Myers, M.G., and Hope-Gill, H.F.: Effect of D- and DL- propranolol on glucose-stimulated insulin release. Clin. Pharmacol. Ther., *25*:303–308, 1979.

138. Nathan, D.M., Singer, D.E., Hurxthal, K., et al.: The clinical information value of the glycosylated hemoglobin assay. N. Engl. J. Med., *310*:341–346, 1984.

139. Okun, R.: Effectiveness of prazosin as initial antihypertensive therapy. Am. J. Cardiol., *51*:644–650, 1983.

140. Olshan, A.R., O'Connor, D.T., Cohen, I.M., et al.: Baroreflex dysfunction in patients with adult-onset diabetes and hypertension. Am. J. Med., *74*:233–242, 1983.

141. Otero, M.L., Pinilla, C.F., Claros, N.M., et al.: The effect of long-term therapy of essential hypertension with atenolol and chlorthalidone on carbohydrate tolerance. Primary Cardiology, *6*:(Suppl. I):193–194, 1983.

142. Parsons, W.B., Jr., and Morledge, J.H.: Antihypertensive effect of a new imidazoline compound (clonidine) and chlorthalidone, individually and in combination. Am. J. Cardiol., *26*:258–261, 1970.

143. Participating Veterans Administration Medical Centers: Low doses vs. standard dose of reserpine. A randomized, double-blind, multiclinic trial in patients taking chlorthalidone. J.A.M.A., *248*:2471–2477, 1982.

144. Pell, S., and D'Alonzo, C.A.: Some aspects of hypertension in diabetes mellitus. J.A.M.A., *202*:104–110, 1967.

145. Perry, H.M., Jr.: Some wrong-way chemical changes during antihypertensive treatment: Comparison of indapamide and related agents. Am. Heart J., *106*:251–257, 1983.

146. Persson, I., and Eskobr, P.: Carbohydrate tolerance during beta adrenergic blockade in hypertension. Eur. J. Clin. Pharmacol., *5*:151–153, 1973.

147. Petru, M.A., Crawford, M.H., Kennedy, G.T., et al.: Long-term efficacy of high-dose diltiazem for chronic stable angina pectoris: 16-month serial studies with placebo controls. Am. Heart J., *109*:99–103, 1985.

148. Podolsky, S., and Pattavina, C.G.: Hyperosmolar nonketotic diabetic coma. A complication of propranolol therapy. Metabolism, *22*:685–693, 1973.

149. Prout, T.E.: Diabetes mellitus. *In* Harvey, A.M., et al. (eds.): The Principles and Practice of Medicine. Edition 2. New York, Appleton-Century-Crofts, 1980, pp. 795–815.

150. Raftos, J., Bauer, G.E., Lewis, R.G., et al.: Clonidine in the treatment of severe hypertension. Med. J. Aust., *1*:786–793, 1973.

151. Ram, C.: Diuretics in the management of hypertension. Postgrad. Med., *71*:155–168, 1982.

152. Rapaport, M.I., and Heard, H.F.: Thiazide-induced glucose intolerance treated with potassium. Arch. Intern. Med., *113*:405–408, 1964.

153. Rehbinder, D., and Deckers, W.: Stoffwechseleffekte des catapres an naunynschmiedebergs. Arch. Pharmak. Exp. Pathol., *261*:162–175, 1968.

154. Robinson, D., Nilsson, C., Leonard, R., et al.: Effect of loop diuretics on carbohydrate metabolism and

electrolyte excretion.. J. Clin. Pharmacol.,
21:637–646, 1981.

155. Roginsky, M.S.: Long term evaluation of timolol maleate combined with hydrochlorothiazide for the treatment of patients with essential hypertension: A cooperative multicenter study. Curr. Ther. Res., 27:374–383, 1980.

156. Röjdmark, S., Andersson, D.E.H., Hed, R., et al.: Effect of verapamil on glucose response to intravenous injection of glucagon and insulin in healthy subjects. Horm. Metab. Res., 12:285–290, 1980.

157. Root, H.F., and Sharkey, T.P.: Arteriosclerosis and hypertension in diabetes. J. Intern. Med., 9:873–882, 1936.

158. Rowe, J.W., Tobin, J.D., Rosa, R.M., et al.: Effects of experimental potassium deficiency on glucose and insulin metabolism. Metabolism, 29:498–502, 1980.

159. Runyan, J.W.: Influence of thiazide diuretics on carbohydrate metabolism in patients with mild diabetes. N. Engl. J. Med., 267:541–543, 1962.

160. Sagal, J., Colwell, J.A., Crook, L., et al.: Increased platelet aggregation in early diabetes mellitus. Ann. Intern. Med., 82:733–738, 1975.

161. Samarthji, L.A.L., Tolis, G., Martin, J.B., et al.: Effect of clonidine on growth hormone, prolactin, luteinizing hormone, follicle-stimulating hormone and thyroid-stimulating hormone in the serum of normal men. J. Clin. Endocrinol. Metab., 41:827–832, 1975.

162. Scandellari, C., Zaccaria, M., De Palo, C., et al.: The effect of propranolol on hypoglycemia. Observations in five insulinoma patients. Diabetologia, 15:297–301, 1978.

163. Selzer, H.S., and Allen, E.W.: Inhibition of insulin secretion in diazoxide diabetes. Diabetes, 14:439A, 1965.

164. Senft, G., Sitt, R., Losert, W., et al.: Hemmung der insulinin kretion durch alpha-Receptoren stimulierende Substanzen Naunyn Schmiedeberg. Arch. Pharmacol. Exp. Pathol., 260:309–323, 1968.

165. Shapiro, A.P., Benedek, T.G., and Small, J.L.: Effect of thiazides on carbohydrate metabolism in patients with hypertension. N. Engl. J. Med., 265:1028–1033, 1961.

166. Shikama, H., and Ui, M.: Adrenergic receptor and epinephrine-induced hyperglycemia and glucose tolerance. Am. J. Physiol., 229:962–966, 1975.

167. Siperstein, M.D.: Type II diabetes: Some problems in diagnosis and treatment. Hosp. Pract., 20:55–63, 1985.

168. Siperstein, M.D., Foster, D.W., Knowles, H.C., Jr., et al.: Control of blood glucose and diabetic vascular disease. N. Engl. J. Med.,296:1060–1062, 1977.

169. Smet, G., Hoobler, S., Sanbar, S., et al.: Clinical observations on a new antihypertensive drug 2-(2-6-dichlorphenylamine)-2-imidazoline hydrochloride. Am. Heart J., 77:473–478, 1969.

170. Somers, G., Devis, G., VanObberghen, E., et al.: Calcium antagonists and islet function. II. Interaction of theophylline and verapamil. Endocrinology, 99:114–124, 1976.

171. Sosenko, J.M., Breslow, J.L., Miettinen, O.S., et al.: Hyperglycemia and plasma lipid levels: A prospective study of young insulin-dependent diabetic patients. N. Engl. J. Med., 302:650–654, 1980.

172. Spivack, C., Ocken, S., and Frishman, W.H.: Calcium antagonists: Clinical use in the treatment of systemic hypertension. Drugs, 25:154–177, 1983.

173. Sung, P.K., Samet, P., and Yeh, B.K.: Effects of clonidine and chlorthalidone on blood pressure and glucose tolerance in hypertensive patients. Curr. Ther. Res., 13:280–285, 1971.

174. Taniguchi, H., Murakami, K., and Morita, S.: Calcium antagonist (diltiazem) for reversal of hypoglycemic symptoms in insulinoma. Lancet, 2:501, 1977.

175. Tasker, P.R.W., and Mitchel-Heggs, P.F.: Non-ketotic diabetic pre-coma associated with high dose furosemide therapy. Br. Med. J., 1:626–627, 1976.

176. Thenot, A.: The place of indapamide in the treatment of arterial hypertension. Curr. Med. Res. Opin., 8:140–143, 1983.

177. Toivonen, S., and Mustala, C.: Diabetogenic action of furosemide. Br. Med. J., 1:920–921, 1966.

178. Tweeddale, M.G., Ogilvie, R.I., and Ruedy, J.: Antihypertensive and biochemical effects of chlorthalidone. Clin. Pharmacol. Ther., 22:519–527, 1977.

179. Veterans Administration Cooperative Study Group on Antihypertensive Agents: Effects of treatment on morbidity in hypertension. III. Influence of age, diastolic pressure and prior cardiovascular disease. Further analysis of side effects. Circulation, 45:991–1004, 1972.

180. Veterans Administration Cooperative Study Group on Antihypertensive Agents: Comparison of propranolol and HCTZ for the initial treatment of hypertension.. I. Results of short term titration with emphasis on racial differences in response. J.A.M.A., 248:1996–2003, 1982.

181. Veterans Administration Cooperative Study on Antihypertensive Agents: Comparison of propranolol and hydrochlorothiazide for the initial treatment of hypertension. II. Results of long term therapy. J.A.M.A., 248:2004–2001, 1982.

182. Veterans Administration Cooperative Study Group on Antihypertensive Agents: Efficacy of nadolol alone and combined with bendroflumethiazide and hydralazine for systemic hypertension. Am. J. Cardiol., 52:1230–1237, 1983.

183. Veterans Administration Cooperative Study Group on Antihypertensive Agents: Low-dose captopril for the treatment of mild to moderate hypertension. I. Results of a 14 week trial. Arch. Intern. Med., 144:1947–1953, 1984.

184. Wada, S., Nakayama, M., and Masaki, K.: Effects of diltiazem hydrochloride on serum lipids: Comparison with beta blockers. Clin. Ther., 5:163–173, 1982.

185. Wales, J.K., Viktoria, J.K., and Wolff, F.W.: The effect of hydrochlorothiazides in normal subjects receiving high carbohydrate diets. Am. J. Med. Sci., 254:499–504, 1967.

186. Walker, B.R., Hare, L.E., and Deitch, M.W.: Comparative antihypertensive effects of guanabenz and clonidine. J. Int. Med. Res., 10:6–14, 1982.

187. Weber, M.A., Drayer, J.I.M., and Kaufman, C.A.: Differing attributes of diuretics and centrally-acting agents as first-line antihypertensive treatment: Evaluations of hydrochlorothiazide and guanabenz. Cardiovasc. Rev. Rep., 4:343–352, 1983.

188. Weller, J.N., and Borondy, P.E.: Effects of benzothiadiazine drugs on carbohydrate metabolism. Metabolism, 14:708–714, 1965.

189. Whitworth, J., and Kincaid-Smith, P.: Diuretics or beta blockers first for hypertension? Drugs, 23:394–402, 1982.

190. Wilkins, R.: New drugs for the treatment of hypertension. Ann. Intern. Med., 50:1–10, 1959.

191. Wolff, F.W., Parmley, W.W., White, K., et al.: Drug induced diabetes. J.A.M.A., 185:568–574, 1963.

192. Wollman, G.L., Gifford, R.W., Jr., and Tarazi, R.C.: Antihypertensive drugs: Clinical pharmacology and therapeutic use. Drugs, *14*:420–460, 1977.

193. Woosley, R.L., and Nies, A.S.: Guanethidine. N. Engl. J. Med., *295*:1053–1056, 1976.

194. Wright, A.D., Barber, S.G., Kendall, M.J., et al.: Beta-adrenoceptor-blocking drugs and blood sugar control in diabetes mellitus. Br. Med. J., *1*:159–161, 1979.

195. Yeh, B.K., Nantel, A., and Goldberg, L.: Antihypertensive action of clonidine.. Arch. Intern. Med., *127*:233–237, 1971.

196. Zatuchni, J., and Kordasz, F.: The diabetogenic effect of thiazide diuretics. Am. J. Cardiol., *7*:565–567, 1961.

197. Zilversmit, D.B.: Atherogenesis: A postprandial phenomenon. Circulation, *60*:473–485, 1979.

Room S-1125
Vanderbilt University Medical Center
Nashville, Tennessee 37232

Left Ventricular Hypertrophy as a Risk Factor

*Edward D. Frohlich, M.D.**

The concept of risk factors is not new to cardiovascular diseases. A number of factors have been identified that predispose the patient with atherosclerosis to increased risk of cardiovascular morbidity and mortality. Among these are hypertension, hyperlipidemia, diabetes mellitus, obesity, and smoking. Additional risk factors are found in those patients who are older, of the male gender, and black and who have hyperuricemia.[3,31,37,38,41,58,63,75]

These risk factors have been identified through a number of prospective epidemiologic studies that have subsequently identified additional cardiovascular factors that impart additional risk.[31,37,38,40,63,75] One of these factors is the presence of left ventricular hypertrophy.[2,40,57] This discussion concerns primarily left ventricular hypertrophy and those related factors that impart enhanced risk of still greater cardiovascular morbidity and mortality.

IS LEFT VENTRICULAR HYPERTROPHY A RISK FACTOR?

At first thought, one would not expect that the development of hypertrophy of a muscle should impose additional risk. Why should this be different for the cardiovascular system, and why should this be different for the presence of left ventricular hypertrophy?

At present, all evidence seems to indicate that left ventricular hypertrophy in hypertension is an adaptive structural phenomenon that accompanies the ever-progressing rise in arterial pressure associated with the increased total peripheral resistance, the hemodynamic hallmark of systemic arterial hypertension.[13,15–17,23] Most authorities would agree that the development of ventricular hypertrophy serves only to maintain the performance of the heart as it is facing an increased afterload imposed by the hypertensive disease.[18,67,69] Moreover, this increased performance of the heart against the rising afterload maintains normal systemic perfusion. Why then should there be enhanced risk? Several major factors come to mind that predispose the patient with cardiac enlargement to enhanced risk, and they are directly associated with left ventricular hypertrophy (Table 1).

The first of these factors is the concept that was introduced earlier: Hypertension is a predisposing risk factor for coronary artery disease. It would be logical to conclude, then, that the increased risk associated with left ventricular hypertrophy could be attributed to the long-standing systemic arterial hypertension. As a result, the associated accelerated atherogenesis and coronary arterial atherosclerosis would enhance the increased risk.[11,82] Thus, the patient with left ventricular hypertrophy must have had long-standing hypertension, and the coexistence of the two clinical diseases is potentiative for accelerating the atherogenic proclivities of that patient. This is the first explanation that comes to mind concerning this enhanced risk.

A second explanation for the postulated risk associated with left ventricular hypertrophy is the coexistent development of myocardial fibrosis. It is clear that increased cardiac mass,

*Alton Ochsner Distinguished Physician and Vice President for Academic Affairs, Alton Ochsner Medical Foundation; Professor of Medicine and Physiology, Louisiana State University; Adjunct Professor of Pharmacology, Tulane University, New Orleans, Louisiana

Table 1. *Factors Associated with Left Ventricular*
          Hypertrophy That May Impart Enhanced Risk

1. Hypertension-accelerated atherogenesis
2. Associated myocardial fibrosis
3. Coronary arterial insufficiency
4. Increased predisposition to develop cardiac dysrhythmias
5. Increased predisposition to sudden death
6. Greater predisposition to congestive heart failure as a consequence of less functional reserve

whether or not it is associated with concentric muscular hypertrophy of the left ventricle, need not be produced solely by increased muscle mass. Increased collagen tissue deposition may also occur.[72] Nevertheless, associated with increased muscle mass (with or without additional collagen tissue) is an increased demand for blood flow to the myocardium, and this may be limited by the associated coronary arterial disease that may occur.[8]

Still another abnormality associated with developing left ventricular hypertrophy might be an increased predisposition of the myocardium to develop cardiac dysrhythmias, of both atrial and ventricular origin.[2,8,39,40,57,78] Indeed, this has been shown from our earliest studies demonstrating atrial enlargement in hypertension,[78] even when obvious left ventricular hypertrophy cannot be demonstrated by the chest radiograph or the electrocardiogram. Thus, evidence of reduced left ventricular compliance can be shown by the presence on the electrocardiogram of left atrial abnormality.[5,7,28,78] These patients with only electrocardiographic evidence of left atrial abnormality and enlargement have an increased prevalence of supraventricular and ventricular dysrhythmias,[78] and when left ventricular hypertrophy is clinically evident, the increased number of ectopic ventricular beats is highly significant,[57] as will be discussed later.

Of course, a major explanation for the enhanced risk imposed on patients with left ventricular hypertrophy is the already utilized adaptive functional capacity and, with it, the reduced intrinsic ability of the myocardium to adapt further to the increasing afterload.[38] Hence, the functional and structural capabilities of the myocardium to adapt further are that much diminished, and with this reduced adaptability of an already hypertrophied ventricle, there is less potential reserve. Therefore, the patient with left ventricular hypertrophy has a greater predisposition for congestive heart failure and coronary artery disease than the patient with hypertension without left ventricular hypertrophy.

The balance of this discussion will be concerned with the three major factors that I believe impart an increased risk of greater cardiovascular morbidity and mortality to the patient with hypertension and left ventricular hypertrophy: the greater predisposition for cardiac dysrhythmias; the more advanced stage of cardiac impairment hemodynamically; and certain additional nonhemodynamic factors that may be associated with the development of left ventricular hypertrophy and, hence, greater cardiovascular risk. Because most patients with systemic arterial hypertension demand pharmacologic therapy for control of arterial pressure, questions exist as to the role of the drug therapy in the maintenance or regression of the status of left ventricular hypertrophy. Further questions exist concerning the implications of this therapy for ameliorating or accelerating overall cardiovascular risk.

CARDIAC DYSRHYTHMIAS

A number of prospective clinical studies have demonstrated that untreated patients with hypertension and left ventricular hypertrophy do, in fact, have an increased risk of cardiovascular morbidity and mortality.[2,40,57] Because patients with hypertension, with or without cardiac enlargement, have a greater risk for the development of coronary artery disease, they have a greater predisposition for atherosclerosis and the associated risk of coronary heart disease.[42,65,74]

Over and above these findings, however, are studies from a variety of laboratories that have reported that patients with hypertension, particularly if they were treated with diuretics and have the attendant hypokalemia, are predisposed to increased cardiac irritability and sudden death.[33,34,36,51,59] Recent studies from our laboratory have shown that untreated patients with hypertension and left ventricular hypertrophy by electrocardiographic criteria who had 24-hour Holter recordings demonstrated an increased number of left ventricular premature beats than patients with hypertension who were also untreated but who did not have left ventricular hypertrophy or normotensive subjects.[57] Thus, patients with ventricular hypertrophy do have increased ventricular irritability, and this state of increased ventricular irritability may predispose them further to other cardiac events, including more severe cardiac dysrhythmias and sudden death in the presence of diuretic-induced hypokalemia or possibly even with hypomagnesemia. Therefore, it is quite conceivable that the increased incidence of sudden death in diuretic-induced electrolyte disturbances may have occurred in patients who already had left ventricular hypertrophy.[60,61] Other studies have refuted the foregoing reports demonstrating that 24-hour Holter recordings did not show increased left ventricular premature beats[49,64]; however, the numbers of patients with left ventricular hypertrophy in these studies may well have been fewer than in the other studies that had demonstrated increased ventricular irritability in hypokalemic hypertensive patients. The conclusions and recommendations that can be drawn at this time must be tentative. First, the question of enhanced ventricular irritability associated with diuretic therapy remains unresolved. However, because the hypertrophied myocardium occurs in a left ventricle that is more irritable, it stands to reason that patients with this abnormality must be watched extremely carefully for hypokalemia. It also follows that the serum potassium should be protected with potassium-sparing agents in order to prevent an increased risk of cardiac ventricular dysrhythmias and sudden death.

HEMODYNAMICS AND LEFT VENTRICULAR PATHOPHYSIOLOGY

The Russian pathophysiologist Meerson reported that there are three stages associated with the development of left ventricular hypertrophy.[52] At first, there is a state of hyperfunction as the left ventricle responds to the increased afterload.[17,18,23] This is followed by a period of greater or lesser duration of stable ventricular hyperfunction, at which time structural changes occur in the left ventricle, represented by a concentric hypertrophy[48] that maintains the performance of the heart for an indeterminate time.[18,23,67,69] However, when this performance cannot be maintained as the hypertensive vascular disease (represented by the increased arterial pressure, total peripheral resistance, and left ventricular impedance) progresses, left ventricular congestive heart failure eventually supervenes.[16,17,23] Thus, when the potential adaptability and functional reserve of the left ventricle become exhausted, the inevitable consequence is the failure of the left ventricular pump.[68] Clearly, these patients with congestive heart failure are at an increased risk.[38]

The development of left ventricular hypertrophy, however, is a subtle one. Initially, this hyperfunction not only is imparted to the left ventricle by the increased hemodynamic afterload but also may be provided by the stimulus imposed by the intrinsic pathophysiologic mechanisms of the hypertensive disease itself. Thus, associated with the early stages in the development of hypertension is some degree of peripheral venoconstriction that serves to redistribute the circulating blood volume from the periphery to the central circulation, thereby increasing venous return.[16,21,79] Moreover, there is increasing evidence emerging that if adrenergic or other factors associated with the development of hypertension are operative, this may also explain the increased myocardial contractility and heart rate that are also found in hypertension at its earliest stages.[6,77] Clearly, one would expect a hyperfunctioning ventricle on the basis of the Starling factors as well as on the basis of increased preload and an increased myocardial contractility, which may be associated with the pressure mechanisms intrinsic to the hypertensive disease itself. Thus, in patients with borderline hypertension, there is evidence of ventricular hyperfunction of the heart (that is, an increased heart rate, cardiac output, and left ventricular ejection) that is associated with a clinical awareness of increased cardiac action.[6,7,13–17,21,25,28,55,77]

Even at these early stages of hypertension, even in the adolescent with mild hypertension, there is evidence of structural changes in individuals who demonstrate greater left ventricular mass and ventricular wall thicknesses than other individuals of the same age. Even adolescent children of hypertensive parents have bigger and thicker left ventricles than normotensive children of the same age, race, and sex whose parents are normotensive. These children have pressures in the upper quintile, and their pressures track at higher levels than those of their peers who are children of parents who are normotensive.[4] As hypertensive disease progresses, this can be determined structurally and functionally. Structural changes of left ventricular hypertrophy can be demonstrated by echocardiography, and these changes may be associated with early impairment of contractility (as evidenced by a reduced ejection fraction, fiber shortening rate, and left ventricular ejection rate).[5–7,28] Clinically, although these individuals may not demonstrate electrocardiographic or roentgenographic evidence of ventricular hypertrophy, the electrocardiogram may demonstrate left atrial enlargement that is highly concordant with auscultatory evidence of an atrial diastolic gallop rhythm.[28,78] These two clinical findings (that is, left atrial abnormality and a fourth heart sound) represent the atrial response to a hypertrophying, less compliant left ventricle, and as hypertrophy progresses, left ventricular contractility becomes impaired.[7,28] These patients are already at increased risk because they have less functional reserve, and they also possess characteristics of increased ventricular irritability.[57,78] It follows from the preceding discussion that there is sufficient hemodynamic evidence available to demonstrate that with progressive development of left ventricular hypertrophy, the patients are at an increased functional risk, and that this hemodynamic risk is independent of the electrical activity of the heart or the coexistent development of atherosclerosis.

OTHER FACTORS ASSOCIATED WITH HYPERTROPHY

The major hemodynamic factors associated with the development of left ventricular hypertrophy have already been discussed. A number of other factors that are associated mechanistically with the development of hypertension also favor the development of ventricular hypertrophy. Infusion of catecholamines in subpressor doses will produce ventricular hypertrophy.[30,76] Infusion of isoproterenol will produce ventricular hypertrophy and myocardial fibrosis independent of a rise in arterial pressure.[30] Other studies have demonstrated that myocytes will increase protein synthesis simply with the addition of angiotensin II to tissue culture of adult cardiac myocytes.[43] Thus, the intrinsic pathogenetic mechanisms producing the hypertension may, by themselves, favor the development of hypertrophy.

Differences have also been demonstrated between white patients and black patients in the development of left ventricular hypertrophy,[9,32] and it is already known that the black patient has a greater risk of development of morbidity and mortality than the white patient not only from complications of hypertension but also from myocardial infarction and congestive heart failure.[12,29,50,71,80] Recent studies from our laboratory[9] and others[32] have demonstrated that in the black patient, there is a highly significant correlation between the height of arterial pressure and total peripheral resistance and left ventricular mass, findings that were not demonstrated in white patients. In these studies, blood pressures of the patients were matched with respect to age, race, and sex. Nevertheless, it may be possible that the black individual sustains a higher integrated pressure over a 24-hour period than the white individual. Thus, racial factors may be related to the pathogenesis of hypertrophy and its morbidity and mortality consequences. Further studies are clearly in order to elucidate these racial differences.

A number of other studies have demonstrated that aging itself is associated with the development of increased cardiac mass and ventricular wall thicknesses,[47] and this factor is independent of whether or not hypertension exists. Still another factor that seems to be related to hypertrophy is the sex of the patient. In animal studies, spontaneously hypertensive female rats developed less hypertrophy than male rats at any level of development of hypertension,[26] and this relationship of the sex of the animal also predisposes the animal to a reduced ventricular mass with pharmacologic therapy.[70] Clinical studies have also suggested that the female patient may have less severe disease, and prospective and retrospective epidemiologic studies have confirmed these findings.[42] Whether this is related to the presence of left ventricular hypertrophy, however, is not known.

A number of coexistent diseases are associated with increased risk. Some of these diseases impart additional disease to the left ventricle. The first and foremost of these is obesity, a condition that frequently coexists with hypertension.[24,53] Recent studies from our laboratories have demonstrated that hypertension without obesity is characterized by an increased left ventricular afterload, and this is associated with concentric hypertrophy.[24,56] In obese normotensive individuals, there is an increased left ventricular preload that results from the expanded circulating and cardiopulmonary volume associated with obesity.[53] Thus, there is a dual left ventricular load in obesity hypertension: an increased afterload associated with the hypertension and an increased preload associated with the volume expansion of obesity.[24,56] These loads favor a dimorphic structural change in the left ventricle that may account for the increased morbidity and mortality associated with patients with hypertension and coexistent obesity.

Other diseases frequently coexist with hypertension, including not only atherosclerosis and its associated coronary artery disease, but also diabetes mellitus and gout.[37,42,63,65,74,75] Each of these is associated with myocardial fibrosis and ventricular changes. More recently, we have demonstrated in untreated patients with hypertension that the higher their uric acid level, the lower their renal blood flow and the higher their intrarenal vascular resistance.[54] Furthermore, we have recently reported in patients with un-complicated essential hypertension that those patients with echocardiographic evidence of ventricular enlargement (but with normal elec-trocardiograms and chest roentgenograms) had systemic and renal hemodynamic function that was normal.[44] In contrast, if these patients dem-onstrated only slightly reduced renal blood flow or slightly elevated serum uric acid levels, they already demonstrated some significant degree of left ventricular enlargement; thus, it would seem that the heart responds earlier to structural hemodynamic changes in hypertension. Our present thinking is that the hyperuricemia rep-resents the early coexistent findings of nephro-sclerosis and vascular disease but that structural evidence of ventricular hypertrophy occurs even before impairment of renal blood flow or rising serum creatinine level. Thus, a number of as-sociated clinical and physiologic factors may be related to the development of left ventricular hypertrophy. Each of these factors may favor an increased risk of cardiovascular morbidity and mortality that is independent of the elevated arterial pressure.

PHARMACOLOGIC THERAPY OF HYPERTENSION AND ITS RELATIONSHIP TO LEFT VENTRICULAR MASS

A new and exciting area of experimental and clinical research concerns the role of antihyper-tensive drug therapy in the regression of left ventricular mass. Although not directly related to this discussion, certain findings are worth con-sideration. The findings that have been dem-onstrated to date indicate that not all drugs that control arterial pressure are associated with a reduced cardiac mass, even though these agents may produce the same reduction in arterial pres-sure.[16,17] For example, agents such as hydrala-zine and minoxidil decrease arterial pressure and left ventricular afterload but do not reduce cardiac mass.[66,73] In contrast, other agents such as methyldopa, the angiotensin-converting en-zyme inhibitors, and some of the calcium-entry blockers will cause a regression of left ventric-ular hypertrophy.[1,10,35,45,66,81]

Initial experimental research seemed to in-dicate that those agents that reduced pressure and reflexively stimulated cardiac adrenergic ac-tivity may have promoted and maintained the developed left ventricular hypertrophy. In con-trast, other agents that inhibited adrenergic ac-tivity or the renin-angiotensin system caused

regression of the left ventricular mass.[16,17,27,73] A clear-cut explanation for these findings has not yet been forthcoming, as two agents having the same pharmacologic effect and physiologic ac-tion on adrenergic activity, methyldopa and clonidine, had disparate effects.[35,66] Thus, in an-imal studies, spontaneously hypertensive rats treated for 3 weeks with methyldopa demon-strated a regression of left ventricular hypertro-phy, whereas in similar animals treated with clonidine, which has the same pharmacologic and hemodynamic effects, ventricular hypertro-phy failed to regress. Only when the clonidine dose was increased threefold, thereby stimulat-ing peripheral alpha-adrenergic receptors that increased arterial pressure and total peripheral resistance, was there evidence of a regression of left ventricular hypertrophy.[66] Experimental studies have confirmed a regression of ventric-ular mass not only in the hypertrophied left ven-tricle but also in normotensive animals without a hypertrophied ventricle.[45,66] Thus, there seems to be a number of factors, over and above the hemodynamic effects of the drugs, that may pro-duce a regression of ventricular mass.[16,17,20,27]

These studies, which have also been con-firmed in humans, require further explanation and clinical elucidation. If drugs do produce a regression of left ventricular mass while con-trolling pressure, it is fair to ask the following question: Will the heart perform as well follow-ing regression of mass, particularly if the drug is discontinued by the patient? Under these cir-cumstances, arterial pressure would not increase slowly and progressively but immediately and precipitously,[19] and it may be asked legitimately whether the ventricle with regressed ventricular hypertrophy performs as well at a higher pres-sure load.[22] Clearly, sufficient evidence is not available at this time. The only evidence that is available from prospectively designed studies is from the experimental laboratories. In these studies, our laboratory and others have dem-onstrated that the heart with regressed left ven-tricular hypertrophy is able to perform as well in pumping a volume load,[46] but these studies were all conducted at arterial pressures that were at the normal levels. In recent studies from our laboratory, the left ventricle was subjected to regression of mass by pharmacologic therapy and then challenged by an increased pressure load by placing a snare around the ascending aorta.[62] The ventricle performed as well as when pressure was not elevated; however, when pres-sure was elevated, a function curve indicative of cardiac failure was observed. Further studies are definitely in order to determine function and performance of the left ventricle of a heart that has undergone regression of ventricular hypertrophy.

CONCLUSION

Major risk factors have been identified that enhance the chances of cardiovascular morbidity and mortality from coronary artery disease. These studies have demonstrated that hypertension, hyperlipidemia, obesity, diabetes mellitus, smoking, and hyperuricemia enhance risk. In addition, other factors, including advancing age, male sex, and black race of the patient, increase that risk. A new risk that has been reported from prospective clinical studies is the development of left ventricular hypertrophy. This discussion has provided a concept from clinical and experimental studies that demonstrate that the increased risk emanates from loss of hemodynamic function with progressively decreasing adaptability; the role of hypertension in accelerating the atherosclerosis process; development of abnormal cardiac rhythm secondary to ischemia and fibrosis; the inherent predisposition to ventricular dysrhythmias and sudden death; risks from associated diseases; and, in fact, the paradoxic risk of beneficial pharmacologic therapy.

REFERENCES

1. Amodeo, C., Kobrin, I., Ventura, H.O., et al.: Immediate and short-term hemodynamic effects of diltiazem in hyperension. Circulation, 73:108–113, 1986.
2. Anderson, K.P.: Sudden death, hypertension and hypertrophy. J. Cardiovasc. Pharmacol., 6:S498–S503, 1984.
3. Build and Blood Pressure Study 1959. Vols. I and II. Chicago, Society of Actuaries, 1959.
4. Culpepper, W.S., Scott, P.C., Messerli, F.H., et al.: Cardiac status in juvenile borderline hypertension. Ann. Intern. Med., 98:1–7, 1983.
5. Dreslinski, G.R., Frohlich, E.D., Dunn, F.G., et al.: Echocardiographic diastolic ventricular abnormality in hypertensive disease: Atrial emptying index. Am. J. Cardiol., 47:1087–1090, 1981.
6. Dreslinski, G.R., Messerli, F.H., Dunn, F.G., et al.: Patterns of left ventricular adaptation in borderline and mild essential hypertension: Echocardiographic findings. Chest, 80:592–595, 1981.
7. Dunn, F.G., Chandraratna, P., de Carvalho, J.G.R., et al.: Pathophysiologic assessment of hypertensive heart disease with echocardiography. Am. J. Cardiol., 39:789–795, 1977.
8. Dunn, F.G., and Frohlich, E.D.: Hypertension and angina pectoris. In Yu, P.N., and Goodwin, J.F. (eds.): Progress in Cardiology. Volume 7. Philadelphia, Lea and Febiger, 1978, pp. 163–196.
9. Dunn, F.G., Oigman, W., Sundgaard-Riise, K., et al.: Racial differences in cardiac adaptation to essential hypertension determined by echocardiographic indexes. J. Am. Coll. Cardiol., 1:1348–1351, 1983.
10. Dunn, F.G., Oigman, W., Ventura, H.O., et al.: Enalapril improves systemic and renal hemodynamics and allows regression of left ventricular mass in essential hypertension. Am. J. Cardiol., 3:447–450, 1984.
11. Dustan, H.P.: Atherosclerosis complicating chronic hypertension. Circulation, 50:871–879, 1974.
12. Entwisle, G., Apostolides, A.Y., Hebel, J.R., et al.: Target organ damage in black hypertensives. Circulation, 55:792–796, 1977.
13. Frohlich, E.D.: Haemodynamics of hypertension. In Genest, J., Koiw, E., and Kuchel, O. (eds.): Hypertension: Physiopathology and Treatment. New York, McGraw-Hill, 1977, pp. 15–49.
14. Frohlich, E.D.: The adrenergic nervous system and hypertension. Mayo Clin. Proc., 52:361–368, 1977.
15. Frohlich, E.D.: Hemodynamic factors in the pathogenesis and maintenance of hypertension. Fed. Proc., 41:2400–2408, 1982.
16. Frohlich, E.D.: Hemodynamics and other determinants in development of left ventricular hypertrophy: Conflicting factors in its regression. Fed. Proc., 42:2709–2715, 1983.
17. Frohlich, E.D.: The heart in hypertension. In Genest, J., Kuchel, O., Hamet, P., et al. (eds.): Hypertension: Physiopathology and Treatment. Edition 2. New York, McGraw-Hill, 1983, pp. 791–810.
18. Frohlich, E.D.: Cardiac hypertrophy: Stimuli and mechanisms. In Sleight, P. (ed.): Scientific Foundations of Cardiology. London, William Heinemann Medical Books Ltd., 1983, pp. 182–190.
19. Frohlich, E.D.: Clinical conference: Hypertensive cardiovascular disease. A pathophysiological assessment. Hypertension, 6:934–939, 1984.
20. Frohlich, E.D.: Changes in hypertrophy by treatment in hypertension: Results of experimental research. In Proceedings of the International Symposium on Hypertension. Cologne, Germany, February 1985. New York, Springer-Verlag, in press.
21. Frohlich, E.D., Kozul, V.J., Tarazi, R.C., et al.: Physiological comparison of labile and essential hypertension. Circ. Res., 27:55–69, 1970.
22. Frohlich, E.D., Messerli, F.H., Pegram, B.L., et al.: Hemodynamic and cardiac effects of centrally acting antihypertensive drugs. Hypertension, 6:II-76–II-81, 1984.
23. Frohlich, E.D., Messerli, F.H., Re, R.N., et al.: Mechanisms controlling arterial pressure. In Frohlich, E.D. (ed.): Pathophysiology: Altered Regulatory Mechanisms in Disease. Edition 3. Philadelphia, J.B. Lippincott Company, 1984, pp. 45–81.
24. Frohlich, E.D., Messerli, F.H., Reisin, E., et al.: The problem of obesity and hypertension. Hypertension, 5:III-71–III-78, 1983.
25. Frohlich, E.D., and Pfeffer, M.A.: Adrenergic mechanisms in human and SHR hypertension. Clin. Sci. Mol. Med., 48:225s–238s, 1975.
26. Frohlich, E.D., Pfeffer, M.A., and Pfeffer, J.M.: Systemic hemodynamics and cardiac function in spontaneously hypertensive rats: Similarities with essential hypertension. In Strauer, B.E. (ed.): The Heart in Hypertension. Berlin, Heidelberg, and New York, Springer-Verlag, 1981, pp. 53–71.
27. Frohlich, E.D., and Tarazi, R.C.: Is arterial pressure

the sole factor responsible for hypertensive cardiac hypertrophy? Am. J. Cardiol., *44*:959–963, 1979.

28. Frohlich, E.D., Tarazi, R.C., and Dustan, H.P.: Clinical-physiological correlations in the development of hypertensive heart disease. Circulation, *44*:446–455, 1971.

29. Gillum, R.F.: Pathophysiology of hypertension in blacks and whites. A review of the basis of racial blood pressure differences. Hypertension, *1*:468–475, 1979.

30. Gordon, A.L., Inchiosa, M.A., Jr., and Lehr, D.: Isoproterenol induced cardiomegaly: Assessment of myocardial protein content, actomyosin ATPase and heart rate. J. Mol. Cell. Cardiol., *4*:543–557, 1972.

31. Gordon, T.: Blood Pressure of Adults by Race and Area, United States 1960–62. Hyattsville, Maryland, National Center for Health Statistics, 1964; DHEW Publication No. (PHS) 1000 (series 11; no. 5).

32. Hammond, I.W., Alderman, M.H., Devereux, R.B., et al.: Contrast in cardiac anatomy and function between black and white patients with hypertension. J. Natl. Med. Assoc., *76*:247–255, 1984.

33. Holland, O.B., Nixon, J.V., and Kuhnert, L.: Diuretic-induced ventricular ectopic activity. Am. J. Med., *70*:762–768, 1981.

34. Hollifield, J.W., and Slaton, P.E.: Thiazide diuretics, hypokalemia and cardiac arrhythmias. Acta Med. Scand. (Suppl.), *647*:67–73, 1981.

35. Ishise, S., Pegram, B.L., and Frohlich, E.D.: Disparate effects of methyldopa and clonidine on cardiac mass and haemodynamics in rats. Clin. Sci., *59*(Suppl. 6):449s–452s, 1980.

36. Johansson, B.W. (ed.): Electrolytes and cardiac arrhythmias. Acta Med. Scand. (Suppl.), *647*:1–177, 1981.

37. Kannel, W., Brand, N., Skinner, J., et al.: Relation of adiposity to blood pressure and development of hypertension: The Framingham Study. Ann. Intern. Med., *67*:48–59, 1967.

38. Kannel, W.B., Castelli, W.P., McNamara, P.M., et al.: Role of blood pressure in the development of congestive heart failure: The Framingham Study. N. Engl. J. Med., *287*:781–787, 1972.

39. Kannel, W.B., Doyle, J.T., McNamara, P.M., et al.: Precursors of sudden death. Circulation, *51*:606–613, 1975.

40. Kannel, W.B., Gordon, T., and Offutt, D.: Left ventricular hypertrophy by electrocardiogram. Prevalence, incidence and mortality in the Framingham Study. Ann. Intern. Med., *71*:89–105, 1969.

41. Kannel, W.B., Gordon, T., and Schwartz, M.H.: Systolic vs diastolic blood pressure and risk of coronary heart disease: The Framingham Study. Am. J. Cardiol., *27*:335–346, 1971.

42. Kannel, W.B., and Sorlie, P.: Hypertension in Framingham. *In* Paul, O. (ed.): Epidemiology and Control of Hypertension. Miami, Florida, Symposia Specialists, 1975, pp. 553–592.

43. Khairallah, P.A., Sen, S., and Tarazi, R.C.: Angiotensin protein biosynthesis and cardiovascular hypertrophy. (Abstract.) Am. J. Cardiol., *37*:148, 1967.

44. Kobrin, I., Frohlich, E.D., Ventura, H.O., et al.: Renal involvement follows cardiac enlargement in essential hypertension. Arch. Intern. Med., in press.

45. Kobrin, I., Sesoko, S., Pegram, B.L., et al.: Reduced cardiac mass by nitrendipine is dissociated from systemic or regional haemodynamic changes in rats. Cardiovasc. Res., *3*:158–162, 1984.

46. Kuwajima, I., Kardon, M.B., Pegram, B.L., et al.: Regression of left ventricular hypertrophy in two-kid-

47. Lakatta, E.G.: Alterations in the cardiovascular system that occur in advanced age. Fed. Proc., *38*:163–167, 1979.

48. Linzbach, A.J.: Heart failure from the point of view of quantitative anatomy. Am. J. Cardiol., *5*:370–382, 1960.

49. Madias, J.E., and Gavras, H.P.: Nonarrhythmogenicity of diuretic-induced hypokalemia. Its evidence in patients with uncomplicated hypertension. Arch. Intern. Med., *144*:2171–2176, 1984.

50. McDonough, J.R., Garrison, G.E., and Hames, C.G.: Blood pressure and hypertensive disease among Negroes and whites. Ann. Intern. Med., *61*:208–228, 1964.

51. Medical Research Council Working Party on Mild to Moderate Hypertension: Ventricular extrasystoles during thiazide treatment: Substudy of MRC Mild Hypertension Trial. Br. Med. J., 2:1249–1253, 1983.

52. Meerson, F.Z.: The myocardium in hyperfunction and heart failure. Circ. Res., *25*(Suppl. II):II-1–II-163, 1969.

53. Messerli, F.H., Christie, B., de Carvalho, J.G.R., et al.: Obesity and essential hypertension: Hemodynamics, intravascular volume, sodium excretion, and plasma renin activity. Arch. Intern. Med., *141*:81–85, 1981.

54. Messerli, F.H., Frohlich, E.D., Dreslinski, G.R., et al.: Serum uric acid in essential hypertension: An indicator of renal vascular involvement. Ann. Intern. Med., *93*:817–821, 1980.

55. Messerli, F.H., Frohlich, E.D., Suarez, D.H., et al.: Borderline hypertension: Relationship between age, hemodynamics, and circulating catecholamines. Circulation, *64*:760–764, 1981.

56. Messerli, F.H., Sundgaard-Riise, K., Reisin, E., et al.: Dimorphic cardiac adaptation to obesity and arterial hypertension. Ann. Intern. Med., *99*:757–761, 1983.

57. Messerli, F.H., Ventura, H.O., Elizardi, D.J., et al.: Hypertension and sudden death: Increased ventricular ectopic activity in left ventricular hypertrophy. Am. J. Med., *77*:18–22, 1984.

58. Metropolitan Life Insurance Company: Blood Pressure: Insurance Experience and Its Implications. New York, Metropolitan Life Insurance Co., 1961.

59. Morgan, D.B., and Davidson, C.: Hypokalemia and diuretics: An analysis of publications. Br. Med. J., *280*:905–908, 1980.

60. Multiple Risk Factor Intervention Trial Research Group: Baseline rest echocardiographic abnormalities, antihypertensive treatment and mortality in the Multiple Risk Factor Intervention Trial. Am. J. Cardiol., *55*:1–5, 1985.

61. Multiple Risk Factor Intervention Trial Research Group: Multiple Risk Factor Intervention Trial. Risk factor changes and mortality results. J.A.M.A., *248*:1465–1477, 1982.

62. Natsume, T., Kardon, M.B., Pegram, B.L., et al.: Assessment of cardiac performance in regressed left ventricular hypertrophy with captopril in spontaneously hypertensive rats. (Abstract.) J. Am. Coll. Cardiol., *5*:414, 1985.

63. Ostrander, L.D., Jr., Francis, T., Jr., Hayer, N.S., et al.: The relationship of cardiovascular disease to hyperglycemia. Ann. Intern. Med., *62*:1188–1198, 1965.

64. Papademetriou, V., Fletcher, R., Khatri, I.M., et al.: Diuretic-induced hypokalemia in uncomplicated sys-

temic hypertension: Effect of plasma potassium correction on cardiac arrhythmias. Am. J. Cardiol., 52:1017–1022, 1983.

65. Paul, O.: Epidemiology of hypertension. *In* Genest, J., Koiw, E., Kuchel, O. (eds.): Hypertension: Physiopathology and Treatment. New York, McGraw-Hill, 1977, pp. 613–630.

66. Pegram, B.L., Ishise, S., and Frohlich, E.D.: Effect of methyldopa, clonidine and hydralazine on cardiac mass and hemodynamics in Wistar-Kyoto and spontaneously hypertensive rats. Cardiovasc. Res., 16:40–46, 1982.

67. Pfeffer, M.A., Ferrell, B.A., Pfeffer, J.M., et al.: Ventricular morphology and pumping ability of exercised spontaneously hypertensive rats. Am. J. Physiol., 235:H193–H199, 1978.

68. Pfeffer, M.A., Pfeffer, J.M.: Mechanisms of dynamic cardiac performance. *In* Frohlich, E.D. (ed.): Pathophysiology: Altered Regulatory Mechanisms in Disease. Edition 3. Philadelphia, J.B. Lippincott Company, 1984, pp. 5–22.

69. Pfeffer, M.A., Pfeffer, J.M., and Frohlich, E.D.: Pumping ability of the hypertrophying left ventricle of the spontaneously hypertensive rat. Circ. Res., 38:423–429, 1976.

70. Pfeffer, M.A., Pfeffer, J.M., Weiss, A.K., et al.: Development of SHR hypertension and cardiac hypertrophy during prolonged beta-blocking therapy. Am. J. Physiol., 232:H639–H643, 1977.

71. Rostand, S.G., Kirk, K.A., Rutsky, E.A., et al.: Racial differences in the incidence of treatment for end-stage renal disease. N. Engl. J. Med., 306:1276–1278, 1982.

72. Sen, S., and Bumpus, F.M.: Collagen synthesis in development of reversal of cardiac hypertrophy in spontaneously hypertensive rat. Am. J. Cardiol., 44:954–958, 1979.

73. Sen, S., Tarazi, R.C., and Bumpus, F.M.: Cardiac hypertrophy and antihypertensive therapy. Cardiovasc. Res., 11:427–433, 1977.

74. Stamler, J.: Hypertension: Aspects of Risk. *In* Hunt, J.C. (ed.): Hypertension Update: Mechanisms, Epidemiology, Evaluation, Management. Bloomfield, New Jersey, Health Learning Systems, 1980, pp. 22–37.

75. Stamler, J., Stamler, R., Rhomberg, R., et al.: Multivariate analysis of relationship of six variables to blood pressure: Findings from Chicago community surveys. J. Chronic Dis., 28:499–525, 1975.

76. Szakacs, J.E., and Mehlman, B.: Pathologic changes induced by L-norepinephrine: Quantitative aspects. Am. J. Cardiol., 5:619–627, 1960.

77. Tarazi, R.C., Ibrahim, M.M., Dustan, H.P., et al.: Cardiac factors in hypertension. Circ. Res., 34(Suppl. I):I-213–I-221, 1974.

78. Tarazi, R.C., Miller, A., Frohlich, E.D., et al.: Electrocardiographic changes reflecting left atrial abnormality in hypertension. Circulation, 34:818–822, 1966.

79. Ulrych, M., Frohlich, E.D., Dustan, H.P., et al.: Cardiac output and distribution of blood volume in central and peripheral circulations in hypertensive and normotensive man. Br. Heart J., 31:570–574, 1969.

80. U.S. Department of Health, Education and Welfare: Blood pressure of adults by race and area. United States, 1960–1962. National Health Survey, National Center Health Statistics Service, 11:No. 5, 1964.

81. Ventura, H.O., Frohlich, E.D., Messerli, F.H., et al.: Cardiovascular effects and regional blood flow distribution associated with angiotensin converting enzyme inhibition (captopril) in essential hypertension. Am. J. Cardiol., 55:1023–1026, 1985.

82. Wittels, E.W., and Gotto, A.M., Jr.: Atherogenic mechanisms. *In* Frohlich, E.D. (ed.): Pathophysiology: Altered Regulatory Mechanisms in Disease, Edition 3. Philadelphia, J.B. Lippincott Company, 1984, pp. 107–118.

Alton Ochsner Medical Foundation
1516 Jefferson Highway
New Orleans, Louisiana 70121

The Adverse Effects of Hormonal Therapy

*Trudy L. Bush, Ph.D., M.H.S.**

The purpose of this article is to describe the risks and benefits of hormonal therapy in women and to evaluate the health impacts of reducing exposure to hormonal therapy. Generally speaking, hormones (specifically estrogens and progestins) are commonly prescribed for two primary purposes: (1) to prevent conception and (2) for relief of symptoms associated with ovarian failure (menopause).

PHARMACOLOGY

Two major classes of estrogens are used in hormonal therapy. The first are the so-called natural estrogens, which are those agents whose chemical structure occurs in nature, although not necessarily in humans. Natural estrogens that are commonly prescribed include conjugated equine estrogens (Premarin), 17-β-estradiol, and piperazine estrone sulfate.

The second class of estrogens are the synthetic agents, whose chemical structures do not occur naturally. The synthetic estrogens include ethinylestradiol, mestranol, and nonsteroidal agents, including diethylstilbestrol (DES). The natural estrogens are prescribed most frequently for menopausal therapy, whereas the synthetic agents are given for contraceptive purposes.

There are also two major classes of synthetic progestins that are commonly used in therapeutic situations. The first are the 19-nortestosterone (19-nor) derivatives, including norgestrel and norethindrone acetate. Because of their derivation, the 19-nor agents exhibit strong androgenic effects on many biologic systems.

A second class of progestins includes the hydroxyprogesterone derivative medroxyprogesterone acetate (Provera). These agents are less androgenic in their effects than the 19-nor progestins. Recently, natural progestogens, mainly micronized progesterone, have been used in experimental situations.[23] However, these agents are not yet readily available for general use.

Most progestins act as antiestrogenic agents, probably by blocking the synthesis of new cytoplasmic estrogen receptors.[9] In general, the 19-nor progestins are combined with synthetic estrogens in contraceptive therapy, whereas the less androgenic agent, medroxyprogesterone acetate, is cycled with natural estrogens during menopausal therapy.

CONTRACEPTIVE VERSUS MENOPAUSAL THERAPY

Agents prescribed for contraceptive purposes (oral contraceptives) presently contain synthetic estrogens such as mestranol or ethinylestradiol at doses of 30 to 50 μg per day. Oral contraceptives also contain a norprogestin (usually norethindrone or norgestrel) at doses between 1 and 5 mg per day. These agents usually are taken as a combined pill for 25 days of the month. Despite reports of serious adverse effects during the last 20 years, oral contraceptives remain a popular, reliable, and reversible form of birth control for millions of women.

Compared with the formulations used in oral contraceptives, estrogens used for the relief of menopausal symptoms tend to be natural agents (usually Premarin) prescribed at the relatively low doses of 0.625 mg per day to 1.25 mg per

*Assistant Professor of Public Health (Epidemiology), Columbia University School of Public Health, New York, New York

day. The potency of the dose of estrogen used in menopausal therapy is between 10 and 40 per cent of the estrogenic potency of oral contraceptives. Menopausal hormonal therapy is normally prescribed for 21 to 25 days of the month.

As unopposed estrogenic stimulation has been shown to increase the risk of endometrial cancer, a progestin, typically medroxyprogesterone acetate (Provera), is prescribed for menopausal women with intact uteri. When used with estrogens, Provera, 10 mg per day, is usually given during the last 10 days of a 25-day cycle. At present, both unopposed estrogen therapy (for women with prior hysterectomy) and estrogens cycled with progestins are commonly used in medical practice.[10]

BIOLOGIC EFFECTS OF ESTROGENS AND PROGESTINS

Both estrogens and progestins have powerful effects on numerous biologic systems that, in turn, may influence the risk of disease. For example, estrogens have been shown to (1) modify lipid and lipoprotein levels, (2) induce changes in coagulation parameters, (3) influence blood pressure levels, and (4) cause alterations in carbohydrate metabolism. In addition, estrogens have also been shown to modify bone metabolism, induce changes in the urogenital epithelium, alter psychologic and mental status, and cause proliferation of the endometrium.

Progestins influence most of the same systems as estrogens do. However, progestins usually act (after estrogen priming) as estrogen antagonists (for example, lipid and lipoprotein metabolism), although they may also act synergistically with estrogens (for example, carbohydrate metabolism and bone metabolism).

Estrogen Effects. The influence of estrogens on the various biologic parameters appears to be a function of both the type of estrogen used (natural versus synthetic) and the dose of the agent. In general, the synthetic estrogens are more potent (that is, they induce more pronounced changes in the biologic systems) than the natural hormones.[26] Higher doses of either synthetic or natural estrogens induce greater changes than lower doses of the same agents.

Lipid and Lipoprotein Metabolism. It has been known for several decades that oral estrogens have profound effects on lipid and lipoprotein metabolism. Basically, all estrogens tend to lower total cholesterol and low-density lipoprotein (LDL) cholesterol levels and increase high-density lipoprotein (HDL) cholesterol and tri-

glyceride levels. Theoretically, the changes induced in lipoprotein patterns by estrogen use (for example, increased HDL and decreased LDL levels) should protect against the development of coronary heart disease. The estrogenic effect of oral conjugated equine estrogens (at doses of 0.625 mg to 1.25 mg) on lipids and lipoproteins are summarized in Figure 1.[5]

Coagulation Factors. Although it has been suggested that estrogens may induce a hypercoagulable state in susceptible women, unopposed natural estrogens such as those used in menopausal therapy have not been shown to affect hemostatic mechanisms adversely in any consistent way. However, it has been proposed that much of the increased risk of thromboembolic disease among oral contraceptive users may be due to estrogen-induced changes in the coagulation system, leading to an increased risk of thrombus formation.[8]

Blood Pressure. There is no consistent evidence that unopposed, low-dose natural estrogens (used primarily in menopausal therapy) adversely affect blood pressure levels.[41] However, increases in blood pressure have been observed consistently in women using oral contraceptives.[16]

These apparently conflicting effects of estrogen on coagulation and blood pressure may be due in part to (1) the differences in dose and type of estrogen used in menopausal therapy compared with oral contraceptive therapy (low-dose natural estrogen versus high-dose synthetic estrogen) and (2) the effects of the norprogestins found in oral contraceptives.

Glucose Intolerance. Estrogens used in menopausal therapy have been shown to cause a temporary alteration in glucose tolerance that resolves after 3 to 6 months of therapy. Although glucose tolerance is modified by estrogen use, fasting levels of glucose tend to be lower in women using menopausal estrogens.[4] Among oral contraceptive users, oral glucose tolerance also tends to be impaired, and hyperinsulinemia is seen frequently.[42] However, estrogen-induced frank diabetes in women using either oral contraceptives or menopausal estrogens is rare.

Other Effects. In addition to the aforementioned effects, estrogens have also been shown to prevent osteoporosis,[19] urogenital atrophy,[34] and depression[17] and to increase the occurrence of endometrial hyperplasia and carcinoma.[43]

Progestin Effects. Unlike estrogen, relatively few studies have evaluated the effects of opposed or unopposed progestins on biologic parameters that may influence risk of disease. Clearly, given the numbers of women that are exposed to this

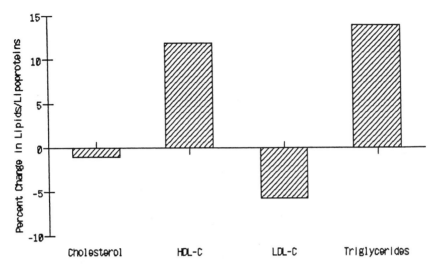

Figure 1. Changes in lipids and lipoproteins induced by conjugated estrogens.

hormone, additional studies of the effects of progestins are urgently needed.

Lipid and Lipoprotein Metabolism. In general, unopposed progestins tend to lower total cholesterol, triglyceride, and HDL levels and to increase LDL levels. Like estrogen, the degree to which a progestin influences lipid and lipoprotein levels may be a function of the type of agent used. For example, the 19-nor agents have the greatest impact on lipid levels, reducing HDL cholesterol by 25 to 30%, whereas medroxyprogesterone acetate has a lesser effect, reducing HDL cholesterol by about 13%.[5] It has been suggested that some of the adverse effect on cardiovascular risk induced by oral contraceptives may be due to the progestin-induced changes in lipoprotein levels.[38] Although it has been suggested recently that natural progesterone does not significantly influence HDL levels,[23] further investigations in this area are needed.

Coagulation Factors. There is presently no evidence that unopposed progestins or progestins cycled with estrogen adversely affect coagulation factors.

Blood Pressure. One report in the literature has suggested that the progestin content of oral contraceptives is associated with increased levels of blood pressure.[31] This report needs to be replicated in additional work.

Glucose Intolerance. Long-term use of the 19-nor progestins or medroxyprogesterone acetate in the postmenopausal period has been associated with significant increases of glucose and insulin levels. However, short-term unopposed

progestin therapy does not appear to alter carbohydrate metabolism.[9]

It has been suggested that the effects of estrogen and progestin on glucose intolerance may be synergistic, that is, may result in greater abnormalities than those seen when only one hormone is administered. Although it has been thought that the abnormalities of glucose tolerance seen in oral contraceptive users was a result of the estrogen content of the pill, a recent study has suggested that the progestin content of oral contraceptives is responsible for these observed effects.[24]

Other Effects. Progestins may interact with estrogen in preventing bone loss and osteoporosis.[6] Progestins also have been used to treat menopausal symptoms and depression[12] and to counter the estrogen-induced proliferation of the endometrium.[10]

HEALTH EFFECTS OF ORAL CONTRACEPTIVES

Adverse Effects

Cardiovascular Diseases. Oral contraceptives were first introduced into medical practice in 1960, and at the time that they were introduced, most formulations contained at least 100 µg of ethinylestradiol or mestranol. Since their introduction, numerous studies have demonstrated consistently that users of oral contraceptives, compared with nonusers, have an increased risk of venous thromboembolism, stroke, and myocardial infarction.[35] Although most researchers would agree that oral contraceptive use increases the risk for cardiovascular disease, a recent overview of the literature questions the validity of reports showing an increased risk in oral contraceptive users.[27]

The discovery that the increased risks of cardiovascular diseases were directly related to the dosage of estrogen in the contraceptive resulted in the current low-dose formulations, that is, oral contraceptives containing 35 to 50 μg of estrogen.

(Nearly all of the studies that show an increased risk of cardiovascular disease with oral contraceptive use were completed when the high-dose formulations were commonly prescribed. However, the risk estimates from these older studies should not be extrapolated to the current oral contraceptive formulations. Additional studies to assess the health effects of low-dose oral contraceptive formulations on the risk of cardiovascular disease are needed.)

Venous Thromboembolism. Early studies have reported a risk of venous thromboembolism in oral contraceptive users to be three to five times the risk in nonusers. Because of this finding, a prior history of venous thromboembolism is an absolute contraindication to oral contraceptive therapy. A recent study has found that users of low-dose oral contraceptives continue to have an increased risk (relative risk = 2.8) of venous thromboembolism compared with nonusers.[25]

Myocardial Infarction. The risk of myocardial infarction among nonsmoking high-dose oral contraceptive users has been shown to be about four times the risk in nonusers. However, among smokers who used oral contraceptives, the relative risk of myocardial infarction is 39 times the risk in nonsmoking nonusers. Age has been shown to be a factor that modifies the effect of oral contraceptive use. For example, among nonsmoking women 30 to 39 years of age, the risk of myocardial infarction due to oral contraceptive use is about 3 per 100,000 high-dose oral contraceptive users per year. However, among heavy smokers 40 to 44 years of age, the risk of myocardial infarction due to oral contraceptive use is 153 per 100,000 high-dose oral contraceptive users per year.[1]

Unfortunately, there are very few reports on the effect of low-dose oral contraceptive formulations on the risk of myocardial infarction. One current study has found no occurrences of myocardial infarction in low-dose users after nearly 38,000 woman-years of follow-up.[25] This low occurrence may be due to several factors, including the effects of a reduced estrogenic con-

tent of oral contraceptives, or to the fact that only healthier women are treated with hormonal contraceptive therapy.

Stroke. Elevated risk for stroke among women using high-dose oral contraceptives has been demonstrated for thrombotic and hemorrhagic strokes and subarachnoid hemorrhages. The risk varies from about 1.5 to 4 times that in nonusers of oral contraceptives.[37] The risk for stroke has been shown to be directly related to the estrogenic content of the contraceptive formulation. However, a recent report comparing low-dose oral contraceptive users with nonusers found no increase in risk of stroke (relative risk = 0.9).[25] Whether the absence of an increased risk in low-dose users is real remains to be seen. The possibility exists that these agents presently are being prescribed only to healthy women.

Current Versus Past Users. In all of the aforementioned studies, the elevated risks of cardiovascular disease were based on current oral contraceptive use. One report has suggested that the excess risk in oral contraceptive users remains after cessation of oral contraceptive therapy.[33] This observation has not been confirmed in other reports and may in fact reflect a bias, for example, that the increased risk observed in ex-users may be the result of an illness that developed while using oral contraceptives and that led them to stop use.[37]

Other Conditions. An older report has suggested that oral contraceptive users have twice the incidence of gallbladder disease than nonusers.[2] However, this finding has not been replicated in other studies. It also has been suggested that liver tumors are increased in oral contraceptive users.[28] However, any association between benign or malignant liver tumors and oral contraceptive use is known to be rare and is hypothesized to be coincidental.[11]

Beneficial Effects

Oral contraceptive use is an effective, acceptable, inexpensive, and reversible form of birth control with a (theoretic) failure rate of less than 1 per cent. The risk of dying from complications of childbirth are 5.5 times higher than the risk of dying from oral contraceptive use. In the United States, oral contraceptives are associated with a death rate of 3.7 per 100,000 per year (1.8 per 100,000 in nonsmokers and 6.5 per 100,000 in smokers), whereas the concurrent maternal mortality rate is 20.6 per 100,000 per year.[29] Although oral contraceptive use is not as safe (with regard to mortality) as the use of barrier methods backed up by abortion,[36] oral contraceptives are more acceptable, convenient, and, in the case of therapeutic abortion, cost-efficient than other contraceptive methods. The mortality risk associated with oral contraceptive use could be substantially reduced if this medication were prescribed only for nonsmokers.

More recently, oral contraceptive use has been shown to be associated with a decreased risk of ovarian cancer[7] and endometrial cancer.[14] In addition, oral contraceptive users, compared with nonusers, have lower rates of benign breast disease,[21] ovarian cysts,[20] anemia,[30] arthritis,[40] and pelvic inflammatory disease.[32]

Oral contraceptive use has not been shown to increase or decrease the risk of breast cancer. This observation is important, as breast cancer is the most common cancer in women, and thus, even a small increase in risk or a small protective effect would have an impact on large numbers of women.

Adverse Effects of Withdrawal of Oral Contraceptives

The major adverse effects of oral contraceptive use are concentrated in two groups of women: those 35 years of age and older and those who smoke. It seems clear that in these individuals, the risk of oral contraceptive use clearly outweighs the benefits, and oral contraceptives should not be prescribed for such women.

However, for women younger than 35 years old with no identifiable risk factors for cardiovascular disease, withdrawal of oral contraceptives may negate any positive effect of these agents. Thus, in nonsmoking women less than 35 years of age, withdrawing oral contraceptive therapy may (1) increase the rate of pregnancy and thus increase the risks associated with abortion, pregnancy, and childbirth; (2) negate any oral contraceptive–induced protective effect on the endometrium and ovaries; (3) negate any protective effect of oral contraceptive use on ovarian cysts and benign breast disease; and (4) negate any protective effect on the development of pelvic inflammatory disease.

The adverse effects of withdrawing oral contraceptives may be substantial in both the short and long terms. For example, in the short term, the risks associated with pregnancy and childbirth are reduced in oral contraceptive users, and the risk of dying is much lower in women using oral contraceptives than in women using no birth control.[29] Long-term beneficial effects have been evaluated, and it has been suggested

that 1700 ovarian cancers and 2000 endometrial cancers were averted in 1982 by the use of oral contraceptives.[13] It also has been estimated that for each 100,000 women using oral contraceptives, 270 fewer surgical procedures for ovarian cysts and breast disease are done each year.[22] In addition, the adverse consequences of pelvic inflammatory disease, including infertility, would not be reduced if oral contraceptives were withdrawn.

Overall, it would seem that the adverse effects of oral contraceptive use outweigh their benefits in older (older than 35 years) women and in women who smoke. However, in younger persons, the beneficial effects (both short-term and long-term) may outweigh the (low) risk of venous thromboembolism and other vascular disorders.

HEALTH EFFECTS OF MENOPAUSAL THERAPY

Adverse Effects

Endometrial Cancer. Estrogen use unopposed by progestin therapy in women with intact uteri has clearly been shown to increase the risk of endometrial adenocarcinoma.[43] Such women have been shown to have three to eight times the risk of developing this cancer than women not using replacement estrogens. The risk seems to be related to both the dose and duration of estrogen therapy.[18] However, the addition of a progestational agent to the estrogen therapy has been shown to protect the endometrium and to reverse any estrogen-induced hyperplastic changes. Thus, current recommendations call for cycling of a progestin with any estrogen therapy in women with intact uteri.[10]

Except for the increase in endometrial cancer, no other adverse effect of unopposed menopausal estrogen therapy has been clearly documented. Despite the widespread use of these agents for more than 40 years, no compelling evidence has been presented that the natural estrogens, prescribed at low doses for relief of menopausal symptoms, increase the risk of (1) vascular disorders (stroke, thromboembolism, myocardial infarction) or (2) cancer (breast, ovary).[4]

Progestins have been prescribed for women with intact uteri since the late 1970s; the only documented adverse effect of estrogen-progestin therapy is uterine bleeding. However, lipid and lipoprotein levels may be affected adversely by the addition of a norprogestin to the estrogen regimen.[5]

Beneficial Effects

Unopposed estrogens used in the menopause have been clearly shown to be effective in alleviating menopausal symptoms (hot flashes, urogenital atrophy, depression) and in preventing osteoporosis, a major cause of morbidity and mortality in aged women.

There is also a growing body of evidence that unopposed estrogen therapy is protective against the development of cardiovascular disease in women. Out of a total of 19 reports that have evaluated menopausal estrogen use and cardiovascular disease, 8 show a significant protective effect (relative risks = 0.3 to 0.7), and 5 additional reports show a reduced risk of disease (relative risks = 0.3 to 0.5). Four studies showed no effect of estrogen use on the occurrence of cardiovascular disease. Only the Framingham Study[39] and a small, flawed case-control study[15] found an increased risk of cardiovascular disease associated with menopausal estrogen use.

It has been hypothesized that any beneficial effect of estrogens on cardiovascular disease may be operating through lipid and lipoprotein mechanisms,[3] that is, estrogens, at the doses used for menopausal therapy, increase HDL levels by about 8 to 10 mg per dl and decrease LDL levels by approximately 10 to 15 mg per dl. Such a change in the lipoprotein profile should be protective against atherosclerotic cardiovascular disease.

The effects of menopausal estrogens cycled with progestins on the occurrence of cardiovascular disease has not yet been evaluated. However, the inclusion of the androgenic norprogestins would reverse and overwhelm any beneficial estrogen-induced changes in lipoprotein levels, that is, HDL levels would be lowered and LDL levels would be increased.[5] The addition of medroxyprogesterone acetate to an estrogen regimen would reverse, but not overwhelm, the estrogen-induced effects on lipoproteins (that is, there would be no net change in lipoprotein levels). Thus, if a protective effect of estrogen on cardiovascular disease is operating by modification of lipoprotein levels, one would expect to see no beneficial effect when medroxyprogesterone acetate is added to the estrogen regimen and perhaps a detrimental effect if a 19-nor progestin is included.

Effects of Withdrawal of Estrogen Therapy

Because estrogens clearly have been shown to be effective in relieving a wide variety of so-matic and psychologic menopausal symptoms, the withdrawal of these agents would mean that millions of women would be without an effective therapy for these conditions. As hot flashes and other disturbances seen in the menopause may be severe, withdrawal of estrogen therapy may cause increased suffering. To date, no other agent has been introduced that is as effective as estrogen in relieving menopausal symptoms.

Withdrawal of estrogen therapy would also eliminate an effective prophylactic therapy for osteoporosis. Although other therapies (calcium consumption, exercise, vitamin D) have been proposed, none has been demonstrated to be as effective as estrogen in preventing both osteoporosis and osteoporosis-induced fractures. Therefore, withdrawal of estrogens may significantly increase the rate of fractures and the morbidity and mortality associated with this condition.

If the association between estrogen therapy and cardiovascular disease is real (that is, if estrogens do protect through changes in the lipoprotein profile), withdrawing estrogen therapy would probably increase the risk of cardiovascular disease in postmenopausal women. This assertion is made for two reasons. First, cardiovascular disease is the major killer of women, and second, the prevalence of estrogen use in postmenopausal women is high (15 to 50 per cent). Removing an agent that may be very protective (that is, the risk estimates suggest that cardiovascular disease is 30 to 50 per cent lower in estrogen users) for a very common disease will have an impact that is discernible.

The major beneficial effect of withdrawing estrogens would be that endometrial cancer would be decreased. As progestins, when cycled with estrogens, have been shown to decrease the risk of endometrial cancer, this advantage is moot.

SUMMARY AND CONCLUSIONS

Estrogen therapy must be cycled with progestin therapy in women with intact uteri in order to prevent uterine cancer. However, these women cannot be expected to benefit (with regard to cardiovascular disease) from any estrogen-induced changes in the lipoprotein profile, as progestins will either negate or overwhelm any estrogen effects. However, such women will definitely benefit from estrogen's effects with regard to menopausal symptoms and bone loss. These clearly beneficial effects of estrogen-progestin therapy are not outweighed by any known risks.

However, in women without uteri (approximately 30 per cent of women), unopposed estrogen therapy in the menopause may protect against cardiovascular disease, as well as have beneficial effects on bone metabolism and menopausal symptoms. In this special case, the beneficial effects of unopposed estrogen therapy clearly outweigh any known risks.

REFERENCES

1. Berendes, H.W.: Health hazards associated with oral contraceptives. *In* Gold, E.B. (ed.): The Changing Risk of Disease in Women. An Epidemiologic Approach. Lexington, Massachusetts, The Collamore Press, 1984, pp. 107–115.
2. Boston Collaborative Drug Surveillance Program: Oral contraceptives and venous thromboembolic disease, surgically confirmed gallbladder disease, and breast tumors. Lancet, *1*:1399–1404, 1973.
3. Bush, T.L., Cowan, L., Barrett-Conner, E., et al.: Estrogen use and cardiovascular mortality: The Lipid Research Clinics follow-up study. (Abstract.) Am. J. Epidemiol., *118*:450, 1983.
4. Bush, T.L., and Barrett-Connor, E.: Noncontraceptive estrogen use and cardiovascular disease. Epidemiol. Rev., 7:80–104, 1985.
5. Bush, T.L., and Miller, V.T.: Beneficial effects of pharmacologic agents used in the menopause. *In* Mishell, D. (ed.): Menopause. Chicago, Year Book Medical Publishers, in press.
6. Christiansen, C.: Prevention of early post-menopausal bone loss: Controlled 2-year study in 315 normal females. Eur. J. Clin. Invest., *10*:273–279, 1980.
7. Cramer, D.W., Hutchinson, G.B., Welch, W.R., et al.: Factors affecting the association of oral contraceptives and ovarian cancer. N. Engl. J. Med., *302*:551–554, 1980.
8. Dugdale, M., and Masi, A.T.: Hormonal contraception and thromboembolic disease: Effects of the oral contraceptives on hemostatic mechanisms. A review of the literature. J. Chronic Dis., *23*:775–790, 1971.
9. Fritz, M.A., and Speroff, L.: The role of progestational agents in hormone replacement therapy. *In* Buchsbaum, H.J. (ed.): The Menopause. New York, Springer-Verlag, 1983, pp. 85–102.
10. Gambrell, R.D., Jr.: The menopause: Benefits and risks of estrogen-progestogen replacement therapy. Fertil. Steril., *37*:457–474, 1982.
11. Goodman, Z.D., and Ishak, K.G.: Hepatocellular carcinoma in women: Probable lack of etiologic association with oral contraceptive steroids. Hepatology, *2*:440–444, 1982.
12. Herrmann, W.M., and Beach, R.C.: Experimental and clinical data indicating the psychotropic properties of progestogens. Postgrad, Med. J., *54*(Suppl. 2):82–87, 1978.
13. Hulka, B.S.: Oral contraceptives. The good news. J.A.M.A., *249*:1624–1625, 1983.
14. Hulka, B.S., Chambless, L.E., Kaufman, D.G., et al.: Protection against endometrial carcinoma by combination-product oral contraceptives. J.A.M.A., *247*:475–477, 1982.
15. Jick, H., Dinan, B., and Rothman, K.J.: Noncontraceptive estrogens and nonfatal myocardial infarctions. J.A.M.A., *239*:1407–1409, 1978.

16. Johansson, S., Vedin, A., and Wilhelmsson, C.: Myocardial infarction in women. Epidemiol. Rev., *5*:67–95, 1983.
17. Klaiber, E.L., Broverman, D.M., Vogel, W., et al.: Estrogen therapy for severe persistent depressions in women. Arch. Gen. Psychiatry., *36*:550–560, 1979.
18. Lifshitz, S., and Bernstein, S.G.: Adenocarcinoma of the endometrium. *In* Buchsbaum, H.J. (ed.): The Menopause. New York, Springer-Verlag, 1983, pp. 103–129.
19. Lindsay, R., Aitken, J.M., Anderson, J.B., et al.: Long-term prevention of postmenopausal osteoporosis by estrogen. Lancet, *1*:1038–1042, 1976.
20. Ory, H.W.: Boston Collaborative Drug Surveillance Program: Functional ovarian cysts and oral contraceptives: negative association confirmed surgically. J.A.M.A., *228*:68–72, 1974.
21. Ory, H.W.: Oral contraceptives and reduced risk of benign breast diseases. N. Engl. J. Med., *294*:419–423, 1976.
22. Ory, H.W.: The health effects of fertility control. *In* Contraception: Science, Technology and Applications. Proceedings of a Symposium, Washington, D.C.: National Academy of Sciences, 1979.
23. Ottosson, U.B., Johansson, B.G., and von Schoultz, B.: Subfractions of high-density lipoprotein cholesterol during estrogen replacement therapy: A comparison between progestogens and natural progesterone. Am. J. Obstet. Gynecol., *151*:746–750, 1985.
24. Perlman, J.A., Russell-Briefel, R., Ezzati, T., et al.: Oral glucose tolerance and the potency of contraceptive progestins, J. Chronic Dis., *38*:857–864, 1985.
25. Porter, J.B., Hunter, J.R., Jick, H., et al.: Oral contraceptives and nonfatal vascular disease. Obstet. Gynecol., *66*:1–4, 1985.
26. Quirk, J.G., Jr., and Wendel, G.D., Jr.: Biologic effects of natural and synthetic estrogens. *In* Buchsbaum, H.J. (ed.): The Menopause. New York, Springer-Verlag, 1983, pp. 55–75.
27. Realini, J.P., and Goldzieher, J.W.: Oral contraceptives and cardiovascular disease: A critique of the epidemiologic studies. Am. J. Obstet. Gynecol., *152*:729–798, 1985.
28. Rooks, R.B., Ory, H.W., Ishak, L., et al.: Cooperative Liver Tumor Study Group: Epidemiology of hepatocellular adenoma: The role of oral contraceptive use. J.A.M.A., *242*:644–648, 1979.
29. Rosenfield, A.: The pill: An evaluation of recent studies. Johns Hopkins Med. J., *150*:177–180, 1982.
30. Royal College of General Practitioners: Oral Contraceptives and Health: An Interim Report from the Oral Contraceptive Study. New York, Pitman Publishing Company, 1974.
31. Royal College of General Practitioners: Oral Contraceptive Study: Effect on hypertension and benign breast disease of progestogen component in combined oral contraceptives. Lancet, *1*:624–628, 1977.
32. Senanayake, P., and Kramer, D.G.: Contraception and the etiology of PID. New perspectives. Am. J. Obstet. Gynecol., *7*:852–856, 1980.
33. Slone, D., Shapiro, S., Kaufman, D.W., et al.: Risk of myocardial infarction in relation to current and discontinued use of oral contraceptives. N. Engl. J. Med., *305*:420–424, 1981.
34. Smith, P.: Postmenopausal urinary symptoms and hormonal replacement therapy. Br. Med. J., *2*:941–945, 1976.
35. Stadel, B.: Oral contraceptives and cardiovascular disease. N. Engl. J. Med., *305*:612–618, 672–677, 1981.

36. Tietze, C.: New estimates of mortality associated with fertility control. Fam. Plann. Perspect., 9:74–80, 1977.

37. Vessey, M.P.: Oral contraceptives and cardiovascular disease: Some questions and answers. Br. Med. J., *284*:615–619, 1982.

38. Wahl, P., Walden, C., Knopp, R., et al.: Effect of estrogen/progestin potency on lipid/lipoprotein cholesterol. N. Engl. J. Med., *308*:862–867, 1983.

39. Wilson, P.W.F., Garrison, R.J., and Castelli, W.P.: Postmenopausal estrogen use, cigarette smoking, and cardiovascular morbidity in women over 50. The Framingham Study. N. Engl. J. Med., *313*:1044–1049, 1985.

40. Wingrove, S.J., and Kay, C.R.: Reduction in incidence of rheumatoid arthritis associated with oral contraceptives. Lancet, *1*:569–571, 1978.

41. Wren, B.G., and Routledge, A.D.: The effect of type and dose of oestrogen on the blood pressure of postmenopausal women. Maturitas, 5:135–142, 1983.

42. Wynn, V.: Metabolic effects of oral contraceptives in relation to coronary heart disease in young women. *In* Oliver, M.F. (ed.): Coronary Heart Disease in Young Women. Edinburgh, Churchill Livingstone, 1978, pp. 129–137.

43. Ziel, H.K.: Estrogen's role in endometrial cancer. Obstet. Gynecol., *60*:509–515, 1982.

Division of Epidemiology
Columbia University School of Public Health
600 W. 168th Street
New York, New York 10032

Negative Effects of Risk Factor Reduction on the Heart

Luis Alcocer, M.D.,* and Ariel J. Reyes, M.D.†

Since 1950, a considerable change in the mortality profile in the United States has been observed.[26] The age-adjusted death rates have fallen 40 per cent, and since 1960, the coronary heart disease mortality rate has decreased steadily and markedly. This decrease is not universal; it is found only in the United States, Canada, and Australia; in contrast, in the same period of time, some countries, such as Ireland, Scotland, the Soviet Union, Denmark, Germany, and some Eastern European nations, registered an increase in the rates of death due to cardiovascular disease.[11,12]

In order to analyze these changes in mortality at least two different aspects must been taken into consideration: (1) improvements in the treatment of cardiovascular diseases and (2) modifications of the risk factors for cardiovascular disease.

Improvement in the treatment of cardiovascular diseases can modify mortality rates by decreasing fatalities in properly treated patients. As the DuPont data suggest,[19] the impact of new drugs, coronary care units, and improved surgical techniques probably lowered the cardiovascular mortality rate, but their precise influence has not been demonstrated quantitatively. As Stamler[27] noted, "Improved treatment is not the only factor influencing the case fatality rates; less serious disease, possibly to improved control of risk factors in the population, may also have played a part."

The modification of the risk factors for cardiovascular disease is probably the main source contributing to the declining mortality rates by means of a decrease in the incidence of coronary heart disease. This probably explains the difference in mortality trends between the United States and the countries that suffered an increase in their cardiovascular mortality rates in the same periods of time.

Control of hypertension and the modification of lifestyles in the United States have become real facts, and the majority of Americans are better informed about the potential value of controlling the major risk factors. The apparently good results of this policy have created the image that the modification of the risk factors can reduce the incidence and severity of coronary heart disease. Yet, the data we do have must be considered with caution, because much of our understanding about the decrease in mortality arises from retrospective investigations. The results of prospective trials on coronary risk factor modification are partial and sometimes controversial. The Multiple Risk Factor Intervention Trial (MRFIT),[18] one of the major efforts in the field, failed to demonstrate a mortality benefit over a 6-year period of active measures to control hypertension, cigarette smoking, and diet.

The Lipid Research Clinics Coronary Primary Prevention Trial findings[23] show a clear reduction in the incidence of mortality due to coronary heart disease after the reduction of total cholesterol levels by means of cholestyramine in men at high risk. However, this was shown in a well-defined group and with cholestyramine treatment only, and the results cannot be extrapolated to other lipid-lowering agents or to the general population.

*Professor of Cardiology, Mexico National University; Chief, Hypertension Clinic, Mexico City General Hospital, Mexico City, Mexico

†Chief of Clinical Research, Fundación Procardias, Montevideo, Uruguay

The role of hypertension treatment in the prevention of coronary disease is elusive. The Veterans Administration Trial[36] showed that hypertension treatment is very effective to prevent both mortality and morbidity related to cerebrovascular disease; however, the effect on prevention of coronary disease was small. The Hypertension Detection and Follow-up Program (HDFP)[9] showed some decrease in mortality due to coronary heart disease and reported a 27 per cent reduction in deaths due to myocardial infarction in the stepped-care treated group. The United States Public Health Service Trial[25] and the Australian Trial[4] showed no change in coronary events.

In two studies, the Oslo Trial[6] and the Multiple Risk Factor Intervention Trial,[18] the number of coronary deaths or coronary events was greater in the treated or special intervention groups than in the placebo or usual care groups. For the first time, these studies call attention to the fact that certain interventions can be not only ineffective but also detrimental.

Some active interventions to modify risk factors paradoxically introduce new risk per se, but benefits in extensive populations vastly offset the proportionally small hazards introduced by these maneuvers. However, in daily practice, this potential source of danger can be crucial in a given patient in whom the new potential risk can be greater than the disease we are trying to prevent or treat.

The identification of patients in whom risk factor modification introduces a new risk should be made before it is decided who, when, and how to treat. In the remainder of this article, we will discuss the clinical profile of these patients, with special reference to the negative effects of risk factor intervention on the heart.

RISK MODIFICATION INTERVENTIONS THAT CAN AFFECT THE HEART

The heart potentially can be affected during reduction of risk factors by the following interventions: (1) inadequate exercise programs, (2) hypolipidemic drugs, (3) anorectic drugs, (4) oral hypoglycemic drugs, and (5) antihypertensive drugs.

Inadequate Exercise Programs. The interest in exercise by the general population has risen dramatically over the past 20 years as a result of epidemiologic evidence that physically active individuals have a low incidence of myocardial infarction[5] and a low mortality from coronary disease.[31]

The findings of several studies support the view that an inverse relationship exists between physical activity and coronary heart disease; however, the type and level of exercise required for protection against coronary heart disease are not well defined. Aerobic exercise, such as jogging, walking, or bicycling, is the type of activity believed to confer this protection. The training effect can be achieved by aerobic exercise of at least 20 minutes, three times weekly, sustained to reach and keep 70 per cent of the maximal heart rate. Whether such a training effect can be associated with the prevention of coronary heart disease is not well known. Furthermore, after a close look at the changes caused by sustained exercise on the heart, a note of concern must be considered.

The incidence of rhythm disturbances in athletes is greater than in the general population; sinus bradycardia occurs twice as frequently, sinus arrhythmia at least 10 times as frequently, first-degree AV block 10 times more frequently, Mobitz I block (second-degree AV block) 8 to 80 times more frequently, Mobitz II block 20 times more frequently, third-degree AV block 170 times more frequently, and atrial fibrillation 15 times more frequently.[8] Although these numbers are impressive, their clinical importance has not been documented.

Hypolipidemic Drugs. The favorable results obtained with the use of cholestyramine in the prevention of coronary heart disease reported by the Lipid Research Clinics Coronary Primary Prevention Trial cannot be extrapolated to other drugs. Moreover, in the Primary Prevention of Ischaemic Heart Disease Using Clofibrate Trial,[20] clofibrate use resulted in a significant decline in suspected and proven myocardial infarction. However, an increase in overall mortality was noted. In the Coronary Drug Project,[29] the use of the drug was associated with a significant increase in new cases of angina and the presence of arrhythmias.

Probucol produces a consistent reduction in high-density lipoprotein,[21] and D-thyroxine has been associated with serious cardiotoxic effects and was withdrawn from the Coronary Drug Project after excessive morbidity and mortality were observed with its use.[10]

Anorectic Drugs. Dextroamphetamine, methamphetamine, benzphetamine, chlorphentermine, diethylpropion, fenfluramine, phendimetrazine, phenmetrazine, and phentermine are drugs used to suppress the appetite. None has proved superior to the first two agents, and their use in a weight reduction program is questionable. Given orally, these drugs cause elevation of systolic and diastolic blood pressure, bradycardia, and potentially lethal arrhythmias.[37]

Some diets, such as low-carbohydrate, high-protein, or high-fat regimens, can produce serious metabolic side effects such as ketoacidosis or modifications of the lipid profile and are probably harmful as well.

The incidence of severe complications caused by the abuse of drugs such as digitalis or thyroid hormones in combination with diuretics and amphetamines as prescribed by ethical physicians is reaching alarming proportions in some countries.

Oral Hypoglycemic Drugs. Atherosclerosis is the most common complication of diabetes. Diabetes mellitus is accompanied by alterations in lipoproteins, prostaglandins, platelets, clotting factors, blood pressure regulation, blood viscosity, and arterial stiffening, all of which can participate in atherogenesis. Many of these changes correlate better with hyperinsulinemia than with hyperglycemia. The normalization of the levels of plasma glucose has not been proved to prevent the development of atherosclerosis. Furthermore, an increased prevalence of myocardial infarction has been reported with the use of oral hypoglycemic agents.[34,35] These reports are controversial and a final conclusion about the usefulness and safety of these drugs has not been obtained at present.

Antihypertensive Drugs. A case against diuretics has been made after the Multiple Risk Factor Intervention Trial suggested that these agents can increase mortality in hypertensive patients with an abnormal previous electrocardiogram.[18] Diuretics are still the most widely used agents for the treatment of hypertension and were recommended as a first-step choice without restrictions in the initial recommendations of the Joint National Committee on Detection, Evaluation, and Treatment of High Blood Pressure.[30]

At present, the nature and importance of this problem are not clear. Attention has been directed to metabolic changes caused by diuretics, especially to potassium and magnesium disturbances. Probably many of these changes are related to high doses used and to the long duration of treatment. Suggestions to reduce doses or to combine the drug with potassium-sparing agents or low-sodium diets sound logical; however, the present evidence is too incomplete to give a decisive answer about whether it is safe to sustain the recommendation to use these agents in the large proportion that has been current until today.

Another unanswered question challenges investigators and continues to attenuate the overriding enthusiasm for treating all mild hypertension aggressively. This question, which surfaced in recent years, is related to the apparently negative change in lipid profile induced by the use of some antihypertensive drugs (Table 1). The changes mentioned are referred to in relatively short-term studies, and no direct proof has been reported that the modification of the lipid profile secondary to antihypertensive treatment can be hazardous to the patient.

Beta-adrenergic blockade and calcium-entry blockade can give rise to a negative inotropic effect on the heart, which becomes of relative importance in failing or diseased hearts. However, in mildly hypertensive patients, this has not been an important problem because these drugs simultaneously reduce afterload, and this effect overrides the negative inotropic action. However, these hazards should be taken into account, particularly at the beginning of the treatment, when the hypertension is not yet controlled.[28]

Beta-blockade reduces the resting heart rate and inhibits the increment in heart rate seen with exercise. These effects can cause problems in patients who perform exercise that requires substantial increments in heart rate, such as jogging. The resting heart rate is decreased by agents without intrinsic sympathomimetic activity. Although agents both with and without intrinsic sympathomimetic activity are equally effective in inhibiting the increments in heart rate seen with exercise,[4] the cardiac output increments of exercise are better preserved with the use of agents with intrinsic sympathomimetic activity.

Table 1. *Effects of Antihypertensive Drugs on Lipid Profile*

DRUG	CHOLESTEROL	TRIGLYCERIDES
Thiazides	+	+
Indapamide	+/−	+/−
Propranolol	0	+
Pindolol	0	+/−
Labetalol	0	0
Prazosin	−	0
Clonidine	−	0
Guanabenz	−	0
Methyldopa	0	0
Reserpine	0	0
Captopril	0	0
Enalapril	0	0
Calcium blockers	0	0

+ = increases; − = decreases; +/− = sometimes increases, sometimes decreases; 0 = no change

MECHANISM OF NEGATIVE CARDIAC EFFECTS OF RISK MODIFICATION INTERVENTIONS

The heart can be affected by the following mechanisms: (1) depression of cardiac function, (2) facilitation of arrhythmogenic mechanisms, (3) left ventricular hypertrophy, and (4) worsening of other coronary risk factors (Table 2).

Depression of Cardiac Function. Beta-blockers in an inverse relation to intrinsic sympathomimetic activity, beta-blockers with membrane-stabilizing action, and calcium-channel blockers such as verapamil or diltiazem exert a negative inotropic action on the cardiac muscle. The mechanism of these actions is presented in Figure 1.

The contractile force of the cardiac muscle depends on the number of contractile sites activated during depolarization, and this number of contractile sites activated is related to the Ca^{++} fixed by troponin during the plateau of the action potential. The number of molecules of Ca^{++} fixed by troponin is dependent on the concentration of myoplasmic Ca^{++}. Several mechanisms control this concentration of the ion; one is the phosphorylation of the sarcoplasmic reticulum as a consequence of activation of a protein kinase by cyclic AMP, which is obtained by the action of adenylate cyclase on ATP. Beta stimulation increases adenylate cyclase, and beta-blockers interfere with this action. Interference

Table 2. *Mechanisms of Negative Effects on the Heart*

DEPRESSION OF CARDIAC FUNCTION
  Beta-blockers without intrinsic sympathomimetic activity
  Beta-blockers with membrane-stabilizing effect
  Calcium-entry blockers such as verapamil

FACILITATION OF ARRHYTHMOGENIC MECHANISMS
  Metabolic changes
    Diuretics, hypolipidemic drugs, oral hypoglycemic drugs, anorectic drugs
  Left ventricular hypertrophy
    Vasodilators
    Inappropriate exercise programs

LEFT VENTRICULAR HYPERTROPHY
  Vasodilators
  Inappropriate exercise programs

WORSENING OF OTHER CORONARY RISK FACTORS
  Hypercholesterolemia
    Diuretics
  Hypertriglyceridemia
    Diuretics and beta-blockers without intrinsic sympathomimetic activity
  Hyperglycemia
    Diuretics
  Hyperuricemia
    Diuretics

is inversely proportional to the intrinsic sympathomimetic activity of the agent.

The final result of beta-blocking activity is a diminution in the velocity and force of contraction, which interferes with systolic function. Diastolic function is altered by beta-blockers because the velocity of relaxation depends on the uptake of Ca^{++} by sarcoplasmic reticulum, and this reuptake is associated with phospholamban, a protein of the sarcoplasmic reticulum that is dependent on a phosphomyosin kinase activated by cyclic AMP during beta stimulation. Under the action of beta-blockers without intrinsic sympathomimetic activity, the heart tends to contract with less force and velocity, and the relaxation takes more time to be completed.[3]

The beta-blockers with membrane-stabilizing activity (that is, propranolol, oxprenolol, pindolol, acebutolol, alprenolol, and metoprolol) depress the myocardium by means of an additional mechanism (exerted only at high doses). The sarcoplasm possesses a bidirectional Na^+-Ca^{++} exchange mechanism, which obtains its energy from the sodium fast inward current. When this current is blocked by a quinidine-like action of the beta-blocker, intracellular Ca^{++} is reduced as a consequence of the shortage of energy in the Na^+-Ca^{++} pump, and a reduction in contractile force results.

Calcium-channel blockers such as verapamil and, to a lesser extent, diltiazem interact with the voltage-dependent Ca^{++} channel during its depolarized inactive phase, causing a "use-dependent" effect on contraction. By inversion of the force-frequency relation,[33] the myoplasmic Ca^{++} during the plateau of the action potential diminishes, generating a negative inotropic effect that is exerted during systole. As phospholamban is not affected, the reuptake of Ca^{++} is normal or relatively increased (because the concentration of Ca^{++} is diminished), and thus, the velocity of relaxation improves. This action is diametrically different from that exerted by beta-blockers and is important, for example, in hypertensive obese patients in whom diastolic volume is augmented[17] and velocity of relaxation is altered.

Facilitation of Arrhythmogenic Mechanisms. The mechanism for increased frequency of rhythm alterations in patients participating in inappropriate exercise programs is not clear; however, isotonic athletes show increased left and right ventricular cavities, with increased left ventricular mass (eccentric hypertrophy).[38] In contrast, isometric athletes tend to develop concentric hypertrophy.[13] Such left ventricular hy-

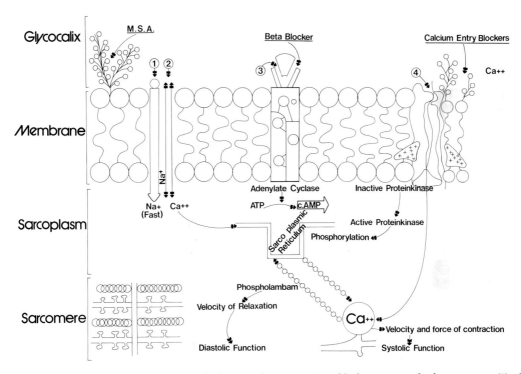

Figure 1. Mechanisms of cardiac contractile function depression. Beta-blockers occupy the beta-receptor (3) of the membrane. Beta-blockers with membrane-stabilizing activity reduce the fast sodium inward current (1), decreasing the energy of the bidirectional Na$^+$–Ca^{++} pump (2). Calcium-entry blockers act on the voltage-dependent calcium channel (4).

pertrophy could explain, at least to some extent, the increased arrhythmogenicity in hypertensive patients with left ventricular hypertrophy, as described previously by Messerli and coworkers.[16]

The presence of rhythm disorders during diuretic treatment has been attributed to alterations in potassium metabolism.[7] More recently, the importance of magnesium turnover alterations has been emphasized. In high doses, thiazide and loop diuretics promote loss of potassium, especially in patients on high-sodium diets or in those who are volume-depleted. However, the incidence of reduction of kalemic values or total body potassium found by various researchers is variable, and the development of rhythm disorders correlates poorly with these parameters. Nonetheless, the role of low intracellular potassium in the genesis of severe arrhythmias is well documented.

Patients with serum potassium levels less than 2.5 mEq per liter are prone to severe rhythm disturbances; patients with serum potassium levels between 2.5 and 3.5 mEq per liter depend on the ability of Na^+-Ka^+ ATPase to pump K^+ from extracellular to intracellular space. This system is magnesium-dependent; thus, if the magnesium level is normal, the intracellular content of K^+ is preserved. However, if the magnesium level is diminished, as occurs with some diuretic treatment, the function of the Na^+-K^+ ATPase becomes impaired, the intracellular K^+ decreases, and the production of severe arrhythmias is facilitated (Fig. 2).

Figure 3 shows the probable mechanisms for the production of arrhythmias and the increased risk of sudden death in patients treated with diuretics. Some types of diuretics[21] promote an excessive loss of magnesium, particularly in the presence of stress, high-phosphate or high-fat diets, high alcohol intake, high soft water consumption, or protein or vitamin D deficiencies. Low serum magnesium levels promote catecholamine release, which in turn worsens magnesium loss.[22]

Na^+-K^+ ATPase is blocked in the presence of low Mg^+; therefore, the intracellular concentration of K^+ diminishes, and Ca^{++} and Na^+ rise with modifications of the myocardial action potential. Arrhythmias and coronary spasm are facilitated by electrolyte imbalance and catecholamine-enhanced activity, and the risk of sudden death increases (Fig. 3).

Left Ventricular Hypertrophy. Exercise and some antihypertensive drugs, such as arteriolar vasodilators, can promote an increase in left ventricular mass. However, in the case of an inappropriate left ventricular muscle mass or dilatation, systolic wall stress will be increased, and ventricular systolic function is impaired.

In patients with severe concentric hypertrophy, as in hypertensive cardiomyopathy of the elderly,[32] or in the lean hypertensive,[15] the use of vasodilators can be contraindicated, because they promote more ventricular hypertrophy and, in some cases, produce severe hypotension.

Reversal of left ventricular hypertrophy is observed with several agents.[2] One might argue

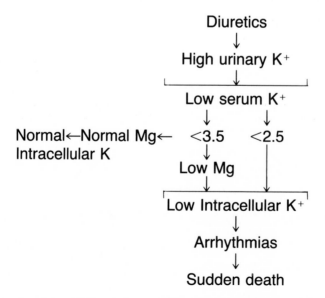

Figure 2. Mechanisms of production of abnormal intracellular potassium concentrations. The intracellular concentrations of potassium are related to serum potassium levels and to effectiveness of Na-K ATPase, which is magnesium-dependent.

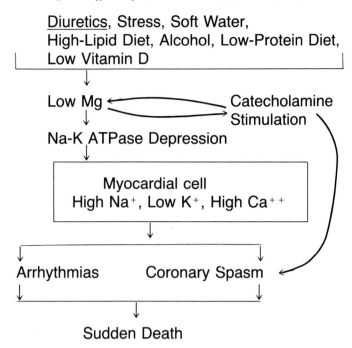

Figure 3. Theoretical explanation for the increased rate of sudden death with the use of diuretics. Both catecholamine imbalance and Na-K ATPase depression can be related to loss of magnesium after the use of diuretics.

that this regression of hypertrophy could occur by substitution of normal muscle by fibrous tissue, although such a mechanism seems less likely.[1]

Worsening of Other Coronary Risk Factors. Diuretics, with the exception of indapamide, increase the very-low-density lipoproteins (VLDL) and triglycerides by 10 to 28 per cent. Beta-blockers without ISA increase triglycerides and VLDL 20 to 60 per cent; the total cholesterol and low-density lipoproteins (LDL) are affected only slightly, and high-density lipoproteins are occasionally reduced slightly.

The action of beta-blockers and diuretics that promotes triglyceride increase is mediated by inactivation of lipase due to alpha-receptor stimulation in the case of diuretics and by a decrease in cyclic AMP in the case of beta-blockers (Fig. 4). Diuretics promote a moderate carbohydrate intolerance by means of catecholamine stimulation, probably related to modifications in Mg^+ turnover. The increase in uric acid caused by diuretics is related to a decrease in distal tubular excretion of uric acid associated with modifications in the turnover of Na^+ and Mg^+

CONCLUSIONS

The issue of the hazards conveyed by risk factor modifications is exceedingly complex and controversial but very important from the clinical point of view, especially in daily practice. It is extremely important to emphasize that all longitudinal studies looking at risk and benefit have shown that, in epidemiologic terms, benefits exceed risks. However, we are very concerned about the tendency to make general recommendations suitable to every patient, without making adjustments to fit each individual, before launching a lifelong treatment.

We should probably temper our enthusiasm for treating all patients with cardiovascular risk factors aggressively. The use of drugs should be considered carefully, their known side effects evaluated, and the risk-to-benefit ratio calculated. Recent information suggests that special attention should be paid to the following clinical situations: (1) use of diuretics in hypertensive patients with an abnormal electrocardiogram; (2) use of arterial vasodilators in elderly hypertensive patients with severe left ventricular hypertrophy; (3) use of arterial vasodilators in lean, young hypertensives; (4) use of beta-blockers in patients who continue to smoke cigarettes; (5) use of beta-blockers without intrinsic sympathomimetic activity in joggers; (6) use of diuretics and probably beta-blockers in patients with an abnormal lipid profile; (7) use of hypolipidemic drugs such as clofibrate, or anorectic drugs in arrhythmia-prone patients; (8) use of oral hypoglycemic drugs for "prevention" of ar-

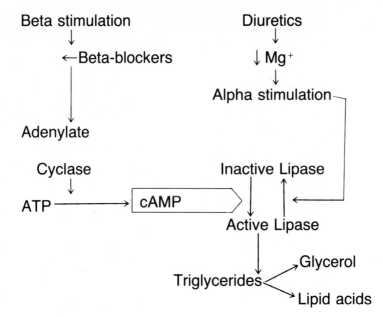

Figure 4. Possible explanation for the triglyceride increase related to the use of diuretics and beta-blockers. Both diuretics and beta-blockers reduce the activity of lipase, an enzyme responsible for triglyceride metabolism.

teriosclerosis; and (9) inappropriate exercise programs or arterial vasodilators in patients with left ventricular hypertrophy.

REFERENCES

1. Alcocer, L., and Aspe, J.: The effect of antihypertensive treatment with methyldopa on left ventricular mass. Royal Society of Medicine, International Congress and Symposium Series, 9:93–97, 1979.
2. Alcocer, L., Aspe, J., and Arce, E.: Left ventricular hypertrophy in hypertension: Considerations regarding its characteristics and its regression. In Velasco, M. (ed.): Arterial Hypertension. Amsterdam, Excerpta Medica, 1980, pp. 240–242.
3. Alcocer, L.: Farmacoterapia antihipertensiva con betabloqueadores. Rev. Med. Hosp. Gral. Mex., 47:273–280, 1985.
4. Frishman, W.H., Kostis, J., Strom, J., et al.: Comparison of pindolol and propranolol in treatment of patients with angina pectoris. The role of intrinsic sympathomimetic activity. In Frishman, W.H.: Clinical Pharmacology of the Beta-adrenoceptor Blocking Drugs. New York, Appleton-Century-Crofts, 1980, pp. 145–162.
5. Froelicher, V.F., and Brown, P.: Exercise and coronary heart disease. J. Cardiac Rehabil., 1:277–288, 1981.
6. Helgeland, A.: Treatment of mild hypertension: A five year controlled drug trial: The Oslo study. Am. J. Med., 69:752–753, 1980.
7. Holland, O.B., Nixon, J.V., and Kuhnert, L.: Diuretic induced ventricular ectopic activity. Am. J. Med., 70:762–765, 1981.
8. Huston, T.P., Puffer, J.C., and Rodney, W.M.: The athletic heart syndrome. N. Engl. J. Med., 313:24–32, 1985.
9. Hypertension Detection and Follow-up Program: I. Reduction in mortality of persons with high blood pressure including mild hypertension. J.A.M.A., 242:2562–2571, 1979.
10. Kuo, P.T., Hayase, K., Kostis, J.B., et al.: Use of combined diet and colestipol in long-term (7–7½ years) treatment of patients with type II hyperlipoproteinemia. Circulation, 59:199–202, 1979.
11. Levy, R.I.: The decline in cardiovascular disease mortality. Annu. Rev. Public Health, 2:49–70, 1981.
12. Levy, R.I., and Moskowitz, J.: Cardiovascular research: Decades of progress, a decade of promise. Science, 217:121–129, 1982.
13. Longhurst, J.C., Kelly, A.R., Gonyea, W.J., et al.: Echocardiographic left ventricular masses in distance runners and weight lifters. J. Appl. Physiol., 48:154–162, 1980.
14. Management Committee: The Australian Therapeutic Trial in Mild Hypertension. Lancet, 1:1261–1267, 1980.
15. Messerli, F.H.: Cardiovascular effects of obesity and hypertension. Lancet, 1:1165–1168, 1982.
16. Messerli, F.H., Ventura, H.O., Elizardi, D.J., et al.: Hypertension and sudden death: Increased ventricular ectopic activity in left ventricular hypertrophy. Am. J. Med., 77:18–20, 1984.
17. Messerli, F.H.: Hemodynamic and cardiac adaptation in essential hypertension. Consequences for therapy. J. Clin. Hypertension, 1:3–14, 1985.
18. Multiple Risk Factor Intervention Trial Research Group: Multiple Risk Factor Intervention Trial. Risk factor changes and mortality results. J.A.M.A., 248:1465–1469, 1982.
19. Pell, S., and Fayerweather, W.: Trends in the incidence of myocardial infarction and in associated mortality and morbidity in a large employed population, 1957–1983. N. Engl. J. Med., 312:1005–1011, 1985.
20. Report from the Committee of Principal Investigators: A cooperative trial in the primary prevention of is-

chaemic disease using clofibrate. Br. Heart J., 40:1069–1073, 1978.

21. Reyes, A.J.: Bases farmacológicas de la terapéutica cardiovascular con diuréticos. Arch. Inst. Cardiol. Mex., 51:291–303, 1981.

22. Reyes, A.J., and Leary, W.P.: Urinary magnesium and zinc excretion after monodosing healthy volunteers with chlorthalidone. Curr. Ther. Res., 32:128–137, 1982.

23. Rifkind, B.: Lipid Research Clinics Coronary Primary Prevention Trial: Results and implications. Am. J. Cardiol., 54:30c–34c, 1984.

24. Simons, L.A., Balasubramanian, S., and Beins, D.M.: Metabolic studies with probucol in hypercholesterolemia. Atherosclerosis, 40:299–305, 1981.

25. Smith, W.M.: Treatment of mild hypertension—results of a ten year intervention trial. U.S. Public Health Service Hospitals Cooperative Study Group. Circ. Res., 40(Suppl. I):98–105, 1977.

26. Stamler, J.: The marked decline in coronary heart disease mortality rates in the United States, 1968–1981: Summary of findings and possible explanations. Cardiology, 72:11–22, 1985.

27. Stamler, J.: Coronary heart disease: Doing the "right things." N. Engl. J. Med., 312:1053–1055, 1985.

28. Tarazi, R.C.: The heart in hypertension. N. Engl. J. Med., 312:308, 1985.

29. The Coronary Drug Project: Clofibrate and niacin in coronary heart disease. J.A.M.A., 213:360–364, 1975.

30. The Joint National Committee on Detection, Evaluation, and Treatment of High Blood Pressure: The 1980 report of the Joint National Committee on Detection, Evaluation, and Treatment of High Blood Pressure. Arch. Intern. Med., 140:1280–1286, 1980.

31. Thomas, G.S., Lee, P.R., Franks, P., et al.: Exercise and Health. The Evidence and the Implications.

Cambridge, Massachusetts, Oelgeschlager, Grunn and Hata, 1981, pp. 23–54.

32. Topol, E.J., Trill, T.A., and Fortuin, N.J.: Hypertensive hypertrophic cardiomyopathy of the elderly. N. Engl. J. Med., 312:277–283, 1985.

33. Triggle, D.J., and Swamy, V.C.: Pharmacology of agents that affect calcium: Agonists and antagonists. Chest, 78(Suppl.):174–179, 1980.

34. University Group Diabetes Program: A study of the effect of hypoglycemic agents on vascular complications in patients with adult-onset diabetes. Diabetes, 19(Suppl. II):474–478, 1970.

35. University Group Diabetes Program: A study of the effects of hypoglycemic agents on vascular complications in patients with adult-onset diabetes. V. Evaluation of phenformin therapy. Diabetes, 24(Suppl. I):65–73, 1975.

36. Veterans Administration Cooperative Study Group on Hypertension: Effects of treatment on morbidity in hypertension. II. Results in patients with diastolic blood pressure averaging 90 through 114 mm Hg. J.A.M.A., 213:1143–1152, 1970.

37. Weiner, N.: Norepinephrine, epinephrine and the sympathomimetic amines. *In* Goodman, A., and Gillman, A. (eds.): The Pharmacological Basis of Therapeutics. New York, Macmillan Publishing Co., 1980, pp. 138–175.

38. Zeppili, S., Sandric, S., Cecchetti, F., et al.: Echocardiographic assessments of cardiac arrangements in different sport activities. *In* Lubich, T., and Venerando, A. (eds.): Sport Cardiology. Bologna, Aulo Gaggi, 1980, pp. 723–734.

Department of Cardiology
Mexico National University
Tuxpan 16, Mexico D.F. 06760

The Modification of Cardiovascular Risk Factors: Ethical Issues

*Allan S. Brett, M.D.**

Over the past several decades, a substantial body of research has focused on risk factors for cardiovascular disease. A more health-conscious public has become aware of the insights generated by this research. In addition, the concept of preventive medicine has grown in popularity and has received increasing attention from the mass media.

When any area of medical theory and practice assumes importance in our society, ethical dimensions emerge and expand accordingly. This is no less true for risk factor intervention than for other areas of medicine. One reason is that the precise effects of many risk factor interventions remain speculative, thus heightening uncertainty. Patients and physicians are more likely to face conflicting choices against a background of medical uncertainty. It follows that ethical issues arise, because ethics may be regarded as the study of rational processes for determining the best course of action in the face of conflicting choices.[2] Furthermore, the genesis and perpetuation of factors such as unhealthy diet, smoking, and high blood pressure are inextricably linked to personal habits and behaviors. To the extent that personal values influence lifestyle, the promotion of changes in lifestyle must be grounded in ethical, as well as medical, principles.

Any discussion of risk factor modification may proceed at two different levels. The first is centered on the physician-patient encounter and is concerned with issues in the treatment of specific patients. The second level is that of the society as a whole; interventions designed to improve the health or welfare of society inevitably raise public policy issues. Naturally these two areas intersect, because private medical decision making occurs in a social, cultural, and political context. In this article, I will discuss both areas after introductory remarks on types of risk factors and sources of uncertainty in risk factor intervention.

TYPES OF RISK FACTORS

Risk factors may be categorized according to differences in their etiology and predisposing characteristics. For example, smoking is a behavior that is learned by imitating others in the social milieu. Self-motivation and encouragement from others are the usual ways that the behavior is changed, although psychologic or pharmacologic therapies are used occasionally as adjuncts. Another category is that of inherited or intrinsic medical conditions, such as hyperlipidemia. The patient bears no responsibility for the initial presence of the condition. Pharmacologic agents are used frequently in this situation in addition to habit-changing strategies (for example, reducing dietary cholesterol). A third category is that of exogenous influences (for example, environmental, social, and occupational influences) over which the patient may or may not have immediate control. Such diverse entities as air pollution and stress may fall into this category; although they may not be pure cardiovascular risk factors, they may affect cardiopulmonary performance. In reality, this type of classification can serve only as a conceptual guideline, because most risk factors have a mul-

---

*Instructor, Department of Medicine, Harvard Medical School; Attending Physician, New England Deaconess Hospital, Boston, Massachusetts

tiplicity of origins. For example, hypertension may have genetic (that is, a strong family history) and behavioral (for example, stress-related) origins. Contributing factors such as salt intake may be partly a function of the sociocultural background and partly a function of individual taste.

The preceding discussion is intended to emphasize the heterogeneity of risk factor origins and the qualitative differences in treatment strategies. Furthermore, risk factors and their corresponding interventions must be approached within the context of individual, family, and society. This complexity makes risk-benefit assessments unusually precarious from both the medical perspective and the ethical perspective.

THE IMPACT OF MEDICAL UNCERTAINTY

The task of integrating an ethical framework with clinical decision making is generally simplified when there are sound data regarding the possible outcomes associated with various interventions. In the study of risk factor modification, researchers face a number of challenging methodologic constraints. These difficulties often tend to limit the applicability of results and increase uncertainty.

One obvious problem is that the pathologic consequences of risk factors may take many years to become clinically obvious. The benefit of a given intervention is accordingly unlikely to be discernible in the short term. However, although studies ideally should continue for many years, there are numerous logistic and economic limitations. For example, three recent studies of the treatment of mild hypertension lasted for 5 years,[6,7,9] even though the adverse effects of hypertension often occur after decades. Either a beneficial result of therapy or a long-term untoward effect of medication could thus be missed. In order to magnify the likelihood of significant results, massive numbers of patients must be studied, and the expense and manpower requirements are raised even further.

A second problem is that control groups may change as a study progresses. This is particularly true because many risk factors demand modifications in behaviors (for example, smoking or diet) that are difficult to monitor. Thus, in the Multiple Risk Factor Intervention Trial (MRFIT), which evaluated the effects of a counseling program to reduce smoking and choles-

terol intake, the "controls" also favorably changed their smoking and eating habits.[10]

A third problem is that of explicitly recording and presenting the adverse effects of interventions, particularly those involving pharmacologic agents. When a reduction in cardiovascular end points, such as myocardial infarction or sudden death, are the goals of therapy, the side effects of therapy may seem trivial by comparison, especially to investigators and physicians. Thus, published reports of pharmacologic risk factor interventions often mention side effects only in passing or tend to minimize their significance. For example, although the results of the Hypertension Detection and Follow-up Program (HDFP) were reported initially in 1979,[7] a detailed review of adverse drug effects was not published until 1985.[3] Approximately 32 per cent of participants stopped medications because of possible or definite side effects. No deaths and very few hospitalizations resulted from these reactions, allowing the authors to "affirm the relative safety of antihypertensive therapy." However, the issue is not only safety but also the relative acceptability (from the patient's point of view) of side effects in exchange for a presumed ultimate benefit of therapy. Even well-intentioned physicians may overtly or unconsciously manipulate patients into accepting the trade-off when the drug is accomplishing its desired effect and side effects are perceived as tolerable by the physician.

A fourth problem is that authors may minimize the distinction between three links in the chain of evidence supporting a risk factor intervention: (1) the epidemiologic evidence that a factor confers risk; (2) the availability of a therapeutic modality that changes the measurable expression of the factor; and (3) the evidence that a measurable change induced by the intervention leads to an improved outcome. Stated another way, reaching a numerical value of a risk factor by virtue of medical intervention is not necessarily equivalent to being at that value in the first place. Reasons might include a failure to modify an underlying and continuing pathologic process, the presence of already irreversible pathologic changes at the time the risk factor is modified, and the existence of drug side effects that negate the beneficial effects of therapy.

For example, even mild hypertension indisputably confers an increased risk of cardiovascular morbidity and mortality,[8] and mildly elevated blood pressure can be lowered relatively easily with medication. However, the effect of this intervention on ultimate outcome remains controversial.[4,13] The presence of suggestive, but not incontrovertible, evidence of efficacy puts the practitioner in an uneasy position. In a medicalized society, physicians may feel uncomfortable in merely observing these high-risk persons.

Finally, the published interpretations of the results of intervention studies and the specific language of those interpretations merit close scrutiny. For example, the Hypertension Detection and Follow-up Program studied "whether total mortality among hypertensive people in the community could be reduced by a rigorous stepped-care approach to the treatment of hypertension, as compared with referral to a usual source of care in the community."[7] Patients were randomized to either special study centers or to their usual sources of medical care. Of particular interest was the finding that in mild hypertension, there was a statistically significant reduction in mortality among patients treated by the stepped-care approach after 5 years. The authors clearly stated their conclusions that mild hypertension should be treated. However, a controversial aspect of the study design was the lack of an untreated control group. Critics have argued that overall improved medical care in the stepped-care group, rather than the antihypertensive therapy, might have been responsible for the difference in mortality.[4] The study does not definitely prove that antihypertensive therapy is beneficial but only that one way of treating mild hypertension may be better than another.

A second highly publicized study, the Multiple Risk Factor Intervention Trial, randomized high-risk men either to a special intervention group (designated SI) that received stepped-care antihypertensive therapy and counseling for smoking and lowering cholesterol intake or to their usual sources of care (designated UC).[10] At 5 years of follow-up, there was no significant improvement in outcome in the study group.

In both studies, much was at stake. Millions of dollars were spent, and the investigators understandably hoped to show beneficial results of their interventions. The failure to provide true untreated controls with mild hypertension seemingly reflects the belief that it would have been unethical not to treat these patients. This belief in turn reflects a strongly held prestudy supposition that treating mild hypertension reduces mortality. In effect, the investigators put themselves in a "can't lose" position. If the study would show a favorable result (as did the Hypertension Detection and Follow-up Program), the investigators could claim success despite the

unorthodox study design. If the study would end unfavorably, as did the Multiple Risk Factor Intervention Trial, the unorthodox design could be blamed:

It may be relevant that multifactor intervention received a less than optimal test owing in part to unexpected declines in risk factor levels and in part to lower-than-expected mortality in the UC group. In regard to the former, the UC men thus constituted to a considerable extent a "treated" group.[10]

Yet the study could still be deemed successful:

In conclusion, we have shown that it is possible to apply an intensive long-term intervention program against three coronary risk factors with considerable success in terms of risk factor changes.[10]

However, the successful modification of risk factors is rather unsatisfying if it does not improve the outcome that was being studied.

ISSUES IN THE PHYSICIAN-PATIENT ENCOUNTER

The preceding sections are intended to highlight the complexities and uncertainties that might influence decisions to modify risk factors. Ultimately, the physician must gather the best available information and individualize it according to the patient's needs and values. The tension between patient autonomy (his or her own conception of his or her best interests) and physician paternalism (the physician's conception of what ought to be done to benefit the patient) requires resolution in each clinical encounter. In the following discussion, I will examine risk factor interventions in this context.

Risk factor interventions differ qualitatively from the treatment of manifest disease in ethically relevant ways. When one treats an existing disease, the benefits are generally identifiable and tangible. In many cases, the relief of symptoms is the most obvious goal. In other cases (for example, a painless breast lump as a first manifestation of cancer), the disease may still be asymptomatic when signs are present. In either situation, the patient immediately becomes assigned to a specific category of disease with a unique set of therapeutic options and outcomes. The patient's values regarding the meaning of illness and his or her tolerance of pain or suffering will influence the treatment decision.

Now consider the modification of risk factors. An entity is identified that may or may not predict or cause disease in a given individual. The entity has little relevance to health apart from its association with later undesirable events. For example, elevated blood pressure readings and cholesterol levels are significant by virtue of their association with pathologic cardiovascular events. In and of themselves, they are asymptomatic in most cases. One is now dealing with a probability of disease conferred by the risk factors rather than with an established disease. Thus, a different set of patient values assumes importance in the decision of whether and how to intervene. These values are related to the patient's perception of his or her vulnerability and his or her aversion to (or acceptance of) risk. One patient may shun medical intervention unless the stakes are immediately obvious and high. Another may seek to maximize medical benefit in the most marginal situation.

When one explores the patient's attitude toward risk, a number of points should be kept in mind. First, the risk factor may increase the probability of a given event in a population but does not identify exactly which individuals in the population will experience the event. Second, the likelihood that a person will benefit from the intervention and the magnitude of that benefit are also probabilistic events. Third, the potential for adverse effects of the intervention is generally probabilistic as well. Fourth, the trade-offs between adverse effects and ultimate benefits must be weighed on a time scale (that is, they may occur at markedly different times after the intervention has been instituted). The preceding contingencies must be synthesized somehow, whether by formal decision analysis[15] or by intuitive judgments.

The example of mild hypertension may be considered in this context. As blood pressure rises, the risk of complications does not appear suddenly at some specific level but rather increases gradually.[8] Thus, the reasons to intervene gradually become more compelling at successively higher levels. It follows that selection of a cutoff for critically elevated blood pressure reflects a value judgment about the point at which a risk is thought to be serious enough to warrant treatment.[5] This point may vary among patients, depending on their aversion to risk, tolerance of treatment side effects, and willingness to invest time, energy, or money in medical care. The situation is more complex when viewed over time. For example, suppose that the most successful antihypertensive regimen causes impotence in a patient; how many years of life with impotence are equivalent to a shorter period without impotence? Finally, when the morbidity and mortality figures themselves reflect considerable uncertainty, as they do for

mild hypertension, the decision-making process is even more difficult.[13]

Another distinction worth considering is that between intervention strategies that modify habits or behaviors and those that use pharmacologic agents. In the former situation, the likelihood of promoting patient autonomy is relatively greater. Even though the physician may encourage the patient to change behaviors (for example, to stop smoking or lose weight), the day-to-day success of the intervention largely depends on the patient's own motivation. In the case of drug therapy, the patient is also presumably free to comply with or reject the physician's advice. However, the patient is relatively more dependent on the physician, who must supply the drug, manipulate the dose, and maintain surveillance for adverse effects.

Furthermore, the patient is usually asymptomatic when the risk factor is discovered. The physician cannot make an asymptomatic person feel any better. Modifications in behavior may entail some inconvenience (for example, pursuing a new diet) or initial frustration (for example, quitting smoking), but they are unlikely to create ongoing harm or discomfort. Drug therapies, on the other hand, usually pose some risk of creating symptoms or even long-term harm.[11] It follows that relatively stronger proof of efficacy should be required for drug therapies as compared with behavioral modifications, because the risks of doing harm are relatively greater when pharmacologic agents are employed.

ETHICAL ISSUES AND PUBLIC POLICY

The preceding discussion is primarily applicable to individual encounters between physicians and patients. However, there are ethical ramifications of risk factor intervention that also extend to public policy.

First, certain risky behaviors affect not only the person indulging in the behavior but also others. If society has a moral obligation to protect its constituents, it has an interest in risky behaviors that encroach upon the health or well-being of others. Conflict arises when individual liberties are pitted against social concerns. One example is the effect of cigarette smoke on nonsmokers who are in close proximity to smokers. A logical solution is to make provisions for the geographic separation of smokers and nonsmokers at the work site or in public places. A more extreme policy is to ban smoking entirely in an institution. At least one hospital has even instituted a policy of not hiring smokers altogether.[16] For even the most ardent antismoking advocates, the latter situation raises serious questions regarding discrimination and civil liberties.

Second, society may have an interest in regulating risk factors simply because improving the health of the population is considered to be a legitimate social good. This goal goes beyond the situation in which the behavior of one person harms another. A noncardiovascular example is legislation requiring the wearing of seat belts in automobiles. Again, a tension is created between proponents of absolute freedom of choice and those who argue that the benefits of preventing highway deaths far outweigh a minimal intrusion on personal liberties. Existing examples are not as forthcoming in the area of cardiovascular risk factors. However, hypothetical situations would be a ban on the sale of cigarettes or legislation requiring reduction in the salt or cholesterol content of processed foods. Less coercive and thus less morally problematic approaches include publicly sponsored educational campaigns promoting healthy behaviors or hypertension screening. Pellegrino argues that health promotion may legitimately become public policy only when certain conditions are met: There should be a compelling body of evidence supporting the effectiveness of an intervention; coercive measures should not be considered unless voluntary measures have failed; and coercive measures, if instituted, should be mild and should entail only trivial inconvenience for the individual.[12]

Third, the economic aspects of risk factor intervention are increasingly important at the public policy level. One might reasonably ask whether society should provide and pay for medical care for those persons who do not modify clearly identified risk factors. After all, the health care costs generated by these individuals are shared by all members of society who pay taxes or insurance premiums. Thus, nonsmokers indirectly finance medical care for those who suffer the complications of smoking. If smoking is considered to be a voluntary behavior, it might be argued that smokers ought to assume financial responsibility for their own health care. Veatch has stated that one way to pay for such care would be to assess a health tax on the product (for example, cigarettes) such that the revenues would approximately cover the anticipated health care expenditures.[14]

What about involuntary risk factors such as hypertension? Although a person is not responsible for acquiring hypertension, does that person nevertheless have a social obligation to undergo antihypertensive therapy? One could respond that such treatment will be cost-effective by reducing later complications and attendant costs to society. It would thus be in the public interest to encourage these individuals to seek treatment when there are sound data to support the efficacy of the intervention. However, it is not clear that more coercive measures can be justified in a democratic society. The best compromise is to identify those persons at highest risk and to give them the opportunity to receive health-related instruction and appropriate treatment.

CONCLUSION

There is no question that the prevention of cardiovascular disease is a worthy goal, but much work must be done to determine which modifications of risk factors consistently result in identifiable reductions in disease, at an acceptable cost in side effects and financial resources. Although it has been established that elimination of smoking and early control of moderate or severe hypertension would contribute to a substantial reduction in cardiovascular disease, it is unclear how much of an impact can be made in other spheres. It just may be that a certain prevalence of cardiovascular disease is an unavoidable concomitant of the lifestyles intrinsic to Western civilization. At present, it would seem medically, ethically, and economically most prudent to identify and offer treatment to those individuals who stand to benefit the most—those whose risk profiles are most clearly amenable to modification. However, the zeal to intervene must be balanced constantly by careful attention to the personal values of patients, the political values of society, and the resources available to the health care system.

ACKNOWLEDGMENT

Several of the ideas in this article were originally developed in an essay in the *American Journal of Medicine*.[1] I thank the editorial staff of the *American Journal of Medicine* for permission to use that material.

REFERENCES

1. Brett, A.S.: Ethical issues in risk factor intervention. Am. J. Med., 76:557–561, 1984.
2. Brody, H.: Ethical Decisions in Medicine. Edition 2. Boston, Little, Brown and Company, 1981.
3. Curb, J.D., Borhani, N.O., Blaszkowski, T.P., et al.:

Long-term surveillance for adverse effects of anti-hypertensive drugs. J.A.M.A. *253*:3263–3268, 1985.

4. Freis, E.D.: Should mild hypertension be treated? N. Engl. J. Med., *307*:306–309, 1982.

5. Guttmacher, S., Teielman, M., Chapin, G., et al.: Ethics and preventive medicine: The case of borderline hypertension. Hastings Cent. Rep., *11*:12–29, 1981.

6. Helgeland, A.: Treatment of mild hypertension: A five year controlled drug trial: The Oslo study. Am. J. Med., *69*:725–732, 1980.

7. Hypertension Detection and Follow-up Program Cooperative Group: Five-year findings of the Hypertension Detection and Follow-up Program. I. Reduction in mortality of persons with high blood pressure, including mild hypertension. J.A.M.A. *242*:2562–2571, 1979.

8. Kannel, W.B.: Some lessons in cardiovascular epidemiology from Framingham. Am. J. Cardiol., *37*:269–282, 1976.

9. Management Committee: The Australian therapeutic trial in mild hypertension. Lancet, *1*:1261–1267, 1980.

10. Multiple Risk Factor Intervention Trial Research Group: Multiple risk factor intervention trial. J.A.M.A. *248*:1465–1477, 1982.

11. Oliver, M.F.: Risks of correcting the risks of coronary disease and stroke with drugs. N. Engl. J. Med., *306*:297–298, 1982.

12. Pellegrino, E.D.: Health promotion as public policy: The need for moral groundings. Prev. Med., *10*:371–378, 1981.

13. Toth, P.J., and Horwitz, R.I.: Conflicting clinical trials and the uncertainty of treating mild hypertension. Am. J. Med., *75*:482–488, 1983.

14. Veatch, R.M.: Voluntary risks to health: The ethical issues. J.A.M.A. *243*:50–55, 1980.

15. Weinstein, M.C., and Fineberg, H.V.: Clinical Decision Analysis. Philadelphia, W.B. Saunders Company, 1980.

16. Wolinsky, H.: When there's no smoke, there's ire. American College of Physicians Observer, *5*:5, 1985.

Department of Medicine
New England Deaconess Hospital
185 Pilgrim Road
Boston, Massachusetts 02215

Index

Note: Page numbers of articles are in **boldface** type.